Master positioning skills!

Over **200** Radiographic positions, procedures and projections

Radiographic Positioning POCKET GUIDE

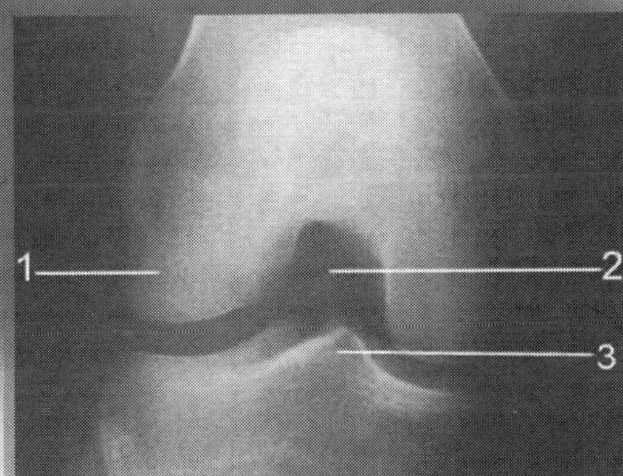

Olive Peart

PELTROVIJAN PUBLISHING

Radiographic Positioning
POCKET GUIDE

Olive Peart M.S. R.T. (R) (M)

Peltrovijan Publishing
P.O. Box 738
Greenbelt, MD 20768-0738
http://www.opeart.com

Radiographic Positioning Pocket Guide

Cover design by Nadine Peart Akindele

PRINTING HISTORY
Peltrovijan Publishing/2020

ISBN-13: 978-1-937143-49-7 Print Edition

Books by Olive Peart

Mammography & Breast Imaging Prep. Program Review.
A comprehensive review for the mammography ARRT registry examination including the history of breast imaging, breast cancer detection, and treatment.

Lange Q & A Mammography Examination.
Everything you need to ace the ARRT Mammography Exam in one complete study package. Includes 450 ARRT-style questions plus two complete practice exams.

Mammography and Breast Imaging: Just the Facts.
The perfect review tool for radiologic technologists certifying or recertifying. The book includes all breast imaging modalities and techniques as well as questions for self-assessment.

Life After High School: Traits that Help and Traits that Hurt
This no-nonsense text explains positive and negative traits that can help or hinder teens in their post high school life. The guide gives readers strategies, helping them to identify the path to success and to avoid the route that often leads to failure.

The Dangers of Medical Radiation
How to protect yourself from medical radiation!

Spanish for Radiology Professionals: An English/Spanish Pocket Guide
Spanish for Radiology Professionals is an English to Spanish translations of often-used, technical terms and radiological instructions. This book is easy to use, even for someone with limited Spanish. The Spanish includes a phonetic spelling guide for easy pronunciation

Table of Content

ACKNOWLEDGMENT

Thanks to many of my past students who helped me in the production of this book.

Thanks also to my husband, family and friends for their help and support.

PREFACE

From its earliest beginning after its discovery in 1895, x-rays were recognized for their amazing ability to penetrate the human body and visualize the skeletal system. Since then, diagnostic imaging has undergone numerous changes in the methods of imaging, developing the image, image display, and image storage. However, throughout the ages there has been little change in the patient positioning aspect of diagnostic radiography. Despite the increasing importance of imaging modalities, such as CT, ultrasound, magnetic resonance (MR) and other molecular imaging studies, it is still essential to visualize the bones, joints and to image the contents of the thorax or abdomen on a two-dimensional image. General radiography often remains the first line of defense in medical diagnosis.

Radiographic imaging typically requires specific skills and positioning techniques. It is the effective use of these positioning skills that makes general radiography such a challenging and rewarding career option. In fact, poor image quality or poor positioning skills is sometimes a factor in the inability of radiographic imaging to diagnosis pathology, leading radiologists or physicians to seek alternative imaging modalities.

Turning to an alternative imaging modality should not be the result of poor image quality or poor positioning skills. It is understood that significant inaccuracies that can occur when the central ray is not perpendicular to the part, the image receptor (IR), the detector or cassette. In trauma situations, or if the patient cannot move, it is the responsibility of the imager to manipulate the central ray and the IR or cassette to produce an accurate representation of the part.

The desired outcome is a quality image and major contributing factor is the imager's competency and positioning skills. However, in addition to knowledge of positioning, another important role of the imaging professional is effective communication. The field of diagnostic radiography can be stimulating, especially from the patient care aspect. Specific verbal skills are necessary and required when interacting with the trauma or seriously ill patient, the intoxicated or mentally challenged patient, and even the overly anxious or the pediatric patient.

Finally, imaging professionals must use radiation wisely, practicing ALARA (As Low As Reasonably Achievable) at all times.

These flash cards will help educators, students, recent graduates and experienced imagers with a comprehensive overview of routine imaging procedures and positioning terminology. Also included is a summary of patient care in radiology, infection control, patient communication and digital technology.

General Policies and Procedures

Importance of Standard Precautions

Radiographic imaging must always be performed using standard precautions and the proper infection control techniques as outlined by the Centers for Disease Control & Prevention (CDC) and the Hospital Infection Control Practices Advisory Committee (HICPAC). Standard Precautions incorporates fluid and body precautions and body substance isolation. Standard Precautions are required whenever there is a possibility of contact with blood, body fluids, secretions, excretions, mucous membranes and nonintact skin. Standard Precautions must be applied to all patients.

Hand washing

Washing hands is a basic infection control technique. Washing hands and cleaning all areas of the x-ray table, erect stand and image plates or detectors before and after contact with the patient. Hand washing must take place even if gloves are worn.

The following are Specific Transmission-Based Precautions. They are applied whenever a patient is infected with a pathogenic organism or a communicable disease, also for patients at risk for infections (immunosuppressed).

Airborne Precautions

- Organisms remain suspended in the air for long periods of time e.g. tuberculosis (TB).
- Infected patients are placed in a negative-pressure isolation room with the door closed.
- Healthcare providers should wear respiratory protection (filtered mask) on entering patient's room.
- Patient leaving room must wear a surgical mask.

Droplet Precautions

- Pathogens spread through large particular droplets expelled when patient coughs, sneezes or talks. Droplets travel about 3 feet (91.5 cm) and infection occurs through contact with mouth, nasal mucosa or conjunctiva.
- Patients are placed in private rooms with doors closed.
- Healthcare provider should wear a mask within 3 feet (91.5cm) of patient.
- Patient should wear mask on leaving the room.

Contact Precautions

- Infections spreads through direct contact with patient or a contaminated object (formite) e.g. bed rails.
- Clean all contaminated equipment after leaving room.
- Health care providers should wear gloves and wash hands before entering and after leaving the room.
- Impervious gown needed only if contact with patient is possible and a face mask is suggested to avoid contaminating the nasal mucosa
- Patients leaving room should wear an impervious gown and face mask.

Clinical History Documentation

The imager must document the clinical history for all patients. Reasons include:

Aids in diagnosis and prevents misdiagnosis.

The radiologist may never see the patient. Clinical documentation is therefore especially helpful. The technologist can locate the actual injury site or foreign body markers be used to indicate the location of a penetrating injury.

Modification of exposure. Additive versus destructive pathologies or the presence of a prostatic device can require changes in the normal technical factors. A clinical history will allow for changes before the exposure.

Ruling out errors.

The wrong body part may be indicated on the requisition or the imaging could be contraindicated because of poor internal preparation, allergies or preexisting medical history. Good clinical history documentation would highlight the error or specific problem and allow corrections.

Legal coding.

In many cases, the clinical history is necessary to determine the correct diagnostic code. This can be critical for medical research and in billing and insurance reimbursement.

Patient Communication

Communicating specific breathing instructions is important in controlling motion. Motion control is critical to producing a high-quality radiograph. There are two types of patient motion.

Involuntary motion

Best controlled by using short exposure times. They are outside of a patient's control and include peristalsis.

Voluntary motion

Best control by communicating instructions clearly, by providing the patient with a warm and comfortable imaging experience, by using support devices when necessary and by using immobilization devices as a last resort.

Breathing instructions are necessary when imaging the thorax and abdomen. It is often not necessary when imaging the skull or extremities. However, even when breathing instruction is not required for imaging, telling a child or anxious adult to stop breathing during an exposure can aid in keeping them still.

General Imaging Rules

Proper use of anatomic side marker

The Right or Left side marker is required on all radiographic images before the exposure

Markers are not legally acceptable if written or digitally applied after the exposure

Markers should not obscure the anatomy or patient's identification information

Palpation to identify landmarks

Applying light pressure with pad of fingers (not the tip/point of fingers and never with the whole hand).

Always advice patient before beginning palpations

Use of grid or Bucky device

Use only when needed. Recommend when imaging parts 10 cm or 4 inches thick or if using over 80 kVp. The exception is chest imaging.

Imaging using a minimum of two (2) projections

Generally, the two projections minimum is taken as near 90-degrees from each other as possible to:

Avoid superimposition of anatomic structures

Allow localization of lesion or foreign bodies

Determine alignment of fractures

Note: Three or more projections are often necessary with accurately visualizing joints

A minimum of two projections, 90-degrees apart are necessary and recommended to show part alignments.

Fig. 1a (schematic drawing mimicking a fracture),
Fig.1b (Lateral radiograph of the part),
Fig.1c (AP radiograph of the part).

Fig 1a

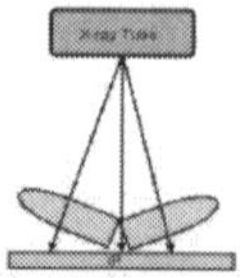

Fig 1b

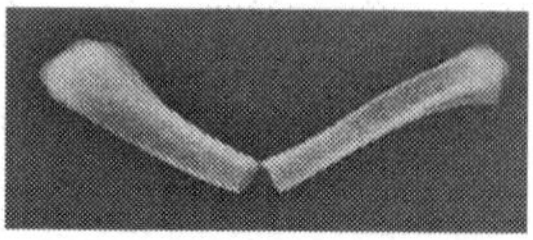

Fig 1c

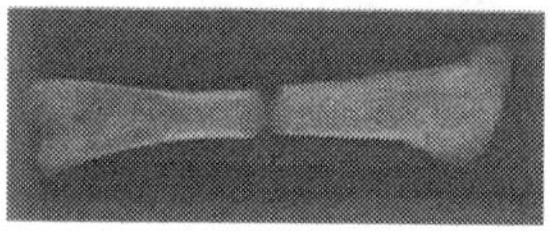

Fig. 1d (schematic drawing mimicking a fracture),
Fig.1e (Lateral radiograph of the part)
Fig.1f (AP radiograph of the part)

Fig 1d

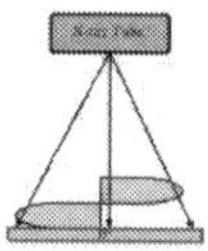

Fig 1e

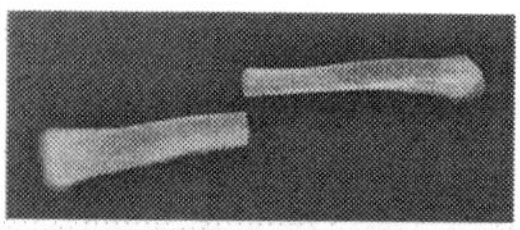

Fig 1f

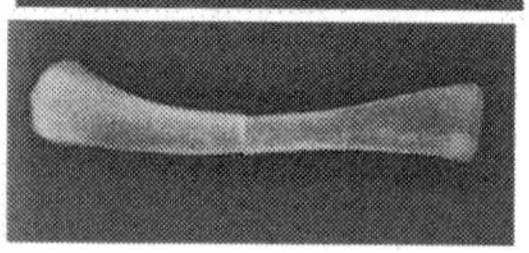

Imaging Information

Cassettes are lightproof devices that hold the film in analog imaging. This terminology is often incorrectly used to refer to the image place in digital imaging.

Films are used to acquire the image, display the image and archive the image in analog imaging.

Image Plate (IP) holds the image receptor in digital **photostimulable phosphor (PSP)** systems also called computed radiography (CR) imaging. In CR the IP replaces the cassette.

Storage phosphor screen (SPS) or photostimulable phosphor (PSP) is placed within the IP. This replaces the film/screen in analog imaging. The IR receives the energy of the x-ray beam. The acquired image can be displayed on a computer monitor and the final image can be archived either as film or on a computer disk.

Image Receptor (IR) received the x-ray. It can be a detector or PSP

Detector is a specialized device that acquires the image in digital flat panel systems or direct radiography (DR), cassettless imaging. The detector is sometimes referred to as the IR.

Anatomical position. All radiographical reference starts from the anatomical position. The patient stands erect, face and eyes directed forward, arms extended by the sides with the palms of hands facing forward, heels together and toes pointing anteriorly.

Viewing radiograph. Patient's right is placed to the viewers left.

Exceptions to viewing rule. Hands & feet are viewed with fingers and toes upwards.

Anode heel effect is the reduction in intensity of the x-ray beam at the anode end of the tube.

Minimizing anode heel effect involves using shorter SID or placing the thicker body part at the cathode and thinner body part to the anode.

Fig 2. The body in the anatomical position

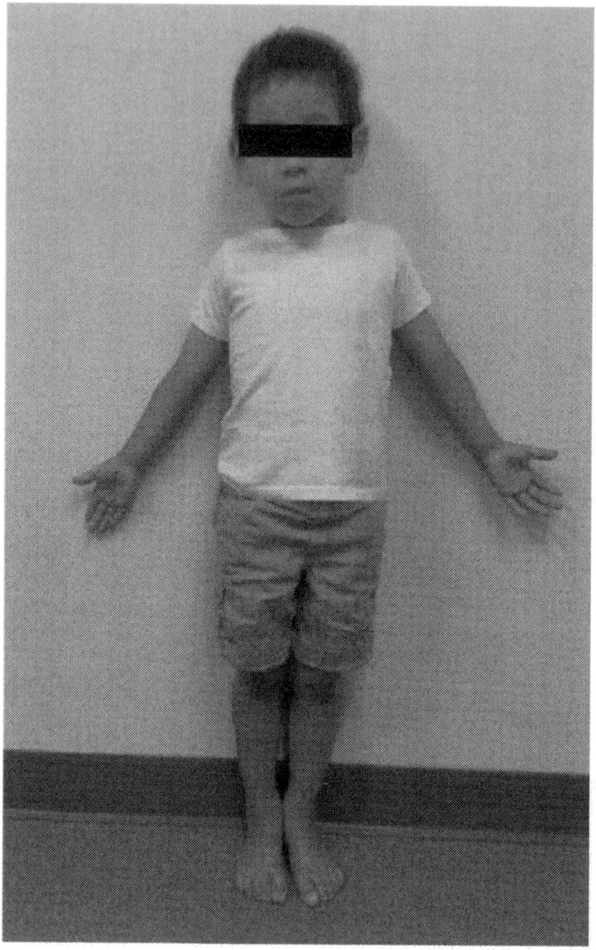

Units of Radiation

Roentgen (R), coulomb/kilogram (C/kg) or (Gy_a)

- Measures radiation exposure in air.

Rad (rad) or Gray (Gy_t)

- Measures the amount of radiation energy absorbed in a medium e.g. body tissue.

Rem (rem) or Seivert (Sv)

- Measures the occupational exposure or dose equivalent–consideration given to the biological effects of various types of radiation.

Skin Entrance Exposure (SEE)

- Measure the exposure to the skin in the region where the radiation first strikes the body.

Effective Dose

- Takes into account the dose to all the organs and their relative risk of become cancerous or the risks of genetic damage to the gonads.

Source to skin distance (SSD)–critical in fluoroscopy imaging

- 15 inches (38 cm) minimum for stationary fluoroscopy units
- 12 inches (30 cm) minimum for mobile fluoroscopy (C-arm)

Somatic effects–Radiation affecting the individual only.
Genetic effects–Radiation affecting future generations of the individual.
Deterministic effects (nonstochastic) effects - High radiation doses produce an early response. All early effects, and most normal tissue late effects are deterministic.
Stochastic effects (probabilistic effects) - Low doses delivered over a long period of time with a late or delayed response. They increase in likelihood as dose increase. Their severity is not dose related

Limiting Radiation to Patient

Minimize repeats–use accurate positioning.
Correct filtration–will remove the low energies before they strike the patient and contribute to skin dose.
Collimation–close collimation will reduce patient dose and improve radiographic quality, especially in digital imaging.
Protective shielding–should be used on all patients whenever possible especially children and potentially reproductive-aged female patients. Shielding is used whenever the gonads are within 5cm or 2 inches of the collimated field and if shielding will not compromise the radiograph.
Selection of correct exposure factors–use high kV and low mAs whenever possible to reduce patient dose. In digital imaging using the 15% rule to reduce the mAs while increasing the kVp will reduce patient dose without affecting image quality.
Patient positioning–using the posteroanterior projection (PA) versus the posteroanterior (AP) will allow reduced radiation to the eyes, breast, thyroids and often the gonads.
Pregnant patients–avoid imaging the fetus especially during the first trimester unless medically necessary.
Personnel protection–provide lead aprons, thyroid shielding or lead gloves if needed, to all personnel in the x-ray room during an exposure. Always practice time, distance and shielding. Doubling your distance from the source of radiation will reduce exposure by ¼.
Technologist should always practice ALARA–As low as reasonably achievable.
The 10-day or LMP (last menstrual period) rule—applies to all radiological examinations involving the pelvis or lower abdomen. Imaging should be scheduled during the first 10 days following the onset of menstruation. The rule is abandoned if imaging is medically necessary.

Radiographic Planes

Sagittal Plane–Divides the body into ANY right and left sections.
Median/Midsagittal Plane (MSP)–Divides the body EQUAL into right and left sections.
Coronal (frontal) Plane–Divides the body into ANY anterior and posterior sections.
Mid Coronal Plane (MCP)–Divides the body into EQUAL anterior and posterior sections.
Horizontal/Transverse Plane–Any horizontal plane at right angle to coronal or sagittal planes.
Oblique Plane–Any plane not classified as a main plane. i.e. slant or deviate from the perpendicular, horizontal, longitudinal or transverse.
Sectional imaging includes:

- Longitudinal sections–A section that is lengthwise in the direction of the long axis or any of its parts, regardless of the body position (erect or recumbent). Sections can be taken in the sagittal or coronal planes.

Body Surfaces

Posterior/dorsal–back
Anterior/ventral–front
Plantar–sole or posterior surface of foot
Palmar–ventral or anterior of hand (palm)
Dorsal can refer to the hand or foot

- Foot–top or anterior surface of foot
- Hand–back or posterior aspect of hand

Spinal Curvature

Lordosis–commonly found in lumbar region or cervical regions (exaggeration of normal curvature)
Kyphosis–commonly found in thoracic region (exaggeration of normal thoracic curvature
Scoliosis–lateral curvature of spine

General Radiographic Terms

SID–The source to image receptor distance.
OID–The object to image receptor distance.
CR–The central ray of the x-ray photon beam leaving the x-ray tube. The beam diverts from the focal spot to strike any object in its path.
Position–Describes the actual patient position in relationship to the x-ray table or IR (can be detector, IP or cassette). Position can also refer to general body position e.g. seated, standing etc. Position and projection are sometimes used interchangeably and incorrectly. Example of correct usage:

- The technologist performed a PA projection of the chest with the patient in the upright position.

View–Used in the U.S. to describe the body part as seen by the IR. In some countries it is used to describe projections.
Lateral–Can be used to describe a patient position, a projection or the relationship between two structures.
Technical factors

- Kilovoltage peak (kVp) controls the energy, the voltage and therefore the penetrability or speed of the electrons leaving the filament.
- Milliampere (mA) controls the quantity or number of electrons produced.
- Exposure time (ms) controls the duration of the exposure in milliseconds.

General Body Positions

Supine– dorsal recumbent), patient lying on back.
Prone– ventral recumbent position), patient lying face down.
Erect– upright, patient seated or standing.
Seated– patient sitting on a chair or stool.
Recumbent– patient lying on the x-ray table, bed or stretcher.
Trendelenburg– patient lying on the x-ray table, bed or stretcher with the head lower than the feet.
Fowlers– patient lying on the x-ray table, bed or stretcher with trunk and head higher than feet.
Sim's position–patient semiprone with left anterior side down and right side raised (left anterior oblique position)
Lithotomy position–patient lying on the x-ray table, bed or stretcher (supine) with knees and hips flexed, thighs abducted and rotated externally. Tights supported with ankle supports.

Radiographic Projections

Projection–Describes the direction of travel of the x-ray bean.
Posteroanterior (PA) projection–CR passes from posterior to anterior aspect of the body.
Anteroposterior (AP) projection–CR passes from anterior to posterior aspect of the body.
PA Oblique projection–Used in describing extremities only. Rotation from the PA. When used, a qualifier, indicating which way the part is rotated (medial or lateral), is required.
AP oblique projection–Used in describing extremities only. Rotation from the AP. When used, a qualifier, indicating which way the part is rotated (medial or lateral), is required.
Lateral (mediolateral or lateromedial projections)–path of the CR based on the patient's anatomic position.

Projection Terms

Axial projection– CR angled along the long axis of the body or body part.
Inferosuperior axial projection–CR enters from below or inferiorly and exits above or superiorly.
Superoinferior axial projection–CR enters superiorly and exits inferiorly.
Tangential–CR touches the structure at the edges, skimming it to produce a profile projection.
Lordotic–CR is horizontal or vertical and the patient is angled to produce an axial projection. E.g. the patient standing AP, leaning backwards with only the shoulders in contact with the IR. A horizontal CR used.
Transthoracic lateral projection–CR travels laterally through the thorax. Requires a qualifying position term (right or left lateral position) e.g. left transthoracic lateral.
Dorsoplantar projections–CR travels from dorsal (anterior) to plantar (posterior) aspect of foot.
Plantodorsal projections–CR travels from plantar (posterior) to the dorsal (anterior) aspect of foot.
Axial plantodorsal projection–angled CR traveling from plantar surface and exiting at the dorsum surface of the foot.

Specific Body Positions

Lateral position–path closest to IR or body part from which the CR exits.
–In extremity imaging it is named for side of the structure the CR enters first then exited e.g. mediolateral.
–In chest imaging it is named for the side nearest the IR.
Oblique–rotation of trunk between lateral and prone or supine position.
Right Posterior Oblique (RPO)–patient recumbent or erect, back to the IR, right side down, left side up.
Left Posterior Oblique (LPO)–patient recumbent or erect, back to the IR, left side down, right up.
Left Anterior Oblique (LAO)–patient recumbent or erect, front to the IR, left side down, right up.
Right Anterior Oblique (RAO)–patient recumbent or erect, front to the IR, right side down, left up.

Decubitus–Imaging of the chest or abdomen with the patient recumbent using a horizontal CR.
Left lateral decubitus–Patient recumbent on left side (lateral), imaging using a horizontal CR.
Right lateral decubitus– Patient recumbent on right side (lateral), imaging using a horizontal CR.
Dorsal decubitus position–Patient recumbent (supine), imaging using a horizontal CR.
Ventral decubitus position–Patient recumbent (prone), imaging using a horizontal CR.

Relationship Terms

Medial–turned toward the median plane or middle of a part/body.
Lateral–turned away from the median plane or middle of a part/body.
Proximal–the part closest to the point of origin or attachment, toward the center of the body.
Distal–the part furthest from the point of origin or attachment, away from the center of body.
Cephalad/cephalic/cranial/superior–angling the CR toward the head, angled up or above.
Caudad/caudal/inferior–angling the CR toward the feet, angled down or below.
Interior/internal– refers to inside the body.
Exterior/external– refers to parts outside an organ, on the outside of the body, on or near outside.
Superficial–refers to parts near the surface of the body or skin.
Deep–refers to parts far from the surface of the body or skin.
Ipsilateral–a part or parts on the same side of the body.
Contralateral–a part or parts on the opposite side of the body.

Terms Related to Movement

Flexion–bending
Hyperflexion–extreme flexion
Extension–straightening of joint
Hyperextension–straightening beyond the normal limits
Ulnar deviation (ulnar flexion)–turn or bend hand and wrist toward ulnar
Radial deviation (radial flexion)–turn or bend hand and wrist toward radius
Dorsiflexion of foot–described the flexion between the lower leg and foot when angle between the two is less than or equal to 90°
Planter flexion of foot–extending the ankle joint or moving foot and toes downwards
Evert/Eversion–turning foot outward at the ankle joint
Invert/Inversion –turning foot inward at the ankle joint
Valgus–bending of part outward or away from midline (e.g. bow-leg)
Varus–bending part inward or toward midline (e.g. knock-kneed)
Terms Related to Movement continued
Medial rotation–rotation of a part or moving anterior aspect of part toward the inside or median plane
Lateral rotation–rotation of part or moving anterior aspect of part toward the outside or away from the median plane
Abduct/Abduction–movement away from the midline of the body
Adduct/Adduction–movement toward the midline of body
Supinate/Supination–the act of turning onto the back, face up
Pronate/Pronation–the act of turning onto the stomach, face down
Elevation–lifting, raising or moving superiorly
Depression–pushing down or moving part inferiorly
Circumduction moving–turning around and around to form a circle. Movement can include flexion, abduction, extension and adduction resulting in a ‘cone’ shaped movement
Rotation–circular movement around a specified axis
Tilt–slanting or movement with respect to the long axis such as moving the body part so that the sagittal plane is not parallel to the long axis of the rest of the body/or support table

External Body Landmarks

Cervical area

C1	Mastoid tip
C2/ C3	Gonion (angle of mandible)
C3/ C4	Hyoid bone
C5	Thyroid cartilage
C7/ T1	Vertebra prominens

Thoracic area

T1	2 in (5 cm) above level of jugular notch
T2/ T3	The jugular notch
T4/ T5	The sternal angle
T7	The inferior angles of scapulae
T9/T10	The xiphoid process

Lumbar area

L1/L2/ L3	The Inferior Costal margin
Navel	Approximately L3 (not accurate because of body habitus)
L4/ L5	Superior aspect of crests

Sacrum and pelvic area

L5/S1	At the Posterior Superior Iliac Spine (PSIS)– dimples in the back
S1/ S2	At the Anterior Superior Iliac Spines (ASIS)
Coccyx	At the upper border of the pubic symphysis & most prominent portion of the greater trochanter

Fig 3a & 3b. External Body Landmarks

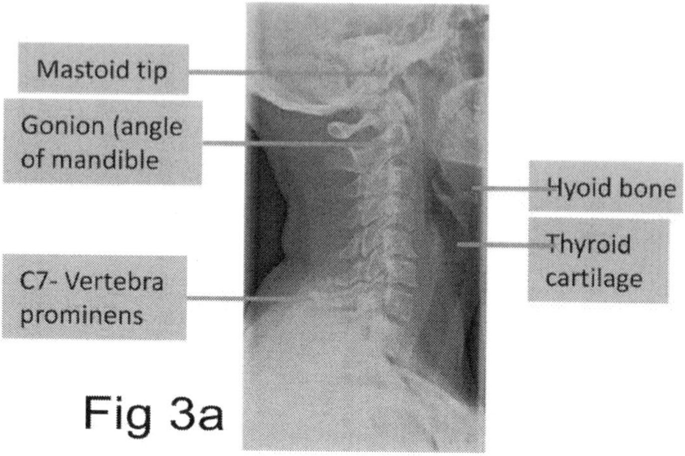

Fig 3a

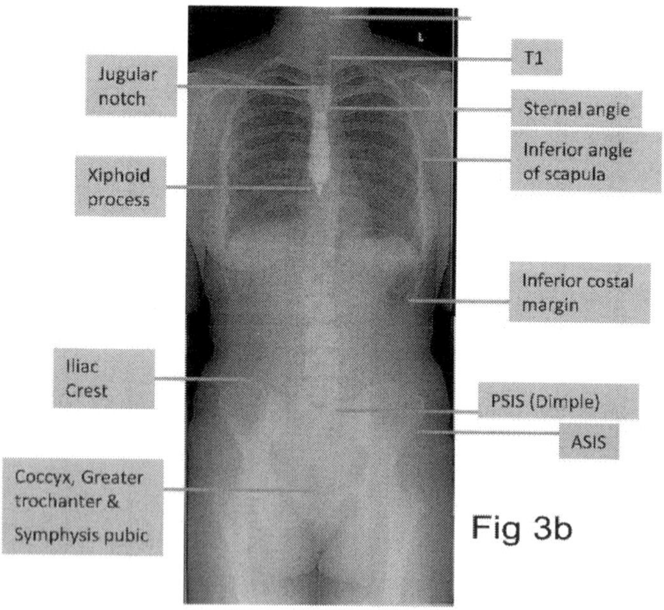

Fig 3b

Factors Controlling Image Quality–Digital

BRIGHTNESS–Intensity of light on monitor. Representing individual pixels in the image (replaces the term density in film-base imaging).

Controlling factors (Note: mAs does not control brightness in digital imaging).

- Processing software–predetermined digital processing algorithms.
- The user can alter the brightness of the digital image after exposure.

CONTRAST–Difference in brightness between light and dark areas of an image.

Controlling factors (Note: Changes in kV has less of a direct impact on image contrast in digital imaging)

- Processing software–predetermined digital processing algorithms.
- User can alter the digital contrast after exposure.

IMAGE NOISE–Random disturbance that obscures or reduces image clarity

- Image noise will present with a grainy or mottled appearance. A high SNR (signal to noise ratio) is best.

Controlling factors reducing image noise

- Increasing the signal, basically the mAs, and therefore the number of photons striking detector.
- Use of grid to minimize scattered radiation and therefore noise.

RESOLUTION–The recorded sharpness or detail of structures on the image (same as for screen film)

Controlling factors

- Acquisition pixel size and display matrix.
- Perceived resolution of image is dependent on the display capabilities of the monitor.

DISTORTION–Misrepresentation of the original object size or shape and can include magnification.

Controlling factors

- SID, OID, central ray alignment, part alignment and CR angulation.

Exposure index–Numeric value representing the exposure the image receptor received.

- The name varies by manufactures. It is called the exposure index, exposure sensitivity or sensitivity (S) number. If the exposure index is outside the recommended range the image may appear acceptable at the technologist's monitor but of poor diagnostic quality on the radiologist monitor. The radiologist's monitor has smaller pixels, superior brightness, and better spatial and contrast resolution.
- It can be directly or indirectly proportional to the radiation striking the IR.

Controlling factor

- Intensity of radiation striking detector.
- mAs, kV, total detector area irradiated and/or objects or part exposed (air versus metal or patient's anatomy).

Deviation Index (DI)– a record of the difference between the ideal exposure and the actual exposure at the detector. DI changes by +1.0 for each +25% (increase in exposure), and by -1.0 for each -20% change. Results are *multiplicative, not additive.* Therefore each step multiplies the previous amount (not the original amount). DI formula: $DI = 10\log_{10}(EI/EI_T)$. Normal DI ranges from -0.5 to +0.5. A +1 DI is overexposure. A -1 DI is underexposure.

Factors Affecting Image Quality–Analog

DENSITY–The overall blackening on the film. Determined by the number of electrons leaving the filament. It is the **Quantity** or **intensity** of the x-ray output.

Controlling factor increasing image density

- Increasing the mA or exposure time (ms) and therefore the mAs (Milliamperage)

RESOLUTION–The recorded geometric sharpness of structures on the image. Other related terms are: detail, recorded detail, image sharpness or definition.

Controlling factor

- A small focal spot size equals less geometric unsharpness
- Increase SID equals less geometric unsharpness
- Decrease OID equals less geometric unsharpness

- Slow film-screen systems, uses smaller crystal size or small screen thickness leading to a higher resolution system
- Motion will produce a blurred image

CONTRAST–The density difference between two adjacent areas of a radiograph or how the densities of two adjacent areas differ. This defines the **quality** of the x-ray beam

- Low contrast image has many density levels (many shades of gray).
- High contrast image has few density levels (mostly black and white).

Controlling factor improving contrast

- Lowering the kVp will increase the differential absorption therefore improving contrast however, higher kVp technique is associated with lower mAs and allows reduced patient dose.

DISTORTION & MAGNIFICATION–Always exists because of the divergent rays and OID. The result is that anatomical structures on the radiograph appear larger or different from the original.

Controlling factors reducing magnification

- Increase SID reduces magnification.
- Reducing OID reduces magnification.

Controlling factors increasing distortion

- Increased distortion occurs when the part is not aligned to the image receptor. Part should be parallel to the detector and beam perpendicular to both.
- Central ray alignment and centering. Central ray should be perpendicular to the long axis of part(IR)

Shapes and Size Distortion—Radiographic Positioning

Fig 4a (schematic diagram showing normal positioning)

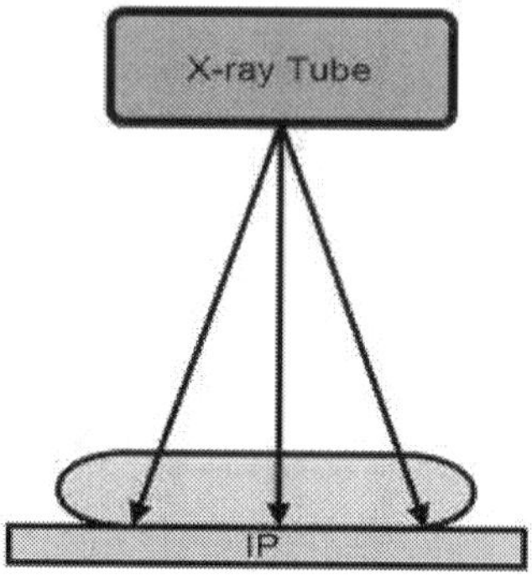

4b (AP radiograph of the part) Shapes and Size Distortion—magnified and angled positioning

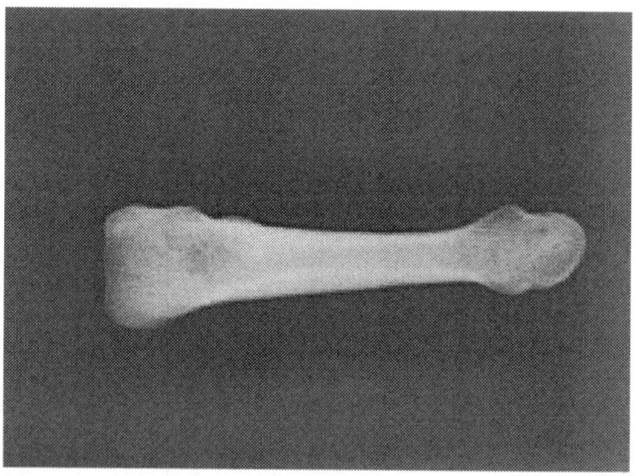

Fig 4c (schematic diagram showing magnified positioning with increase OID)
4d (AP radiograph of the magnified part).
4e (schematic diagram showing part angulation),
4f (AP radiograph of the angled part).

Fig 4c

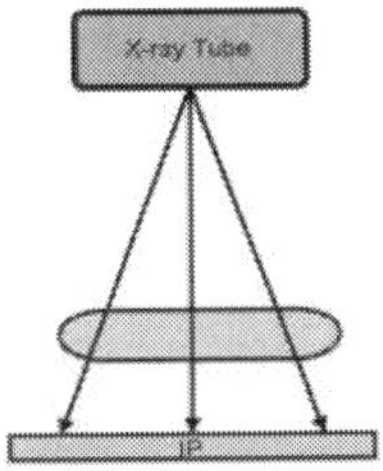

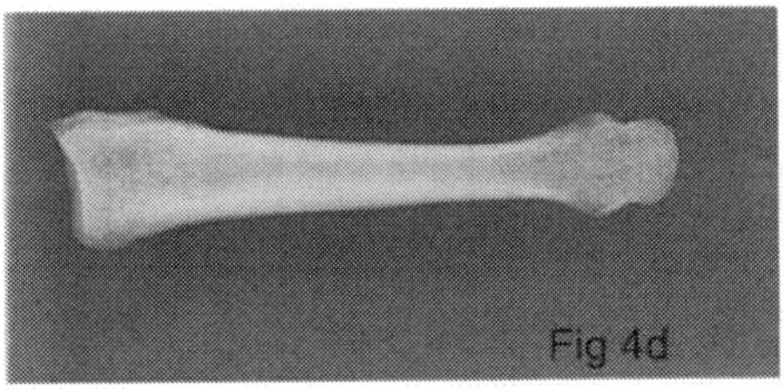

Fig 4d

Fig 4e

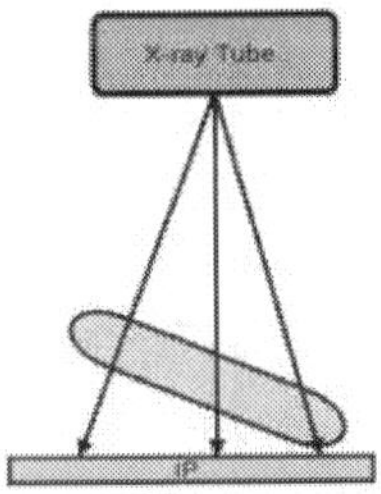

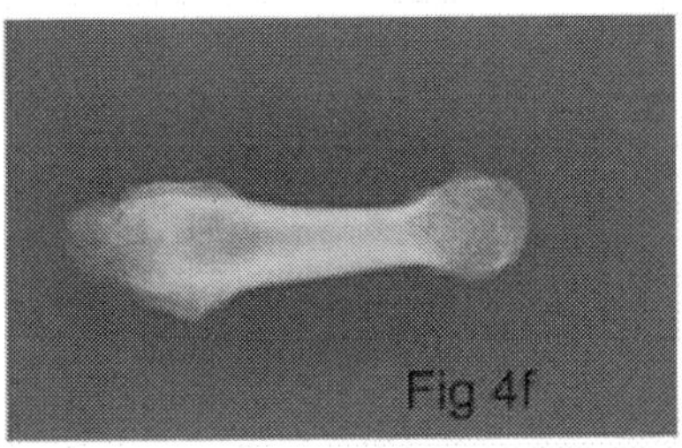

Fig 4f

Chest and Upper Airway Imaging

Breathing instructions for chest imaging

- Second arrested inspiration

External preparations

- Undress to waist–remove bra and any underwear with metallic parts
- Remove long hair braids/ jewelry/ external lines or leads

Radiation protection

- Shielding provided to all patients, especially to children and females of child bearing age
- Gonad shielding always be wrap around shielding to protect against back scatter

Reasons for erect chest

- Assist the diaphragm to its lowest level
- Allow maximum expansion of lungs
- Prevent engorgement and hyperemia of pulmonary vessels
- To demonstrate air/fluid levels

Reasons for recommended SID

- To minimize magnification of image (heart) and increase sharpness of lung structures.

Fig. 4g. SID-SOD-OID relationship

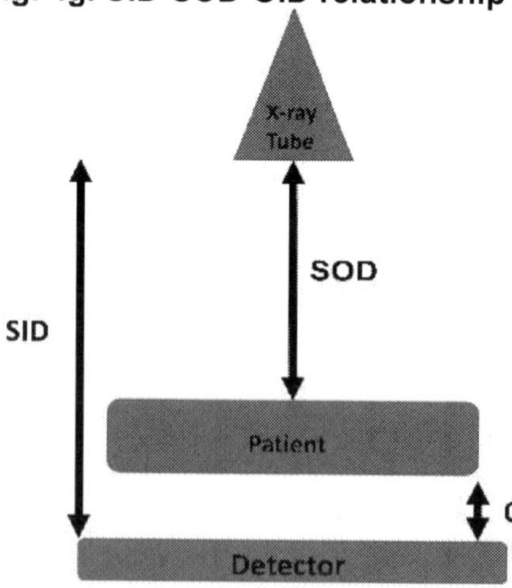

Anatomy of Respiratory System

Main function of the respiratory system–taking in oxygen and removing carbon dioxide from the body.

Structures:

Nasal cavity—internal and external naris (nostril) bounded by bone, cartilage covered skin and lined with mucus membrane

Pharynx or throat, part of both the respiratory and digestive system includes:

Nasopharynx—immediately behind the two nasal cavities

Oropharynx—behind the mouth

Laryngopharynx—from the hyoid bone to the larynx

Larynx or voice box–at the level of C3-C6. It included the thyroid cartilage

Trachea or windpipe—anterior to esophagus from C6 to the carina at T4/5. It branches into the two bronchi

Lungs—Two pairs on either side of the mediastinum

Right lung is shorter and broader has three lobes divided by a horizontal and two oblique fissures

Left lung has two lobes divided by oblique fissures

Two bronchi or main stem bronchi enter the lungs. Bronchial tree ends at the alveoli, air sac at the end of the bronchioles where oxygen and carbon dioxide exchange take place.

Right bronchus is shorter, wider and more vertical–branches into three secondary bronchi

Left bronchus is longer, narrower and more horizontal—branches into 2 secondary bronchi

Mediastinum–between the lungs, includes heart, great vessels, thymus gland trachea and esophagus

Diaphragm– muscle separating thorax from abdomen

Upper Airway–Anteroposterior (AP) projection

SID, Technical factors, Shielding

- 40 inches (100 cm). Grid. 70kVp @ 5-10mAs or middle AEC cell. Gonadal shielding

Patient/part position

- Patient seated, supine or standing facing the x-ray tube

Specific part/body position or rotation

- Chin raised–not hyperextended. Both shoulders at same level. No rotation.

Direction and point of entry of CR

- CR to a C4 for larynx or perpendicular to IR at level of the jugular notch

Fig. 5a. Position. Upper Airway-Anteroposterior (AP) projection

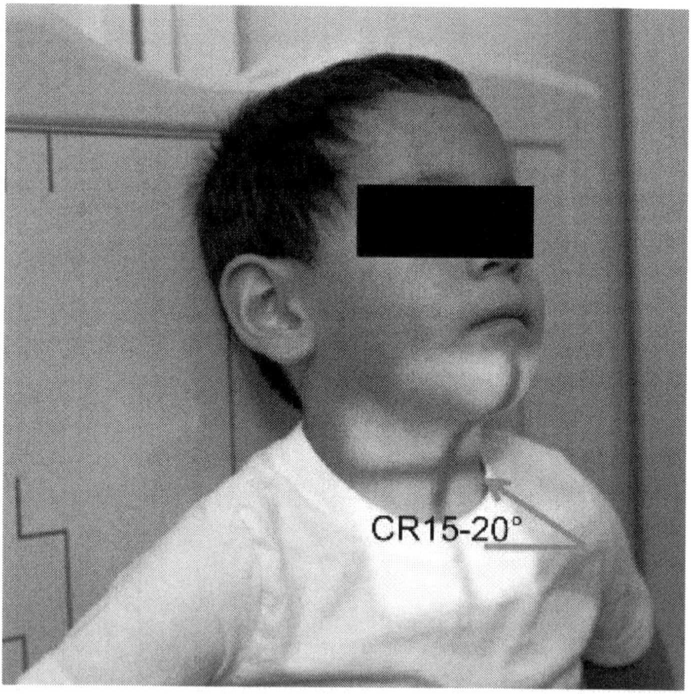

Breathing Instructions (2 methods)

1. Slow deep breaths during exposure–allows the airway to fill with air during exposure and allow a more accurate diagnosis
2. Arrested deep inhalation to ensure air-filled trachea.

Collimation to include or structures demonstrated

- Soft tissue of neck laterally to S/C joint to include from C4 to T6

Image evaluation

- Sternoclavicular joints equidistant from spine.
- Air filled trachea in middle of IR

Fig 5b. Radiograph. Upper Airway-Anteroposterior (AP) position

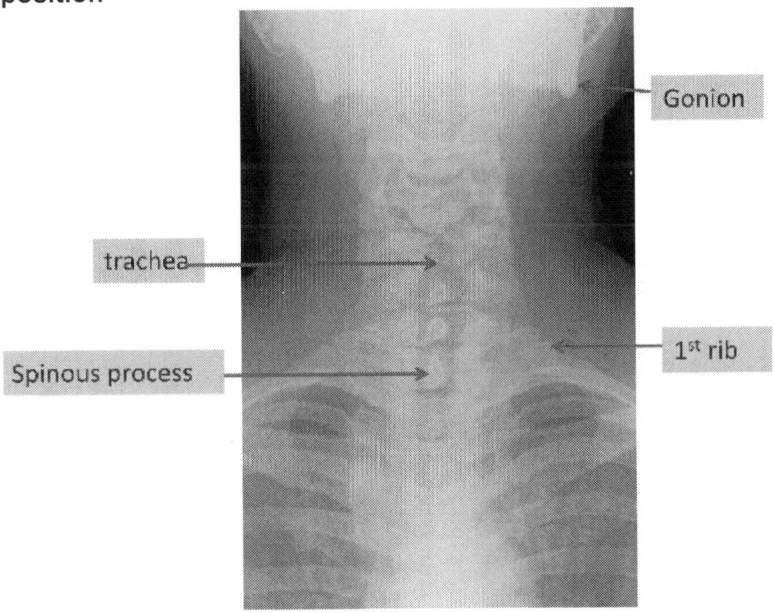

Upper Airway–Lateral

SID, Technical factors, Shielding

- 72inches (183 cm). No Grid. 70 kVp @ 5-10 mAs. No AEC. Gonadal shielding

Patient/part position

- Patient standing or seated–lateral aspect against the wall unit
- Top of IR at level with top of ear

Specific part/body position or rotation

- Chin raised, prevents superimposition over anterior vertebral bodies Shoulders level

Direction and point of entry of CR

- CR to a C4 for larynx or T2/3 at jugular notch to demonstrate upper mediastinum

Fig 6a. Position. Upper Airway- Lateral

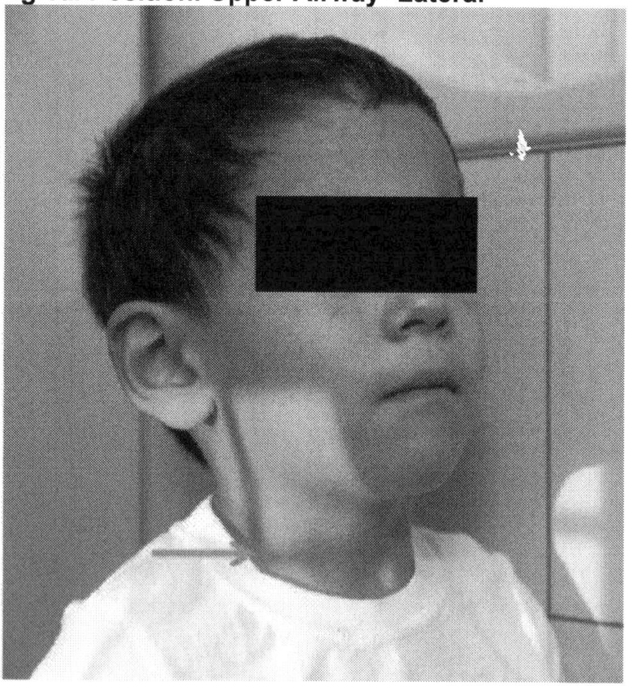

Collimation to include or structures demonstrated

- To include soft tissue of neck from C4 to T7.

Breathing Instructions

- Exposure on deep inhalation to maximize air-filled trachea.

Image evaluation

- True lateral C spine with air filled upper airways seen anteriorly.

Notes:

- Non-Bucky imaging because air-gap removes scatter
- Long SID used to minimize magnification due to increase OID.

Fig 6b. Radiograph. Upper Airway-Lateral

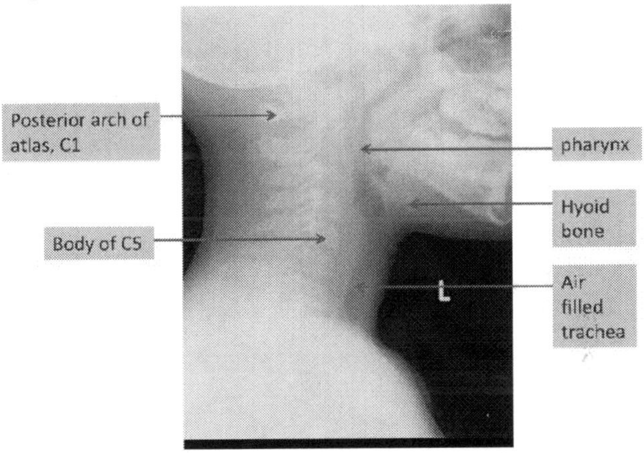

Chest–Posteroanterior (PA) projection

SID, Technical factors, Shielding

- 72inches (183 cm). Grid. 100-110 kVp @ 1.2-5 mAs or lateral AEC cells. Wrap around gonadal shielding.

Patient/part position

- Feet slightly separated with weight equally distributed.

Specific part/body position or rotation

- Top of IR 1½ - 2 inches (3.8-5cm) above the shoulder
- Elevate chin to remove it from apex
- Flex elbow and rest the backs of the hands low on the hips to rotate scapulae laterally and avoid superimposition over lungs

Direction and point of entry of CR

- CR to T7 at inferior angle of scapula

Fig 7a. Position. Chest -Posteroanterior (PA) projection

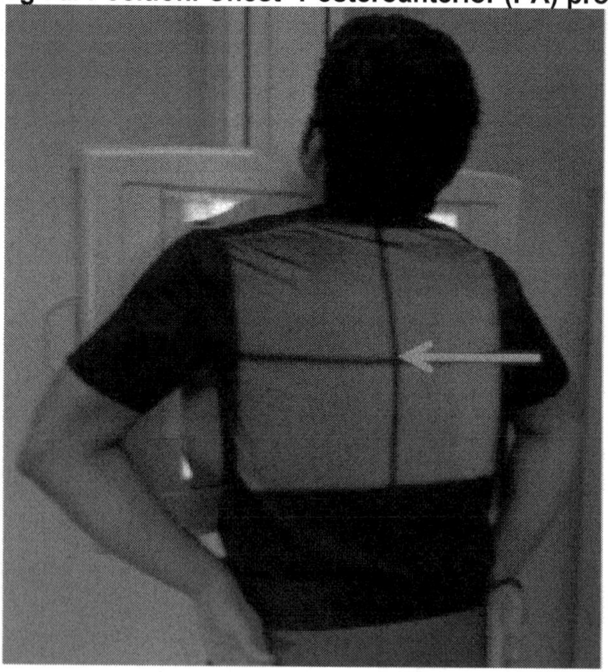

Collimation to include or structures demonstrated

- Apices to base of chest (costophrenic angle) lengthwise. Crosswise to lateral margins of ribs.

Breathing Instructions

- Exposure on second arrested inspiration

Image evaluation

- Lung markings clearly seen. Lungs demonstrated to show 10 posterior ribs.
- Heart adequately penetrated–vascular margins clearly seen.
- Symmetry of sternoclavicular joints, absence of scapulae and chin from lung fields.
- Apices and costophrenic angles seen.
- Thoracic vertebrae seen to the level of bifurcation. (should not be seen further as this would indicate overexposure & can masks lung markings

Fig 7b. Radiograph. Chest- Posteroanterior (PA) projection

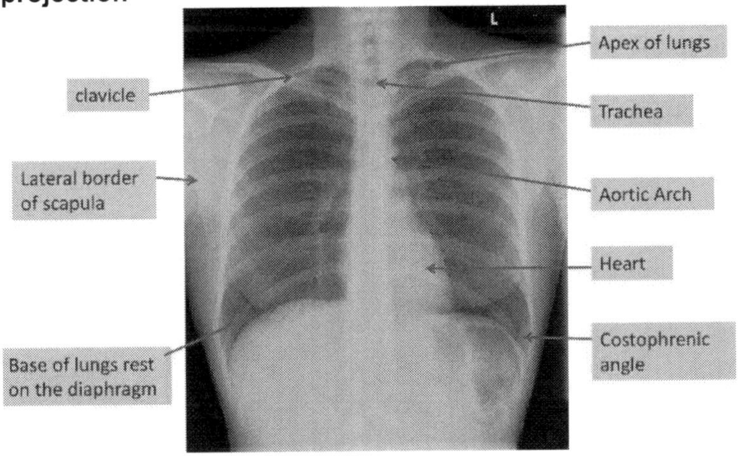

Chest–Lateral projection

SID, Technical factors, Shielding

- 72inches, 183 cm. Grid. 120-130 kVp @ 2-5 mAs or center AEC cell. Wrap around gonadal shielding

Patient/part position

- Place top of IR 1½ to 2 inches (3.8-5cm) above the shoulders with feet separated slightly and weight equally distributed

Specific part/body position or rotation

- Left lateral to place heart closest to IR and minimized heart magnification
- Chin raised, both arms raised above head–flex elbows, grasp opposite elbow with hand

Direction and point of entry of CR

- CR to T7 (level of inferior angle of scapula)

Fig 8a. Position. Chest – Lateral projection

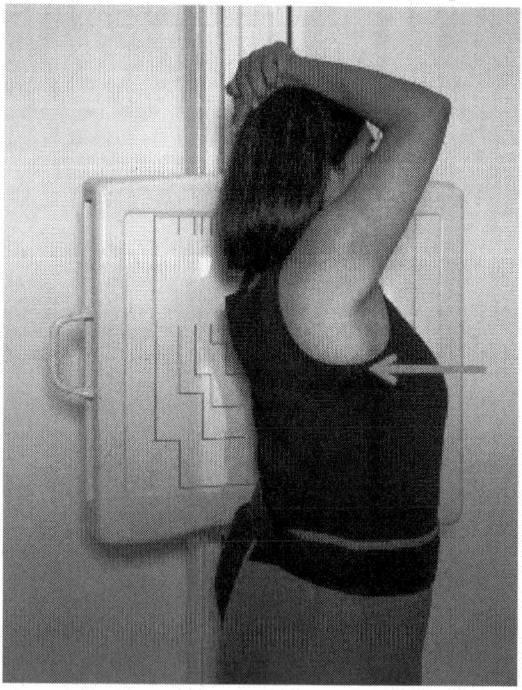

Collimation to include or structures demonstrated

- Apex and lung bases. Sternum and posterior ribs

Breathing Instructions

Second arrested inspiration effort

Image evaluation

- Patient's arm clear of upper lung fields (not superimposed within)
- Both lung apices superimposed with hilar region seen in midline above heart
- Posterior ribs superimposed or within 1cm (0.5inch) if separated
- Spinous process and sternum in profile. Posterior margins of lungs superimposed

Fig. 8b. Radiograph. Chest – Lateral projection

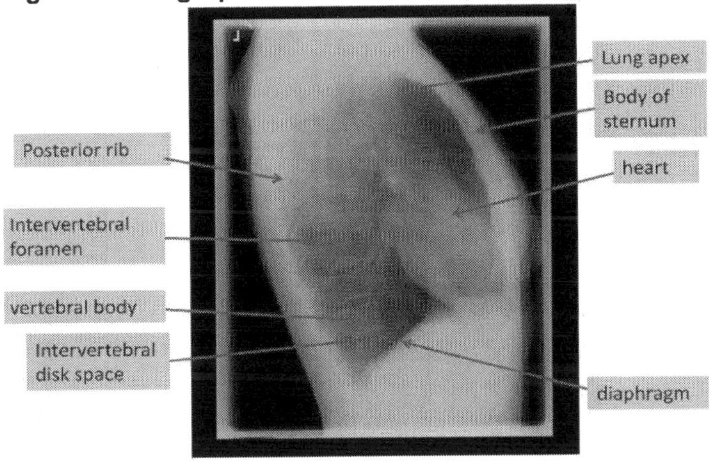

Chest Oblique–Right Anterior Oblique position (RAO)
or Left Anterior Oblique (LAO)

SID, Technical factors, Shielding

- 72inches, 183 cm. Grid. 100-110kVp @ 1.2-5mAs or lateral cells. Wrap around gonadal shielding

Patient/part position for RAO

- Top of IR 1½ - 2 inches (3.8-5cm) above the shoulder
- Patient erect facing the x-ray tube or prone on the x-ray table
- Right side resting on the IR with the left side raised.

Specific part/body position or rotation

- Routine chest obliques uses 45-degrees patient rotation
- If erect, flex left arm to rest on forehead or on top of the wall unit. Keep right arm down or resting the back of hand on hip
- 60-degree rotation uses in cardiac imaging to separate heart and vertebral column.
- 10°–20 ° rotation used to demonstrate pulmonary nodules

Direction and point of entry of CR

- CR to T7

Fig. 9a. Position. Chest – Right Anterior Oblique position, RAO

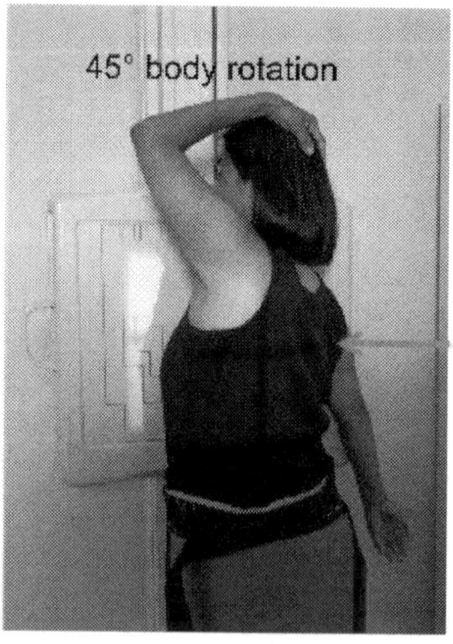

Collimation to include or structures demonstrated

- Apices to base of chest (costophrenic angle) lengthwise
- Crosswise to lateral margins of ribs

Breathing Instructions

- Arrested second inspiration

Image evaluation

- Both lungs, from apex to costophrenic angles.

Note:

- The RAO will show the same image as the LPO
- On the 45-degree LPO, the distance from the outer margin of the ribs to the vertebral column on left side should be equal to twice the distance on the right. Therefore the down side should be twice the distance of the upside

Fig. 9b. Radiograph. Chest – Right Anterior Oblique position, RAO

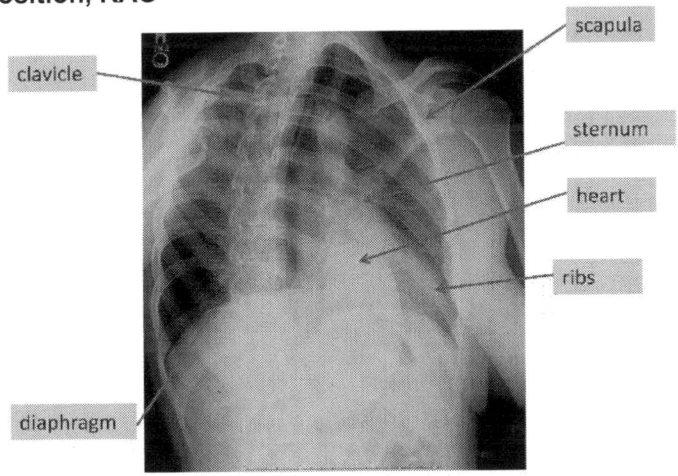

Chest Oblique– Right Posterior Oblique (RPO) or Left Posterior Oblique position (LPO)

SID, Technical factors, Shielding

- 72inches, 183 cm. Grid. 100-110kVp @ 1.2-5mAs or lateral cells.
- Wrap around gonadal shielding

Patient/part position for RPO

- Top of IR 1½ - 2 inches (3.8-5cm) above the shoulder
- Patient supine on x-ray table or erect with back to the x-ray tube
- Right side resting on IR with right side raised

Specific part/body position or rotation

- Routine Chest Obliques uses 45-degrees patient rotation
- On erect, patient oblique with the left arm raised to rest on forehead or top of wall unit. The right arm stays down
- 60-degree patient rotation used in cardiac imaging to separate heart and vertebral column.
- 10°–20 ° rotation used to demonstrate pulmonary nodules

Direction and point of entry of CR

- CR to T7

Fig. 10a. Position. Chest Oblique – Right Posterior Oblique position, RPO

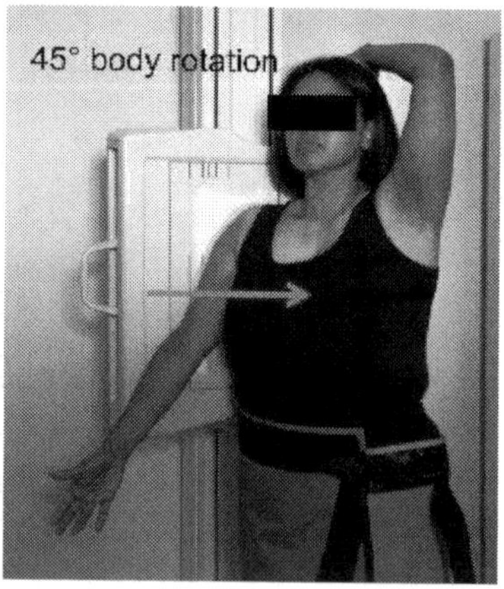

Collimation to include or structures demonstrated

- Apices to base of chest (costophrenic angle) lengthwise.
- Crosswise to lateral margins of ribs.

Breathing Instructions

- Arrested second inspiration

Image evaluation

- Both lungs, from apex to costophrenic angles.

Note:

- The RPO will show the same image as the LAO
- On the RPO, 45-degree oblique, the distance from the outer margin of the ribs to the vertebral column on the downside or right side which is closest to the IR should be equal to two times the distance of the up side or side away from the IR. Therefore the right side will be twice the left

Fig. 10b Radiograph. Chest Oblique- Right Posterior Oblique or Left Anterior Oblique position

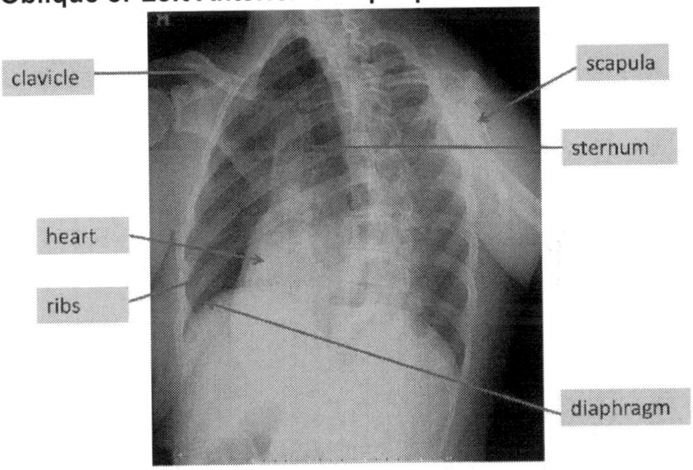

Chest–Lordotic position

SID, Technical factors, Shielding

- 72inches, 183 cm. Grid. 100-110kVp @ 1.2-5mAs or lateral cells. Wrap around gonadal shielding

Patient/part position

- Erect AP with top of IR at level of shoulder

Specific part/body position or rotation

- Patient stands about 1 foot from unit and leans backwards or patient erect using and cephalic tube angulation

Direction and point of entry of CR

- CR to midline at level of midsternum.
- If patient erect AP or supine use 20° cephalic angulation.

Fig 11a. Position. Chest – Lordotic position

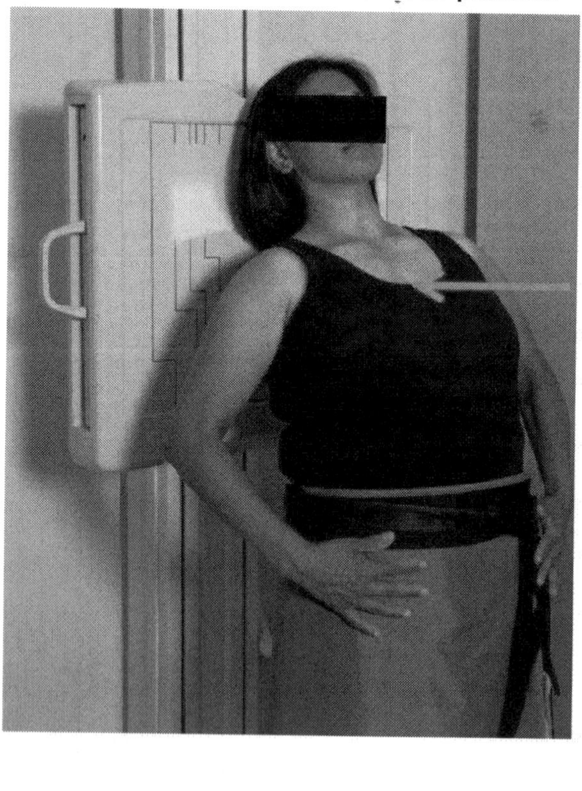

Collimation to include or structures demonstrated

- Apices and lateral margins of ribs.

Breathing Instructions

- Arrested second inspiration effort.

Image evaluation

- Clavicles projected above the thorax
- Medial ends of clavicles slightly superimposed over 1st or 2nd ribs.
- Anterior and posterior ends of 1st ribs should be superimposed

Fig.11b. Radiograph. Chest – Lordotic position

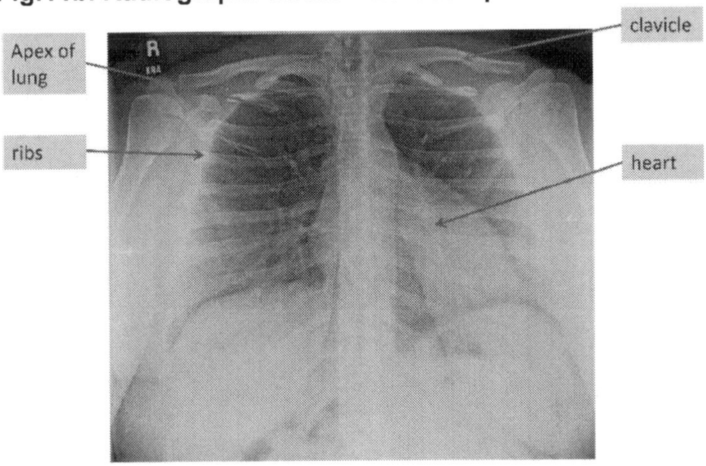

Chest–Decubitus

Left or Right Lateral

SID, Technical factors, Shielding

- 40 inches (100cm). Grid. 100-110kVp @ 1.5-5mAs or lateral cells. Wrap around gonadal shielding

Patient/part position for the left lateral decubitus

- Top of IR 1½- 2 inches (3.8-5cm) above shoulder
- Patient on raised radiolucent sponge or supported higher than the IR

Specific part/body position or rotation

- To demonstrate fluid levels, patient should remain in the lateral recumbent position on table or stretcher for **10 minutes** before exposure
- Patient on left sided with arms raise and legs flexed for balance

Direction and point of entry of CR

- CR to T7

Fig 12a. Position. Chest – Decubitus, Left Lateral

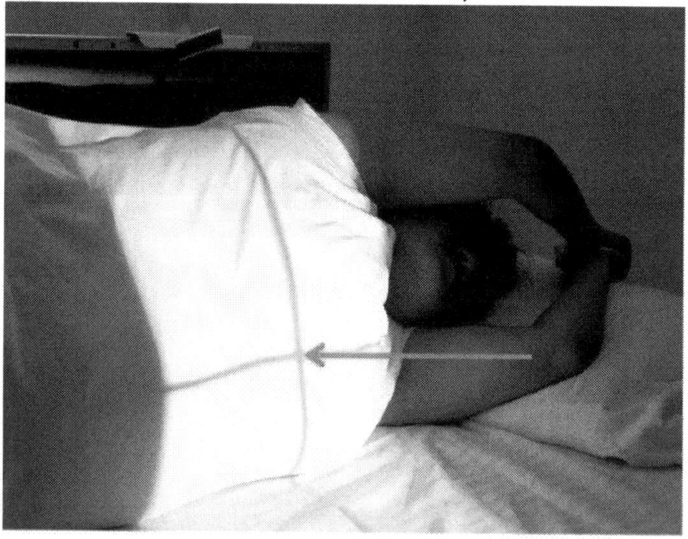

Collimation to include or structures demonstrated

- Apices to base of chest (costophrenic angle) lengthwise. Crosswise to lateral margins of ribs
- AP or PA chest obtained

Breathing Instructions

- Arrested second inspiration

Image evaluation

- Symmetrical sternoclavicular joints
- Clear lung markings with ribs seen through heart shadow
- Vertebrae seen to bifurcation

Notes

- Right or left lateral decubitus performed
- If entire thorax cannot be seen because of patient size image the down side **fluids visualization** or the up side for **air visualization**
- Fluid visualization–affected side placed down.
- Air visualization– affected side placed up

Fig. 12b. Radiograph. Chest – Decubitus, Left Lateral

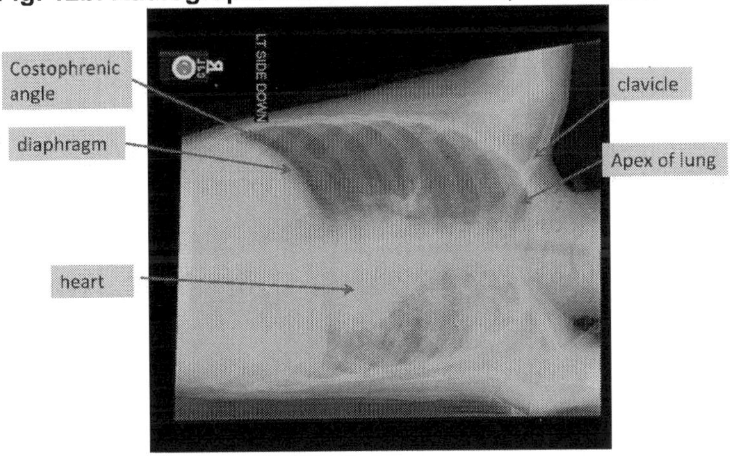

Abdomen Imaging

Patient Preparation includes:

- Internal: not needed unless patient is scheduled for a contrast study
- External: removal of outer clothing, underwear with metallic attachments and long necklaces

Exposure factors

- Low kVp to allow enhancement of inherently low contrast structures
- High kVp (over 100) for contrast studies
- Exposure time of 0.5 sec or less–to minimize breathing and peristaltic motion.

Recommended breathing instructions & reasons

- Arrested expiration relives pressure on the abdominal content.
- Give one second delay after expiration to allow involuntary motion of bowel to cease.

Purpose of supine imaging

- Evaluate the abdominal contents (size and location of organ bowel gas patterns)
- Check tube placements or localize foreign bodies
- Preliminary image prior to the administration of contrast medium
- To rule out residual contrast in the abdomen from a previous exam
- To identify any pathology congenital abnormalities or stones in the kidneys or gallbladder

Purpose of erect imaging

- Bowel obstruction, perforations or to rule out free air in the abdomen

Radiation protection–how/when applied

- Not possible on females
- Gonadal shields on males if such shielding does not obscure essential anatomy as determined by a physician

Divisions of the Abdomen

Four-quadrant division of the abdomen

- RUQ- Right Upper Quadrant,
- LUQ–Left Upper Quadrant,
- RLQ- Right Lower Quadrant,
- LLQ–Left Lower Quadrant

Location of Abdominal Content in 4-Quadrant

Right Upper Quadrant (RUQ)

- Liver, Gall bladder, Hepatic flexure, Duodenum, Head of pancreas, Right Kidney, Right Adrenal Gland

Left Upper Quadrant (LUQ)

- Left Kidney, Left Adrenal Glan, Spleen, Left Splenic Flexure, Tail of Pancreas, Stomach

Right Lower Quadrant (RLQ)

- Ascending Colon, Appendix, Cecum, 2/3 Ileum, Ileocecal Valve

Left Lower Quadrant (LLQ)

- Descending Colon, 2/3 Jejunum, Sigmoid Colon

Nine-region division of the abdomen

- R & L hypochondriac – upper portions below the ribs;
- Epigastric – upper central portion, over the stomach;
- R & L lumbar – middle regions located lateral to the umbilicus & also called R & L lateral regions;
- Umbilical – central region around the navel;
- R & L iliac – lower sides, area of the ilia of pelvis & also called the inguinal regions;
- Hypogastric – below the umbilicus – lower middle region

Fig 13a. Abdomen – The Four Quadrants

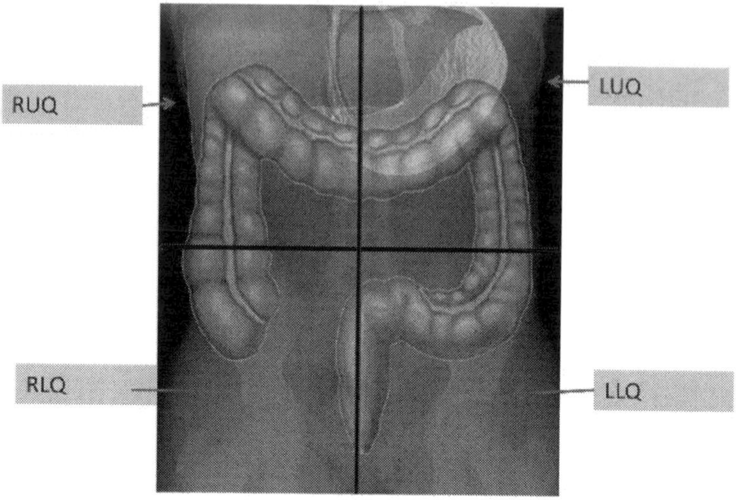

Fig 13b Abdomen – The Nine Region Divisions

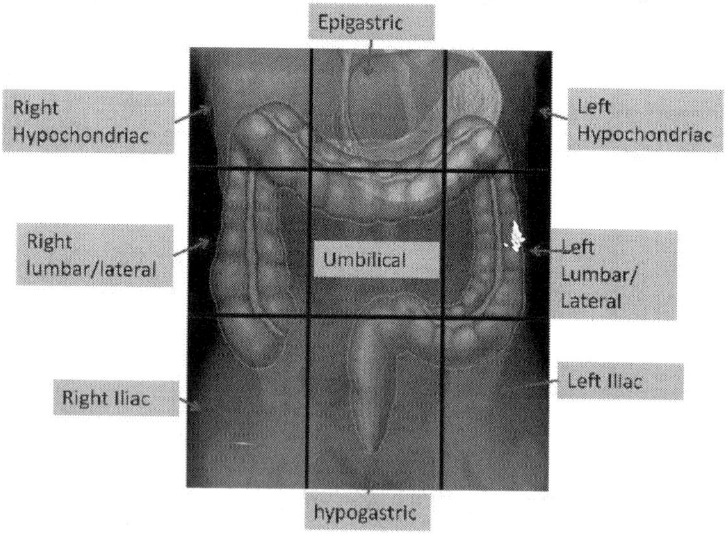

Positioning Considerations & Projection guide

- The symphysis must be included on the supine abdomen radiograph.
- The diaphragm must be included on the erect or decubitus abdomen radiograph.
- Very thin patients may need pad support (if lying for over 20 minutes).
- Pillow under head and knee relieve will stress on back.
- A tall hyposthenic, or asthenic type patients, may require two images lengthwise, one centered lower to include the symphysis pubis and the second centered high to include the upper abdomen and diaphragm.
- A broad hypersthenic-type patient may also require two 35 x 43 cm (14 X 17) images placed crosswise, one centered lower to include the symphysis pubis and the second for the upper abdomen, with a minimum of 3 to 5 cm (1 to 2 inches) overlap.

Projection guide

Obstruction series/acute abdomen:

- Chest, supine & erect abdomen or decubitus

Free air:

- erect or decubitus abdomen

Foreign body series:

- lateral soft neck, PA/AP CHEST, supine abdomen

Aortic aneurysm or foreign body localization

- AP/PA erect or recumbent and lateral or dorsal decubitus

Kidney stones

- AP erect or PA recumbent and oblique

Abdomen–Supine, Anteroposterior (AP) projection

SID, Technical factors, Shielding

- 40 inches (100 cm). Grid.70-80 kVp @ 20-50 mAs or lateral cell. Gonadal shielding on males

Patient/part position

- Patient supine, lying on the x-ray table

Specific part/body position or rotation

- Arms placed at patient's sides, away from body
- Legs extended with support under knees as needed
- No rotation of pelvis or shoulders (ASISs are the same distance from tabletop).

Direction and point of entry of CR

- CR to midline at level of iliac crest can vary by body habitus

Fig. 14a. Position. Abdomen – Anteroposterior (AP) projection

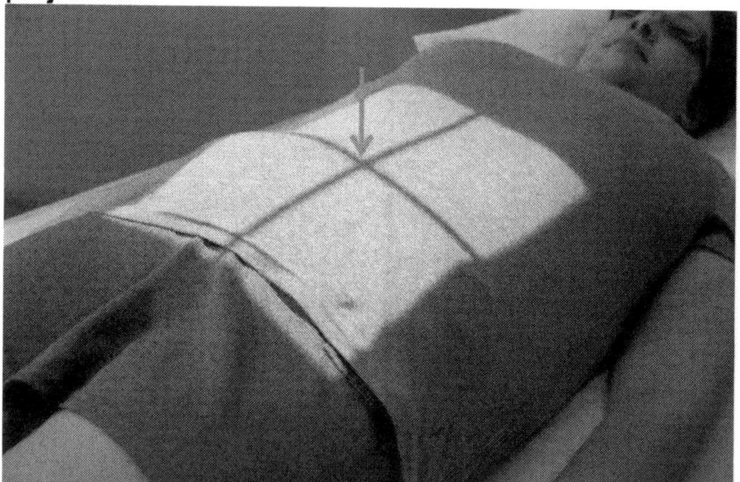

Collimation to include or structures demonstrated

- Collimate to lateral skin margins
- The symphysis must be included

Breathing Instructions

- Arrested expiration

Image evaluation

- No motion, with sharp outline of internal structures
- No rotation of iliac wings and obturator foramina
- Sacrum & coccyx aligned with arch of symphysis pubis
- Ischial spines symmetrical
- Visualization of psoas muscle outlines and lumbar transverse processes
- Outline of liver, kidneys, air filled stomach and fecal/gas patterns

Note

Low kVp (under 80) will enhance the subject contrast

Fig. 14b. Radiograph. Abdomen – Anteroposterior (AP) projection

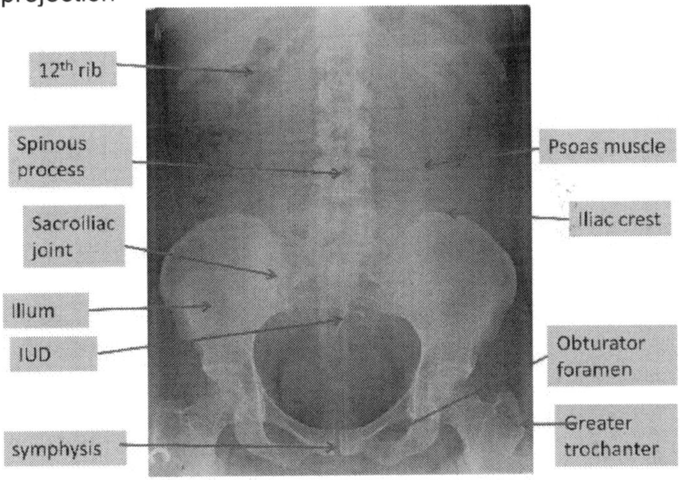

Abdomen–Prone, Posteroanterior (PA) projection

SID, Technical factors, Shielding

- 40 inches (100 cm). Grid.70-80 kVp @ 20-50 mAs or lateral cell. Gonadal shielding on males

Patient/part position

- Prone with midsagittal plane centered to midline of table and IR and /or IR

Specific part/body position or rotation

- Arms placed at patient's sides, away from body
- Legs extended with support under knees if this is more comfortable
- No rotation of pelvis or shoulders. Both ASIS same distance from tabletop

Direction and point of entry of CR

- CR to midline at level of iliac crest can vary by body habitus

Fig 15a. Position. Abdomen – Posteroanterior (PA) projection

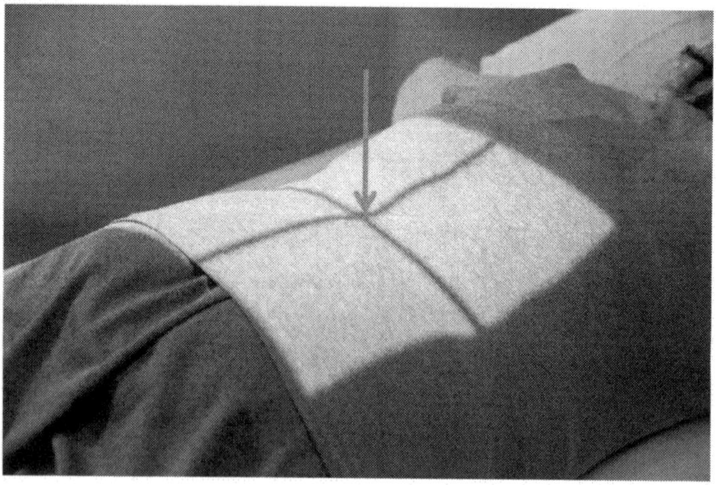

Collimation to include or structures demonstrated

- Collimate to lateral skin margins
- The symphysis must be included

Breathing Instructions

- Exposure on arrested expiration. Give 1 second delay after expiration to allow involuntary motion of bowel to cease.

Image evaluation

- No motion, with sharp outline of internal structures
- No rotation of iliac wings and obturator foramina
- Sacrum & coccyx aligned with arch of symphysis pubis
- Ischial spines symmetrical
- Visualization of psoas muscle outlines and lumbar transverse processes
- Outline of liver, kidneys, air filled stomach and fecal/gas patterns

Note

- Low kVp (under 80 will enhance the subject contrast

Fig. 15b Radiograph. Abdomen - Posteroanterior (PA) projection

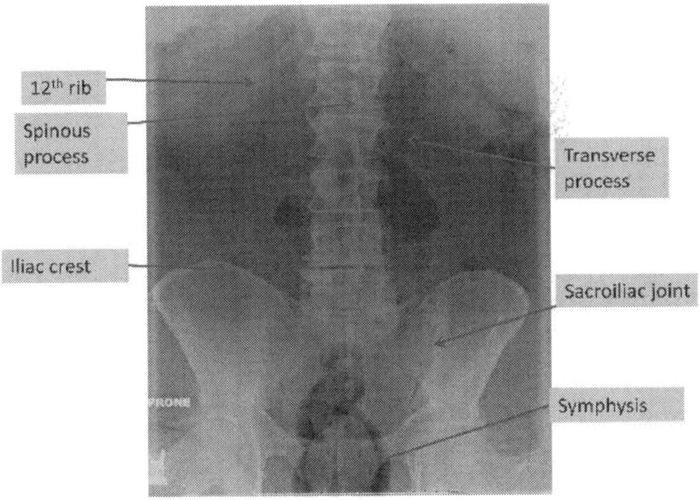

Abdomen–Erect, Posteroanterior (PA) projection

SID, Technical factors, Shielding

- 40 inches (100 cm). Grid.70-80 kVp @ 20-50mAs or lateral cell. Gonadal shielding when possible

Patient/part position

- Erect, standing or sitting with back to the x-ray tube

Specific part/body position or rotation

- Arms placed at patient's sides, away from body
- No rotation of pelvis or shoulders with ASIS symmetrical

Direction and point of entry of CR

- CR perpendicular to and directed to 3 inches (7cm) above the iliac crest with top margin of the IR at the axilla
- Centering can vary according to patient size and build

Collimation to include or structures demonstrated

- Collimate to skin margins and on top and bottom to IR borders
- Imaging must include the diaphragm

Fig 16a. Position. Abdomen – Erect, Posteroanterior (PA) projection

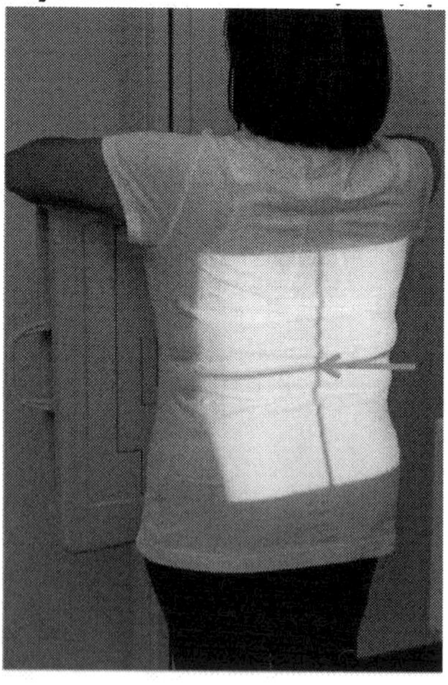

Breathing Instructions

- Exposure on arrested expiration. Give 1 second delay after expiration to allow involuntary motion of bowel to cease.

Image evaluation

- No motion, with sharp outline of internal structures
- No rotation of iliac wings and obturator foramina
- Sacrum & coccyx aligned with arch of symphysis pubis
- Ischial spines symmetrical
- Outline of psoas muscles and lumbar transverse processes
- Outline of liver, kidneys, air filled stomach and fecal/gas patterns

Notes

- Low kVp (under 80 will enhance the subject contrast
- PA imaging will give the patient 90% less gonadal dose then the AP and 50% less breast dose

Fig 16b. Radiograph. Abdomen – Erect, Posteroanterior (PA) projection

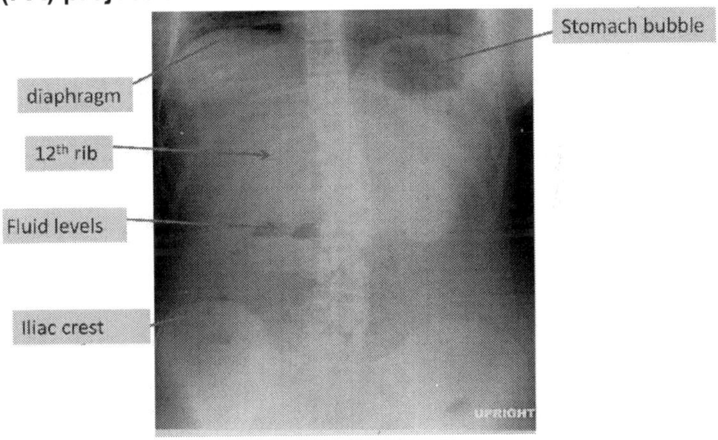

Abdomen–Lateral projection

SID, Technical factors, Shielding

- 40 inches (100 cm). Grid. 80 kVp @ 20-50mAs or middle cell. Gonadal shielding on males

Patient/part position

- Erect or recumbent. MSP parallel to IR

Specific part/body position or rotation

- Arms raised or prayer position
- Legs flexed for balance if recumbent with support between knees for comfort

Direction and point of entry of CR

- CR perpendicular to and directed to center of IR at level of iliac crest
- Centering can vary according to patient size and build

Fig. 17a. Position. Abdomen – Lateral projection

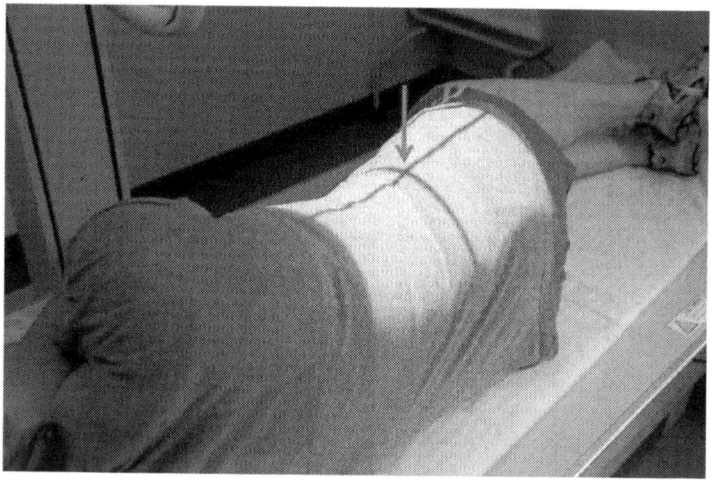

Collimation to include or structures demonstrated

- Collimate closely on sides to lateral skin margins and on top and bottom to IR borders
- Bottom of IR at level with the symphysis pubis

Breathing Instructions

- Exposure on arrested expiration
- Give 1 second delay after expiration to allow involuntary motion of bowel to cease

Image evaluation

- No motion with sharp outline of internal structures
- Superimposed iliac wings

Fig. 17b. Radiograph. Abdomen – Lateral projection

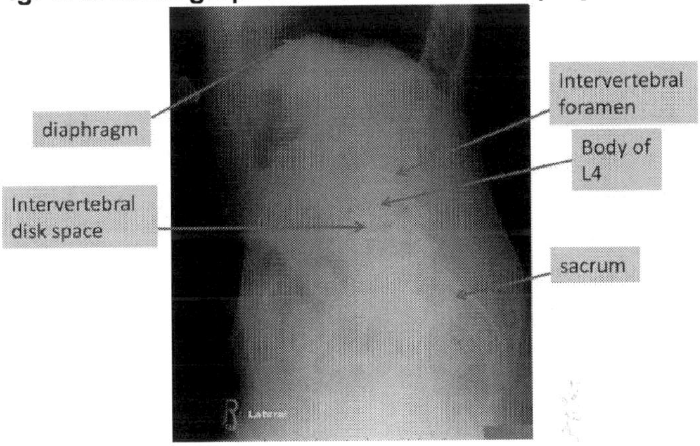

Abdomen–Lateral Decubitus position

SID, Technical factors, Shielding

- 40 inches (100 cm). Grid. 70-80 kVp @ 20-50mAs or lateral cell. Gonadal shielding on males

Patient/part position, left lateral decubitus

- Patient on left side with MSP parallel to IR
- Patient should be in place for at least 10 minutes before exposure.

Specific part/body position or rotation

- Legs flexed for balance with support between knees for comfort

Direction and point of entry of CR

- CR perpendicular to and directed to 3 inches (7cm) above the iliac crest) with top margin of the IR at the axilla

Fig 18a. Position. Abdomen – Lateral Decubitus position

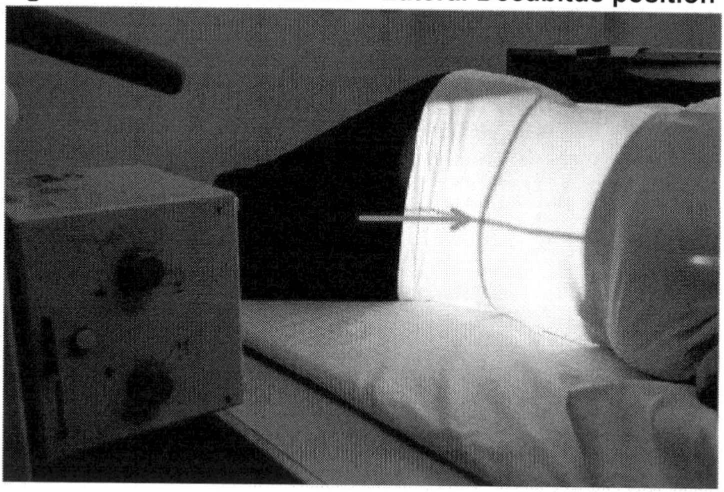

Collimation to include or structures demonstrated

- AP or PA projection obtained
- Collimate closely on sides to lateral skin margins
- Diaphragm must be included in the image

Breathing Instructions

- Exposure on arrested expiration. Give 1 second delay after expiration to allow involuntary motion of bowel to cease.

Image evaluation

- No motion with sharp outline of liver, kidneys, air filled stomach and fecal/gas patterns
- No rotation of iliac wings and obturator foramina
- Sacrum & coccyx aligned with arch of symphysis pubis
- Ischial spines symmetrical
- Visualization of psoas muscle outlines and lumbar transverse processes

Note:

- The left lateral decubitus is more common versus the right to minimize any risk of confusing the stomach bubble with any free air in the abdomen.

Fig 18b. Radiograph. Abdomen – Lateral Decubitus position

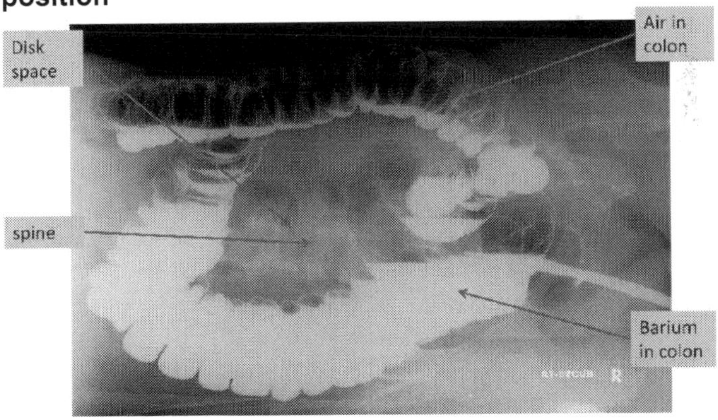

Abdomen–Dorsal Decubitus

SID, Technical factors, Shielding

- 40 inches (100 cm). Grid. 80 kVp @ 20-50mAs or middle cell. Gonadal shielding on males

Patient/part position

- Should be in place for at least 10 min before exposure.

Specific part/body position or rotation

- Supine with midsagittal plane centered to midline of table and IR and /or IR
- Arms placed at patient's sides, away from body
- Legs extended with support under knees if this is more comfortable
- No rotation of pelvis or shoulders
- Both ASIS at the same distance from tabletop

Direction and point of entry of CR

- CR perpendicular to and directed to center of IR (to level of iliac crest) with bottom margin at symphysis pubis
- Centering can vary according to patient size and build

Fig. 19a Position. Abdomen – Dorsal Decubitus

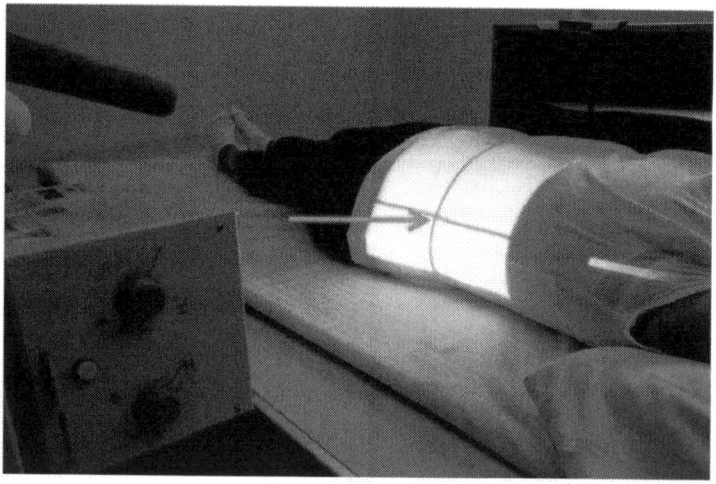

Collimation to include or structures demonstrated

- Collimate closely on sides to skin margins and on top and bottom to IR borders

Breathing Instructions

- Exposure on arrested expiration. Give 1 second delay after expiration to allow involuntary motion of bowel to cease.

Image evaluation

- No motion with sharp outline of internal structures

Fig. 19b. Radiograph. Abdomen – Dorsal Decubitus

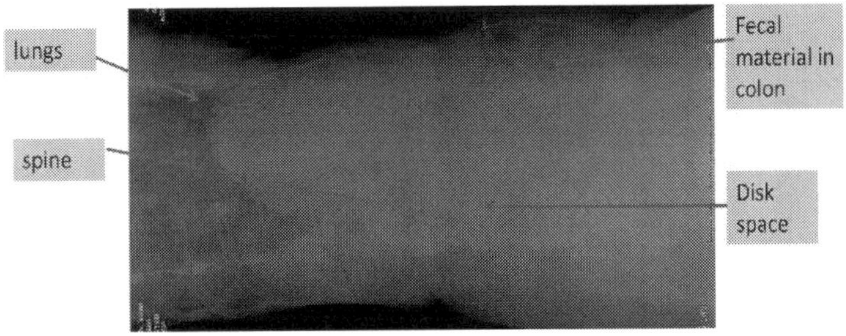

Abdomen–Posterior Oblique, LPO or RPO position Or Anterior Oblique, LAO or RAO position

SID, Technical factors, Shielding

- 40 inches (100 cm). Grid.70-80 kVp @ 20-50mAs or lateral cell. Gonadal shielding on males
  Patient/part position
- Recumbent

Specific part/body position or rotation

- From the prone position rotate the patient 30° to one side
- Bring the opposite arm across the chest
- Use lumbar sponge to support the shoulders and hips
- Flexion of down side knee may cause superimposition of leg over bladder

Direction and point of entry of CR

- CR to midline at level of iliac crest can vary by body habitus

Collimation to include or structures demonstrated

- Collimate to lateral skin margins
- The symphysis must be included

Fig. 20a. Position. Abdomen – Posterior Oblique, LPO position

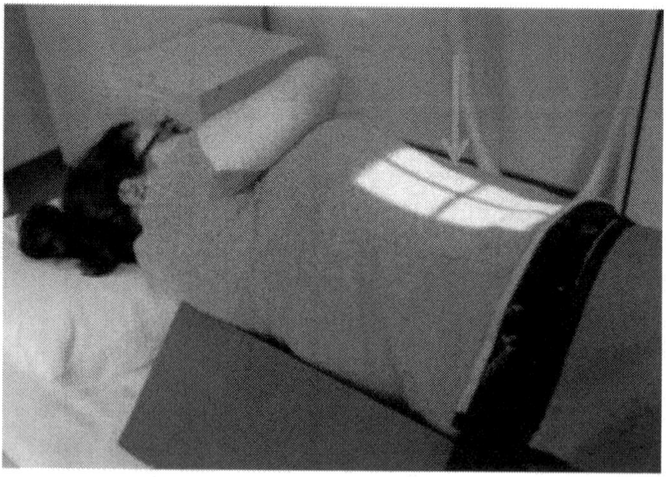

Breathing Instructions

- Exposure on arrested expiration. Give 1 second delay after expiration to allow involuntary motion of bowel to cease.

Image evaluation

- No motion, with sharp outline of internal structures

Note

- Low kVp (under 80 will enhance the subject contrast
- **Obliques** will evaluate displacement of kidney/ureters, calculi, masses
- Demonstrates the elevated kidney parallel with the IR and the downside kidney perpendicular with the IR
- Down ureter will project clear of spine
- RPO shows right ureter and left kidney (Right kidney projected perpendicular and left kidney parallel
- LPO shows left ureter and right kidney. (Left kidney projected perpendicular and right parallel)

Fig. 20b. Radiograph. Abdomen – Posterior Oblique, LPO position

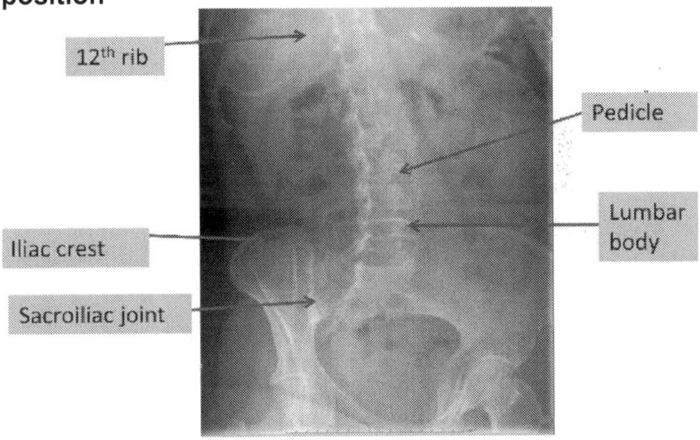

Upper Extremity Imaging

Reducing magnification

- Bucky used increases OID therefore extremities should be imaged tabletop

Breathing instructions

- Not necessary however a child or anxious adult is more likely to keep still when told to stop breathing.

External preparations

- Remove anything metallic from the area of interest

Radiation protection

- Always shield if gonads lie within 5cm or 2 in of the collimated field or primary beam
- Shielding provided to all patients, especially to children and females of child bearing age

Seating of patient

- Patient seated sideways at end of table to reduce radiation to gonads.
- The head, neck and face always turned away from the CR to minimize radiation to eyes and thyroid

Bones of Upper Extremity

Number of bones on each side of the body

Hand–19 bones (excluding the carpals)

- 14 phalanges articulate proximally with the metacarpals –(**metacarpophalangeal joints**) and distally with the second row of the phalanges of each digit –(**interphalangeal joints**)
  - The thumb has 2 phalanges –proximal and distal
  - The other digits have 3 phalanges –proximal, middle and distal
- 5 metacarpals named 1-5
  - The metacarpals articulate with the phalanges proximally, and the with the carpals distally

Wrist –8 carpals

- Proximal row – starting laterally
  - Scaphoid, lunate, triquetrum, pisiform
- Distal row – starting laterally
  - Trapezium, trapezoid, capitate, hamate

Forearm –2 bones

- Radius –on lateral side
  - Radius articulates with the ulna and humerus proximally and with the ulna, scaphoid, lunate and triquetrum distally
- Ulna –on medial side
  - Ulna articulates with humerus and radius proximally, and with the radius distally

Arm –1 bone

- Humerus
  - Humerus articulates proximally with the glenoid cavity of the scapula and distally with the radius and ulna

Finger–Posteroanterior (PA)

SID, Technical factors, Shielding

- 40 inches (100 cm). No Grid. 50 kVp @ 1.3 mAs. No AEC. Gonadal shielding

Patient/part position

- Seated, face turned away with side to the x-ray table to reduce radiation to gonads, eyes and thyroid

Specific part/body position or rotation

- Hand pronated, resting on the IR. Forearm and hand on same level

Direction and point of entry of CR

- Perpendicular to the proximal interphalangeal joint

Fig. 21a Position. Finger – Posteroanterior (PA)

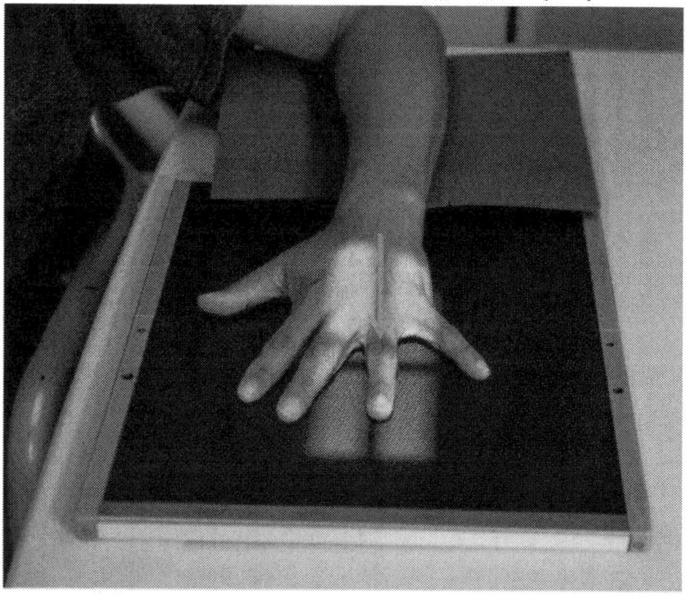

Collimation to include or structures demonstrated

- All phalanges, plus 1/2 of metacarpal

Image evaluation

- Bone trabeculae and soft tissue with symmetrical concavity of shafts of phalanges.
- Open metacarpophalangeal joints (MCP) & interphalangeal joints

Fig. 21b. Radiograph. Finger – Posteroanterior (PA)

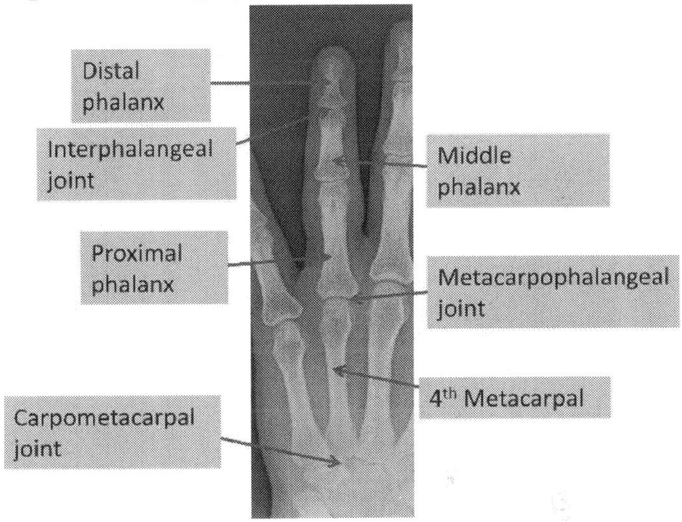

Finger–Oblique

SID, Technical factors, Shielding

- 40 inches (100 cm). No Grid. 50 kVp @ 1.3 mAs. No AEC. Gonadal shielding

Patient/part position

- Seated, face turned away with side to the x-ray table to reduce radiation to gonads, eyes and thyroid

Specific body/part position or rotation

- Finger rotated 45° to tabletop.

Direction and point of entry of CR

- Perpendicular to the proximal interphalangeal joint

Fig. 22a. Position. Finger - Oblique

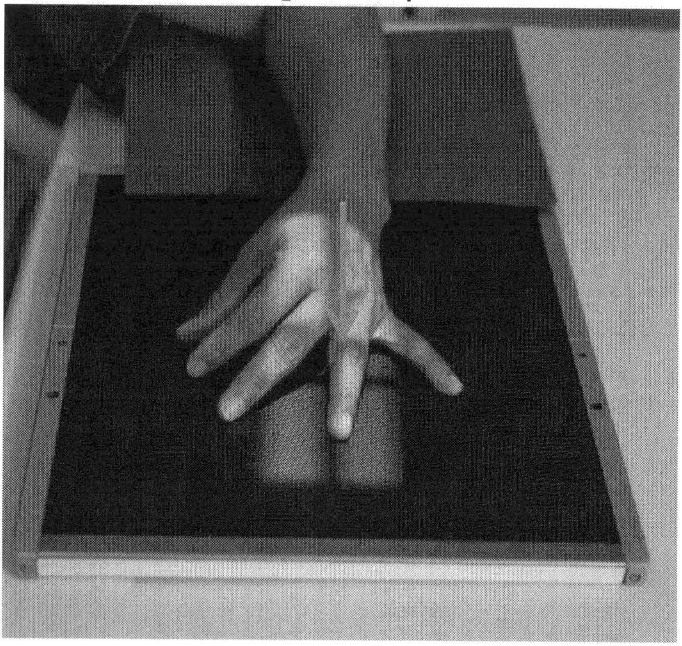

Collimation to include or structures demonstrated

- All phalanges visualized plus 1/3 of metacarpal

Image evaluation

- Bone trabeculae and soft tissue with open MCP & interphalangeal joints.
- Symmetric concavities of both sides of shafts of phalanges

Notes

- Using a radiolucent finger sponge will place fingers parallel with the tabletop to demonstrate joint spaces and prevent foreshortening
- To minimize OID and minimize patient discomfort hand should be internally rotated for 2nd digit and externally rotated of for 3-5th digits.

Fig. 22b. Radiograph. Finger - Oblique

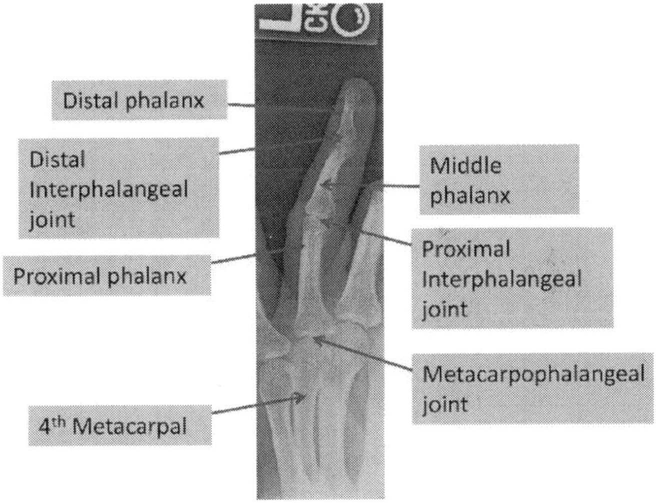

Finger–Lateral

SID, Technical factors, Shielding

- 40 inches (100 cm). No Grid. 50 kVp @ 1.3 mAs. No AEC. Gonadal shielding

Patient/part position

- Seated, face turned away with side to the x-ray table to reduce radiation to gonads, eyes and thyroid

Specific body/part position or rotation

- Rotate hand to lateral position, 90 degrees from the PA. Extend affected finger. Flex other fingers or extend them out of the way.

Direction and point of entry of CR

- Perpendicular to the proximal interphalangeal joint

Fig. 23a. Position. Finger – Lateral

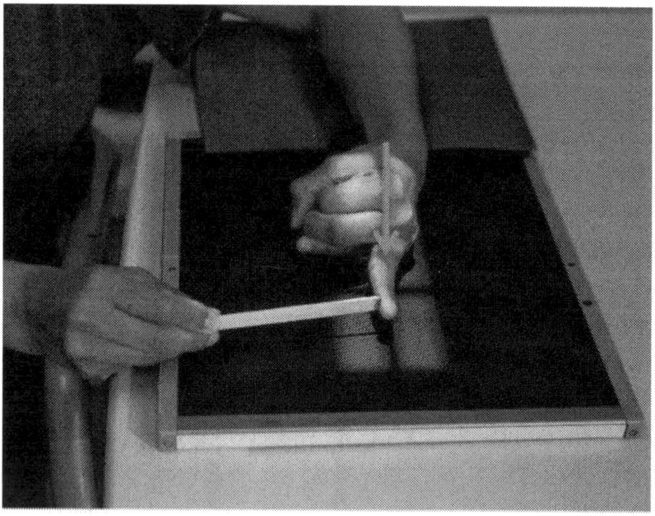

Collimation to include or structures demonstrated

- All phalanges visualized plus 1/3 of metacarpal

Image evaluation

- Bone trabeculae and soft tissue with open MCP & interphalangeal joints.
- Concave anterior shafts

Notes

- To minimize OID and patient discomfort hand should be internally rotated for 2nd digit and externally rotated of for 3-5th digits.
- Using a radiolucent finger sponge will place fingers parallel with the tabletop to demonstrate joint spaces and prevent foreshortening

Fig. 22b. Radiograph. Finger - Oblique

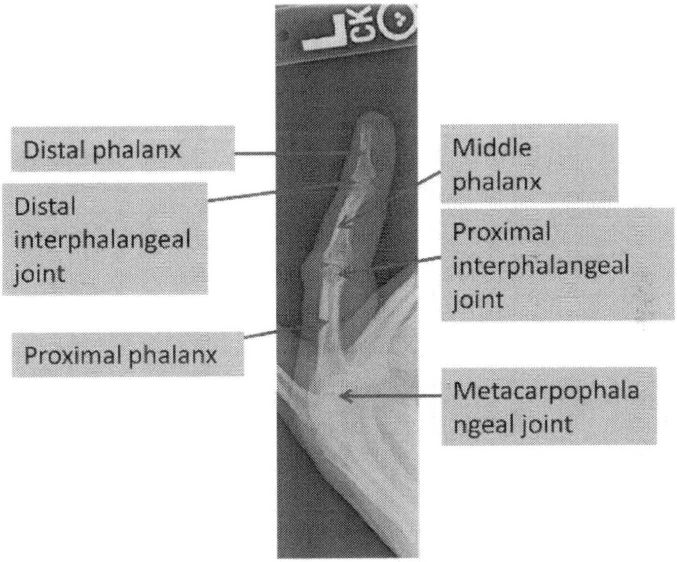

Thumb–Posteroanterior (PA)

SID, Technical factors, Shielding

- 40 inches (100 cm). No Grid. 50 kVp @ 1.3 mAs. No AEC. Gonadal shielding

Patient/part position (PA)

- Seated, face turned away with side to the x-ray table to reduce radiation to gonads, eyes and thyroid

Specific Body/part position or rotation

- Position hand true lateral. Keep thumb extended in true PA position

Direction and point of entry of CR

- Perpendicular to metacarpophalangeal joint

Fig. 24a. Position. Thumb- Posteroanterior (PA)

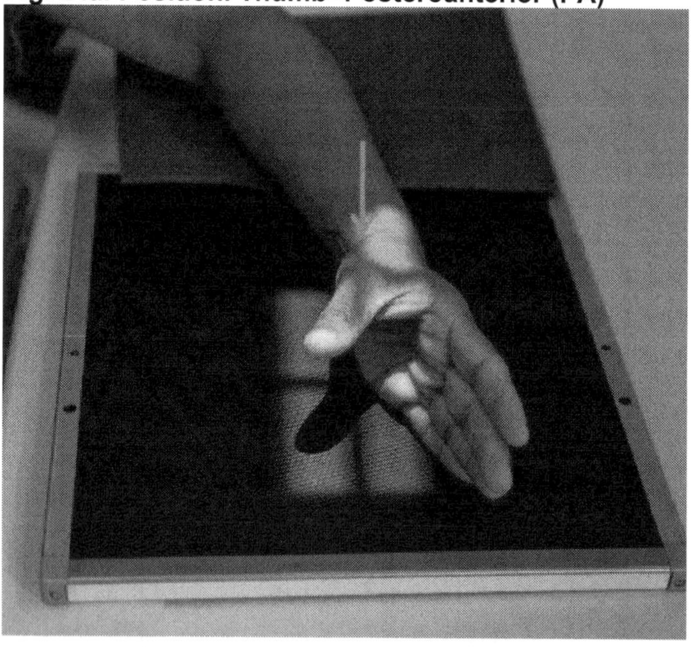

Collimation to include or structures demonstrated

- All phalanges, plus the trapezium or 1 inch (2.5cm) distal radius/ulna

Exposure/image evaluation

- Bone trabeculae and soft tissue with symmetrical concavity of shafts of phalanges.
- Interphalangeal joints open. 1st MCP joint open

Note

- PA is more comfortable for most patients however the AP provides more detail with a smaller OID

Fig. 24b. Radiograph. Thumb- Posteroanterior (PA)

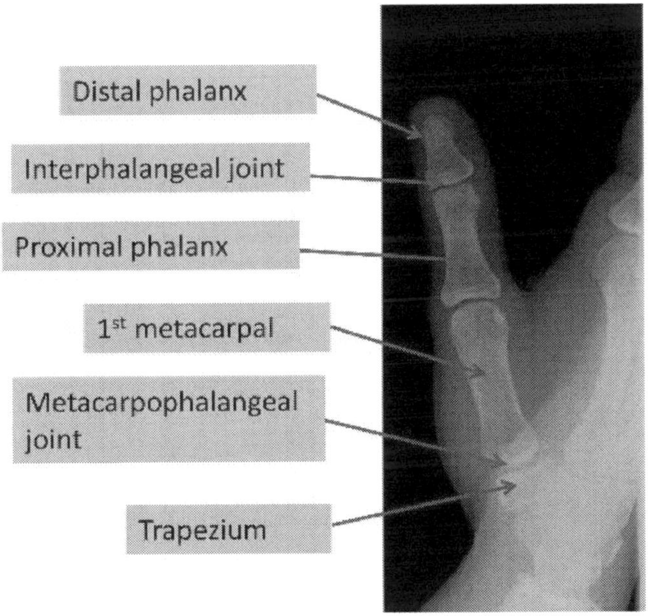

Thumb–Anteroposterior (AP)

SID, Technical factors, Shielding

- 40 inches (100 cm). No Grid. 50 kVp @ 1.3 mAs. No AEC. Gonadal shielding

Patient/part position (AP)

- Seated, face turned away with side to the x-ray table to reduce radiation to gonads, eyes and thyroid

Specific Body/part position or rotation

- Internally rotate hand and wrist to place dorsal surface of thumb on IR
- Slightly elevate forearm and elbow

Direction and point of entry of CR

- Perpendicular to metacarpophalangeal joint

Fig. 25a Position. Thumb – Anteroposterior(AP)

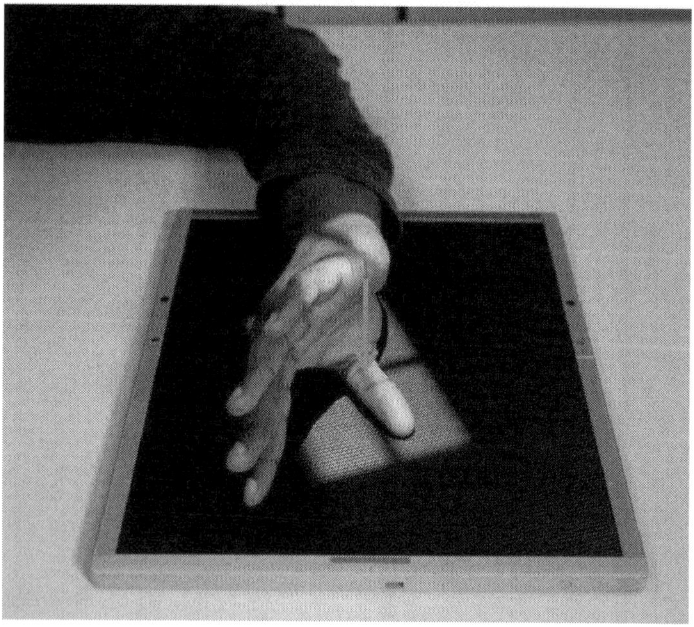

Collimation to include or structures demonstrated

- All phalanges, plus the trapezium or 1 inch (2.5cm) distal radius/ulna

Exposure/image evaluation

- Bone trabeculae and soft tissue with symmetrical concavity of shafts of phalanges.
- Interphalangeal joints open. 1st MCP joint open

Note

- PA is more comfortable for most patients however the AP provides more detail with a smaller OID

Fig. 25b. Radiograph. Thumb – Anteroposterior(AP)

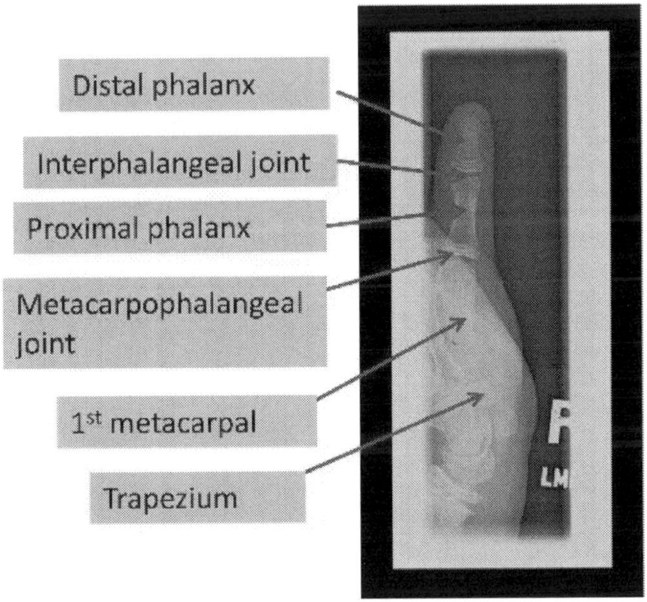

Thumb–Posteroanterior (PA) Oblique

SID, Technical factors, Shielding

- 40 inches (100 cm). No Grid. 50 kVp @ 1.3 mAs. No AEC. Gonadal shielding

Patient /part position

- Seated, face turned away with side to the x-ray table to reduce radiation to gonads, eyes and thyroid

Specific body/part position or rotation

- Pronate hand, separate thumb from fingers
- Thumb is oblique when hand is PA

Direction and point of entry of CR

- Perpendicular to metacarpophalangeal joint

Fig. 26a. Position. Thumb Posteroanterior (PA) Oblique

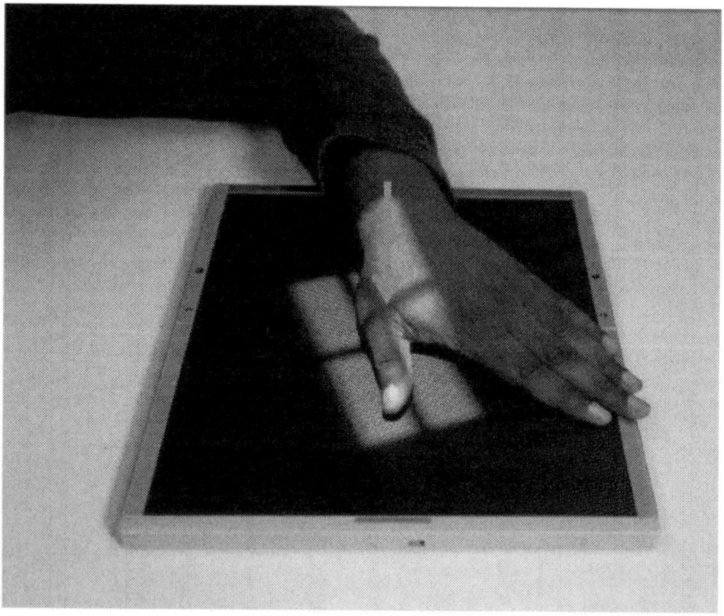

Collimation to include or structures demonstrated

All phalanges and trapezium or 1 inch (2.5cm) of distal radius/ulna

Image evaluation

- Bone trabeculae and soft tissue with the interphalangeal and metacarpophalangeal joints open

Fig. 26b. Radiograph. Thumb Posteroanterior (PA) Oblique

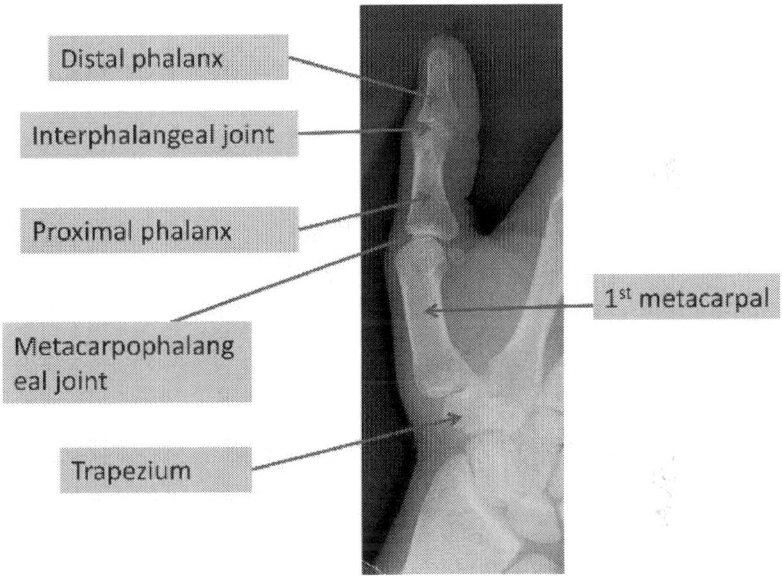

Thumb–Lateral

SID, Technical factors, Shielding

- 40 inches (100 cm). No Grid. 50 kVp @ 1.3 mAs. No AEC. Gonadal shielding

Patient/part position

- Seated, face turned away with side to the x-ray table to reduce radiation to gonads, eyes and thyroid

Specific Body/part position or rotation

- Arch fingers, placing fingertips on IR. Adjust thumb to true lateral position

Direction and point of entry of CR

- Perpendicular to metacarpophalangeal joint

Fig.27a. Position. Thumb – Lateral

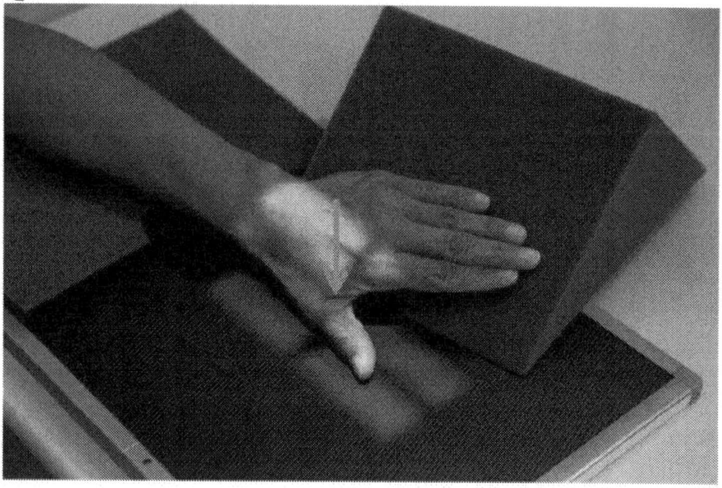

Collimation to include or structures demonstrated

- All phalanges to the trapezium or 1 inch (2.5 cm) of distal radius/ulna

Image evaluation

- Bone trabeculae and soft tissue structures with the interphalangeal (IR) and metacarpophalangeal (MCP) joints open

Fig.27b. Radiograph. Thumb – Lateral

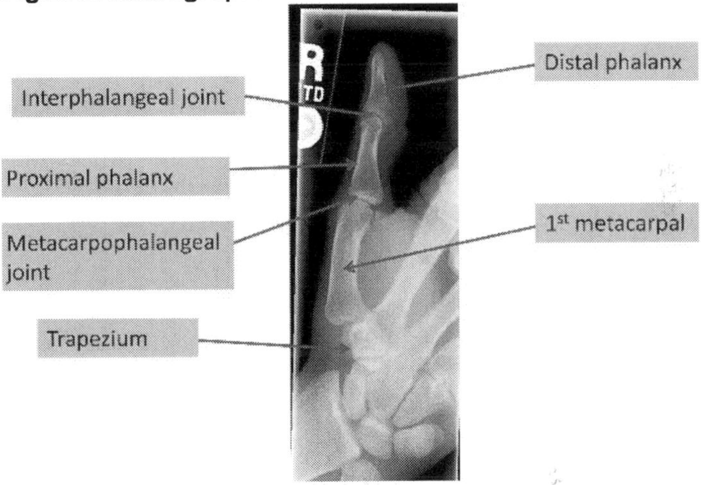

Hand–Posteroanterior (PA)

SID, Technical factors, Shielding

- 40 inches (100 cm). No Grid. 52 kVp @ 1.3 mAs. No AEC. Gonadal shielding

Patient/part position

- Seated, face turned away with side to the x-ray table to reduce radiation to gonads, eyes and thyroid

Specific body/part position or rotation

- Hand flat on the tabletop
- Hand pronated and fingers separated

Direction and point of entry of CR

- Perpendicular to 3rd metacarpophalangeal joint

Fig. 28a. Position. Hand- Posteroanterior (PA)

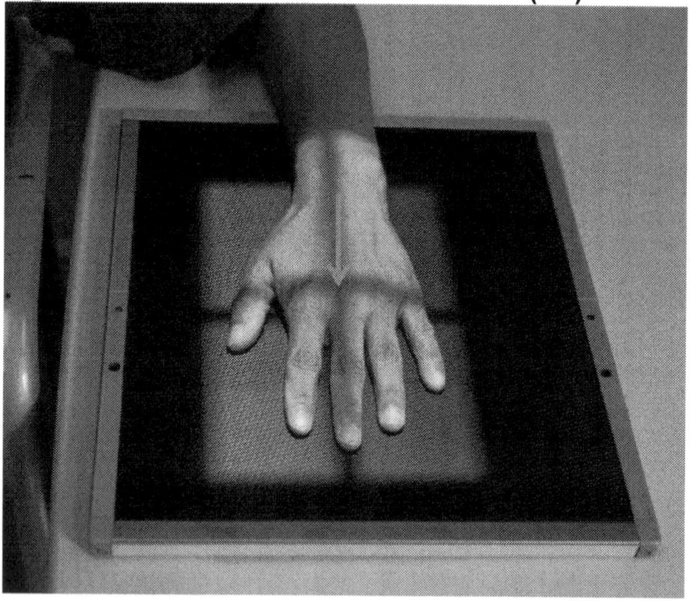

Collimation to include or structures demonstrated

- The carpal, metacarpals and phalanges plus at least 1 inch (2.5cm) distal radius/ulna

Image evaluation

- Bone trabeculae and soft tissue with symmetrical concavity of shafts of metacarpals
- Interphalangeal and metacarpophalangeal joints open and demonstrated

Fig. 28b. Radiograph. Hand- Posteroanterior (PA)

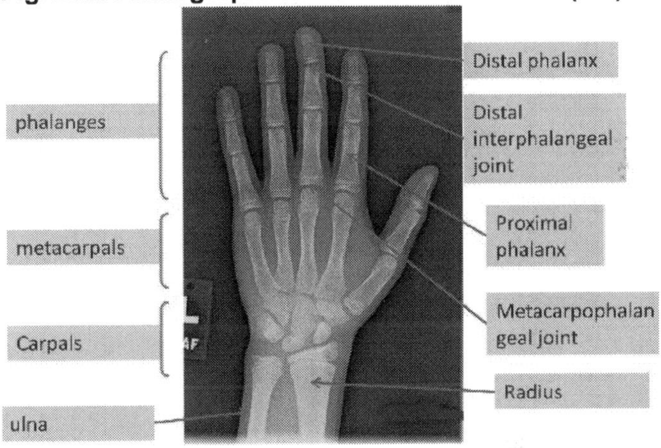

Hand–Posteroanterior (PA) Oblique

SID, Technical factors, Shielding

- 40 inches (100 cm). No Grid. 52 kVp @ 1.3 mAs. No AEC. Gonadal shielding

Patient/part position

- Seated, face turned away with side to the x-ray table to reduce radiation to gonads, eyes and thyroid

Specific part/body position or rotation

- From the PA position hand is rotated 45° to elevate lateral side of hand
- A finger sponge can immobilize if necessary

Direction and point of entry of CR

- Perpendicular to 3rd metacarpophalangeal joint

Fig. 29a. Position. Hand – Posteroanterior (PA) Oblique

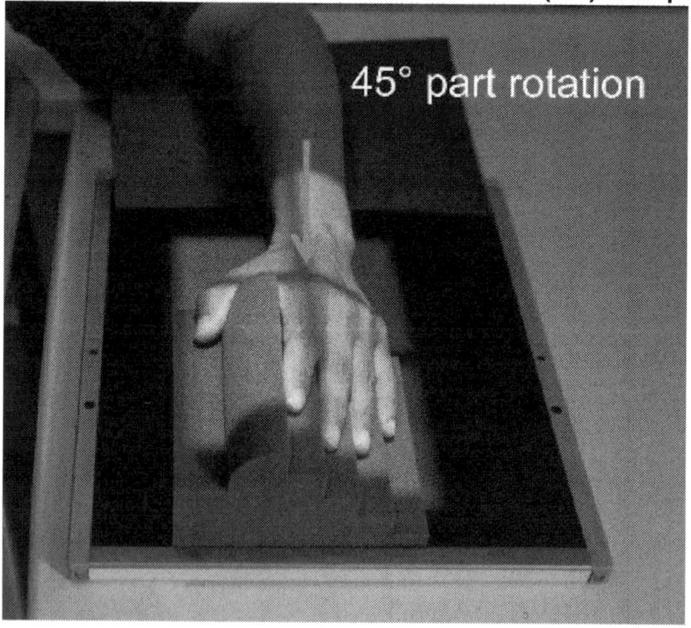

Collimation to include or structures demonstrated

- All phalanges, metacarpals, carpals plus soft tissue and at least 1inch (2.5 cm) distal radius/ulna

Image evaluation

- Bone trabecular and soft tissue details with separation of bases of 1st & 2nd metacarpal
- Superimposition of bases of 3rd through 5th metacarpals
- Slight separation shafts of 3rd through 5th metacarpal.

Note

- The fingers will position parallel to tabletop preventing foreshortening of distal phalanges and closure of interphalangeal joints if a finger sponge support is used

Fig. 29b. Radiograph. Hand – Posteroanterior (PA) Oblique

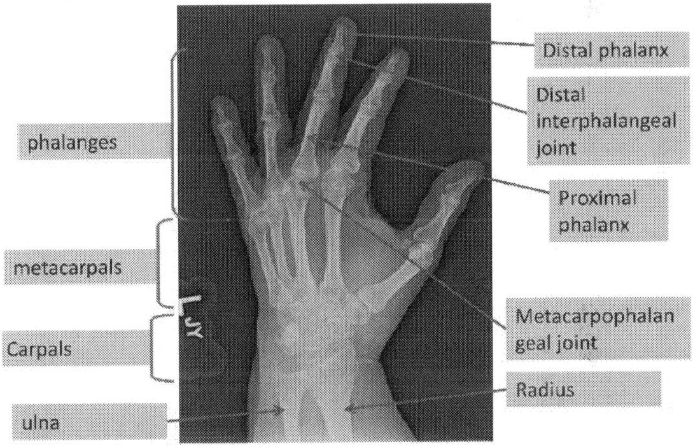

Hand–Anteroposterior (AP) Oblique

SID, Technical factors, Shielding

- 40 inches (100 cm). No Grid. 52 kVp @ 1.3 mAs. No AEC. Gonadal shielding

Patient/part position

- Seated, face turned away with side to the x-ray table to reduce radiation to gonads, eyes and thyroid

Specific part/body position or rotation

- Ball catcher's position–both hands in the AP 45-degree oblique position

Direction and point of entry of CR

- Perpendicular at the level of metacarpophalangeal joints in midline

Fig. 30a. Position. Hands– Anteroposterior (AP)Oblique

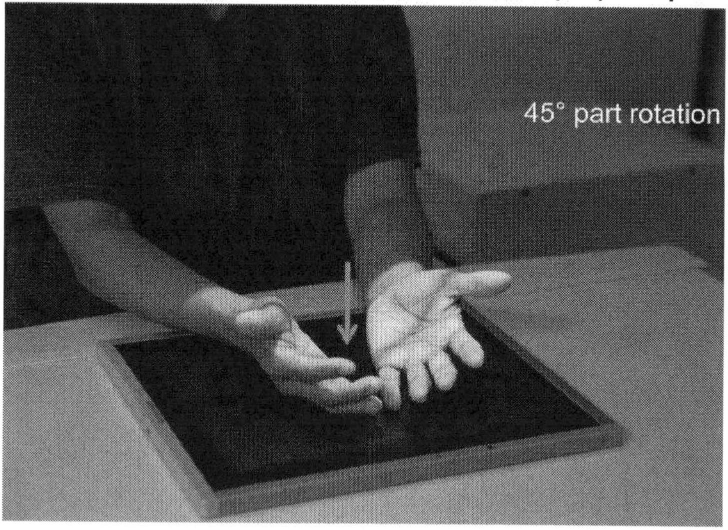

Collimation to include or structures demonstrated

- All phalanges, metacarpals, carpals plus soft tissue and at least 1inch (2.5cm) distal radius/ulna

Note

- This projection is often taken bilateral to demonstrated arthritis

Fig. 30b. Radiograph. Hands– Anteroposterior (AP)Oblique

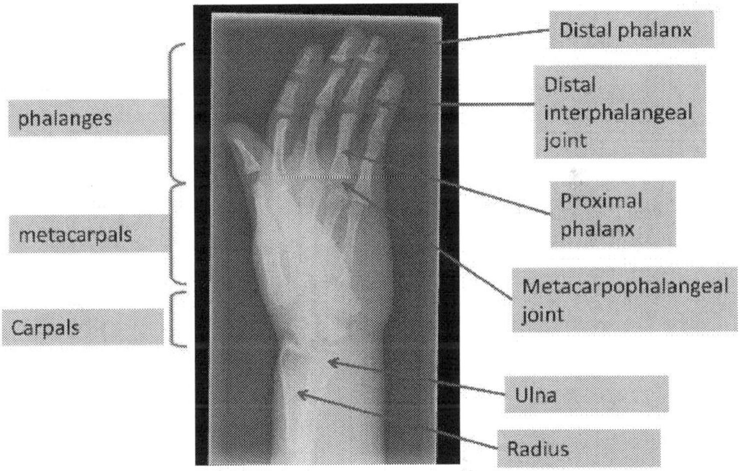

Hand–Lateral, (fan lateral)

SID, Technical factors, Shielding

- 40 inches (100 cm). No Grid. 54 kVp @ 1.3 mAs. No AEC. Gonadal shielding

Patient/part position

- Seated, face turned away with side to the x-ray table to reduce radiation to gonads, eyes and thyroid

Specific part/body position or rotation–fan lateral

- Elbow flexed, forearm on table
- Hand positioned true lateral
- Separate the phalanges

Direction and point of entry of CR

- Perpendicular to the metacarpophalangeal joints

Fig. 21a. Position. Hand – Lateral, Fan Lateral

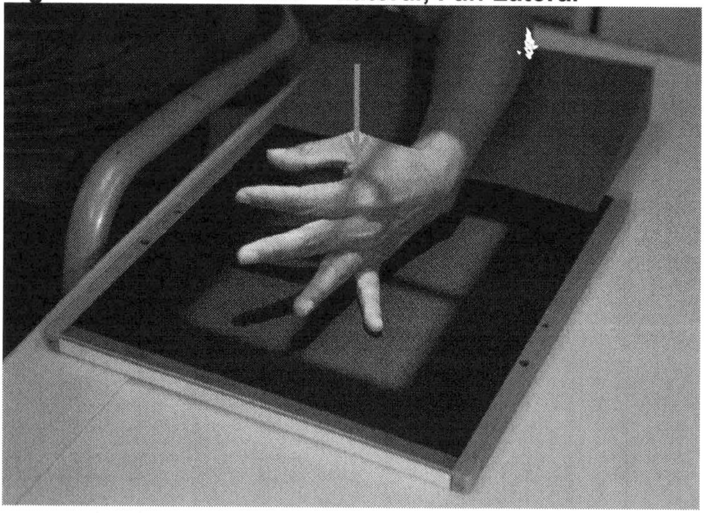

Collimation to include or structures demonstrated

- Phalanges, metacarpals and carpals plus at least 1inch (2.5 cm) of distal radius and ulna

Image evaluation

- Soft tissue and bone trabeculae with superimposed distal radius & ulna
- Separation of phalanges on fan lateral with superimposed metacarpals

Note

- Radiolucent sponge support may be used to separate the digits on fan lateral keeping the phalanges parallel to the tabletop and allowing visualization of the interphalangeal joints.
- This projection can be used to demonstrate the phalanges without superimposition

Fig. 21b. Radiograph. Hand – Lateral, Fan Lateral

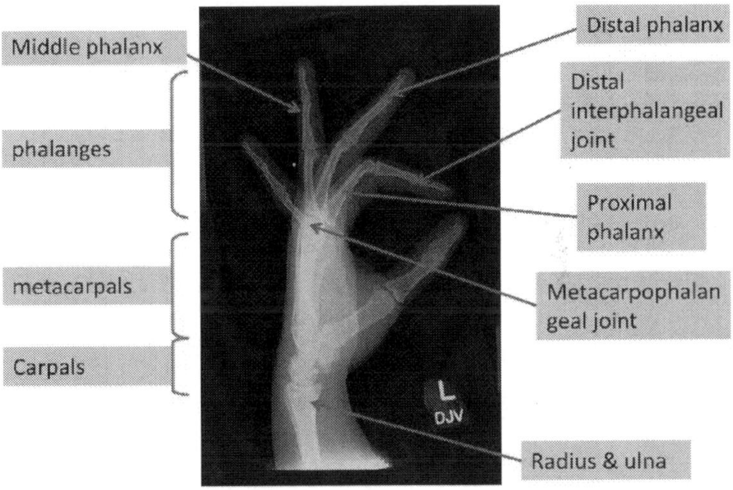

Hand–Lateral, (extension lateral)

SID, Technical factors, Shielding

- 40 inches (100 cm). No Grid. 54 kVp @ 1.3 mAs. No AEC. Gonadal shielding

Patient/part position

- Seated, face turned away with side to the x-ray table to reduce radiation to gonads, eyes and thyroid

Specific part/body position or rotation–lateral in extension

- Elbow flexed, forearm on table
- Rotate hand to true lateral with 5th digit resting on IR
- Digits and metacarpal superimposed

Direction and point of entry of CR

- Perpendicular to the metacarpophalangeal joints

Fig. 32a. Position. Hand – Lateral, Extension

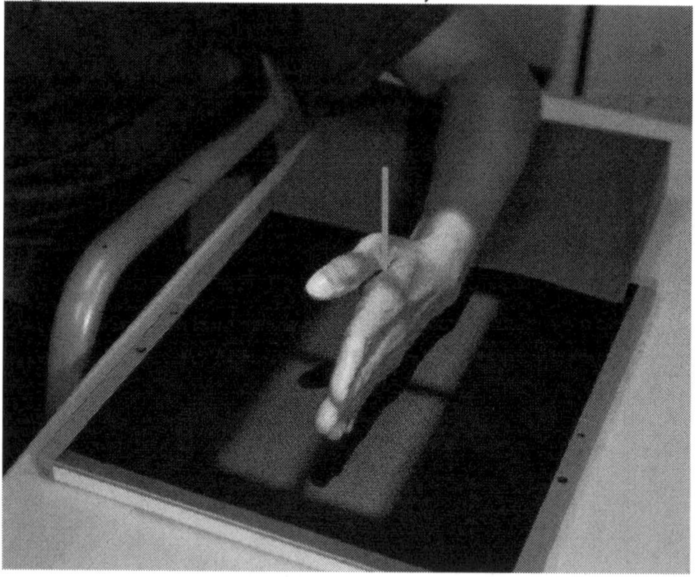

Collimation to include or structures demonstrated

- Phalanges, metacarpals and carpals plus at least 1inch (2.5cm) of distal radius and ulna

Image evaluation

- Soft tissue and bone trabeculae with superimposed distal radius & ulna
- Superimposed metacarpals and phalanges on extension lateral

Note

- This projection can be used to localize foreign bodies.

Fig. 32b. Radiograph. – Lateral, Extension

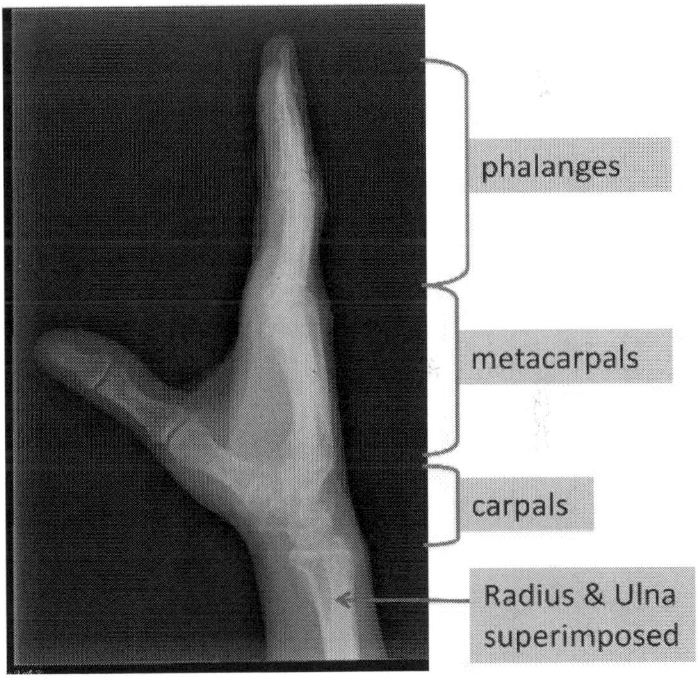

Hand–Lateral, (natural flexion lateral)

SID, Technical factors, Shielding

- 40 inches (100 cm). No Grid. 54 kVp @ 1.3 mAs. No AEC. Gonadal shielding

Patient/part position

- Seated, face turned away with side to the x-ray table to reduce radiation to gonads, eyes and thyroid

Specific part/body position or rotation–lateral in natural flexion

- Elbow flexed, forearm on table. Hand positioned lateral in its natural flexed position

Direction and point of entry of CR

- Perpendicular to the metacarpophalangeal joints

Fig. 33a. Position. Hand – Lateral, Natural Flexion

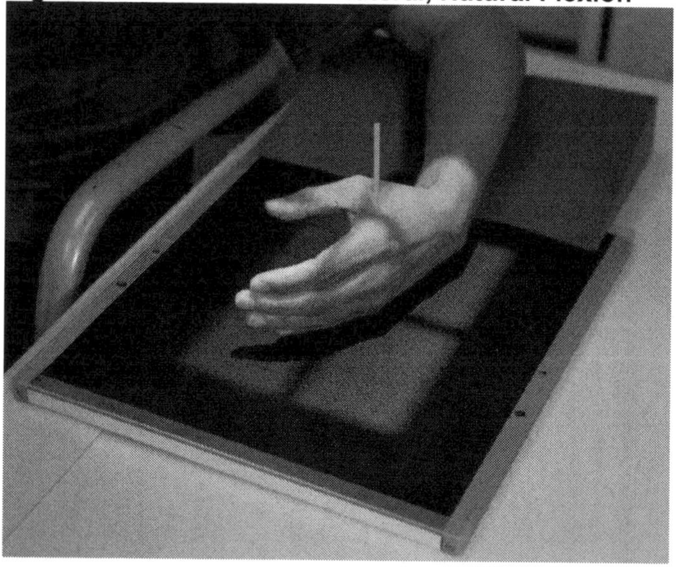

Collimation to include or structures demonstrated

- Phalanges, metacarpals and carpals plus at least 1inch (2.5cm) of distal radius and ulna

Image evaluation

- Soft tissue and bone trabeculae with superimposed distal radius & ulna
- Superimposed metacarpals and phalanges on natural flexion

Note

- Can be used to demonstrate anterior or posterior displacement in fractures of the metacarpals.

Fig. 32b. Radiograph. Hand – Lateral, Extension

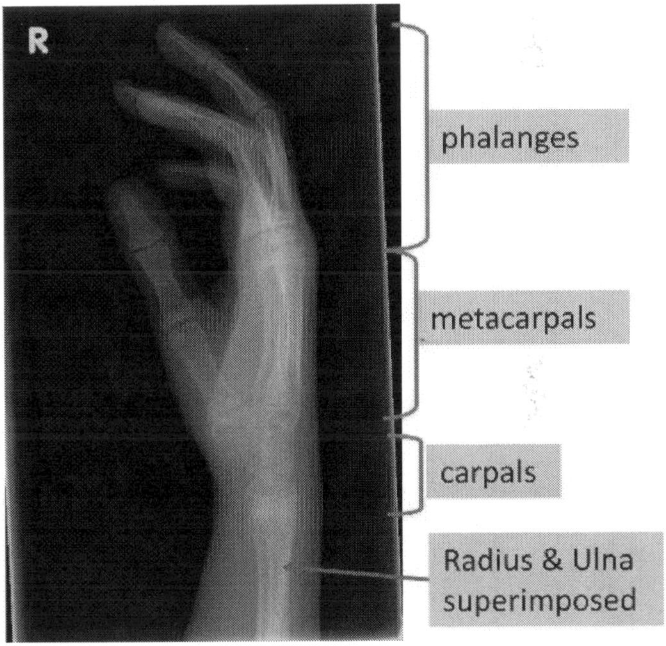

Wrist–Posteroanterior (PA)

SID, Technical factors, Shielding

- 40 inches (100 cm). No Grid. 55 kVp @ 1.6 mAs. No AEC. Gonadal shielding

Patient/part position

- Seated, face turned away with side to the x-ray table to reduce radiation to gonads, eyes and thyroid

Specific part/body position or rotation

- Elbow flexed 90-degrees
- Hand, wrist, elbow and shoulder on same plane
- Hand pronated with fingers arched to reduce OID

Direction and point of entry of CR

- Perpendicular to mid carpal region.

Fig. 34a. Position. Wrist – Posteroanterior (PA)

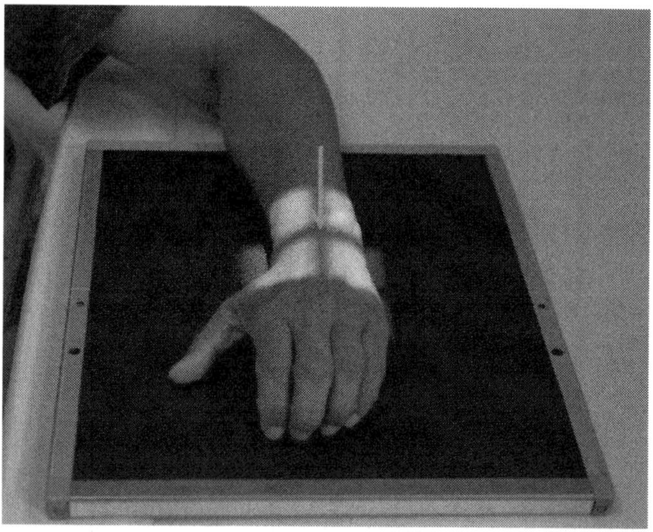

Collimation to include or structures demonstrated

- All the carpals plus 1-2 inches (2-5 cm) distal radius & ulna and the metacarpals

Image Evaluation

- Soft tissue and bony trabeculae with separation of radius and ulna, bony overlap of carpals
- The irregular bone of the carpals will not allow demonstration of intercarpal spaces
- Minimal superimposition of distal radioulnar joint
- Symmetrical concavity of shafts of metacarpals
- Distal ulna positioned slightly rotated

Notes: AP wrist (positioned with fingers arched to reduce OID) will better show intercarpal spaces because of the divergent rays. AP wrist also projects the distal ulna without rotation– true AP

Fig. 34b. Radiograph. Wrist – Posteroanterior (PA)

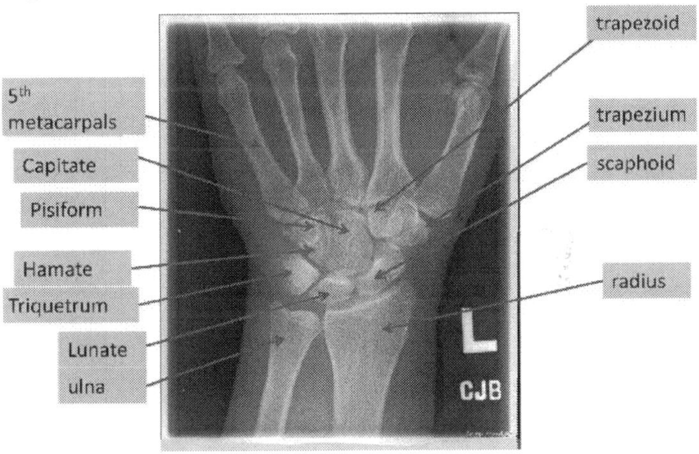

Proximal Row: Scaphoid, lunate, triquetrum, pisiform

Distal Row: Trapezium, trapezoid, capital, hamate

Wrist–Posteroanterior (PA) oblique

Semi-pronation or PA with lateral rotation

SID, Technical factors, Shielding

- 40 inches (100 cm). No Grid. 55 kVp @ 1.6 mAs. No AEC. Gonadal shielding

Patient/part position

- Seated, face turned away with side to the x-ray table to reduce radiation to gonads, eyes and thyroid

Specific part/body position or rotation

- From the PA rotate the wrist 45-degrees (laterally)
- A sponge support will partially flex fingers and maintain 45-degree position

Direction and point of entry of Central Ray/SID

- Perpendicular to mid carpals

Fig. 35a Position. Wrist – Posteroanterior (PA) Oblique

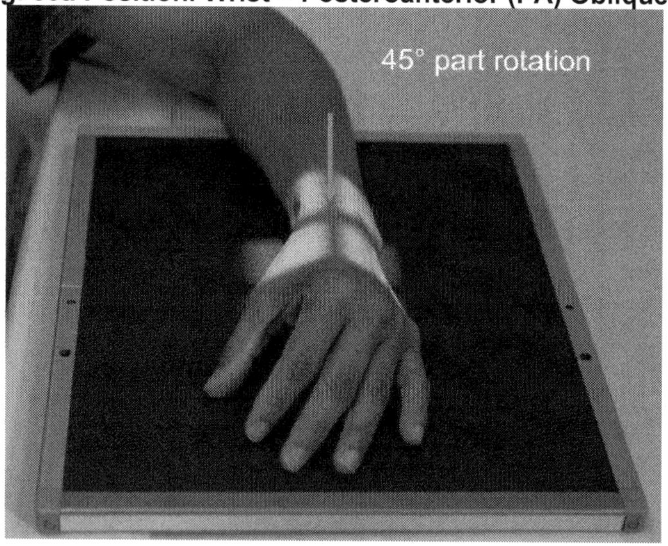

Collimation to include or structures demonstrated

- The carpals with 1-2inches (2-5 cm) of the distal radius & ulna and the metacarpals
- Trapezium and scaphoid visualized

Image evaluation

- Soft tissue and bony trabeculae with the proximal 3rd through 5th metacarpals bases superimposed
- Ulna partially superimposed distal radius

Notes:

- The PA oblique, semi-pronation or lateral rotation demonstrates the scaphoid and lateral carpal bones

Fig. 35b. Radiograph. Wrist – Posteroanterior (PA) Oblique

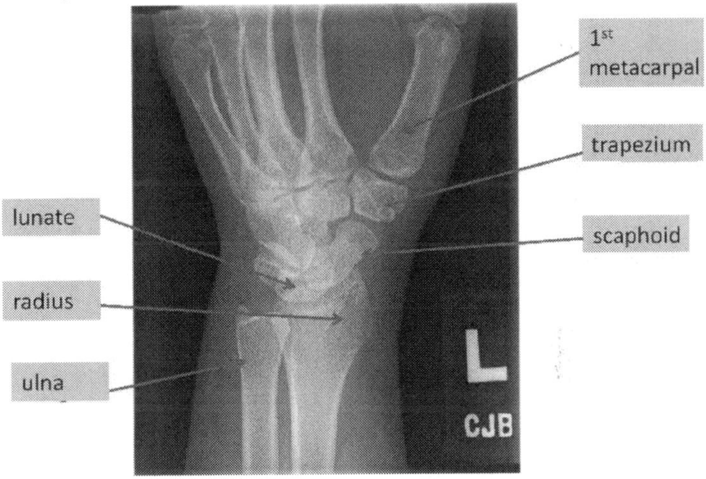

Wrist–Anteroposterior (AP) oblique

Semi-supination or AP with medial rotation

SID, Technical factors, Shielding

- 40 inches (100 cm). No Grid. 55 kVp @ 1.6 mAs. No AEC. Gonadal shielding

Patient/part position

- Seated, face turned away with side to the x-ray table to reduce radiation to gonads, eyes and thyroid

Specific part/body position or rotation

- From the AP rotate the wrist 45-degrees (medially)
- A sponge support will partially flex fingers and maintain 45-degree position

Direction and point of entry of Central Ray/SID

- Perpendicular to mid carpals

Fig. 36a. Position. Wrist – Anteroposterior (AP) Oblique

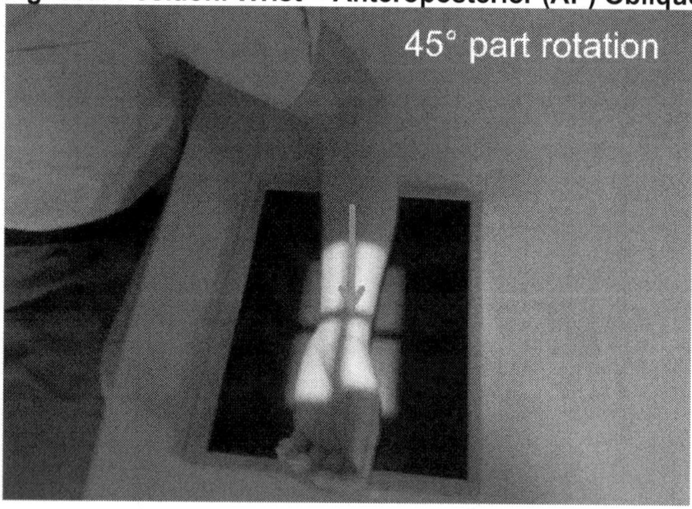

Collimation to include or structures demonstrated

- The carpals with 1-2inches (2-5 cm) of the distal radius & ulna and the metacarpals

Image evaluation

- Soft tissue and bony trabeculae of the medial carpal with the pisiform without superimposition
- Ulna partially superimposed distal radius

Note:

- This projection demonstrates the medial carpal bones

Fig. 36a. Position. Wrist – Anteroposterior (AP) Oblique

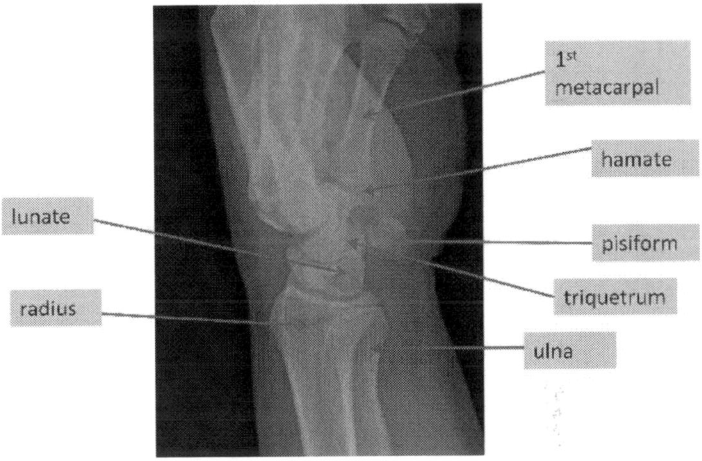

Wrist–Lateral

SID, Technical factors, Shielding

- 40 inches (100 cm). No Grid. 57 kVp @ 1.6 mAs. No AEC. Gonadal shielding

Patient/part position

- Seated, face turned away with side to the x-ray table to reduce radiation to gonads, eyes and thyroid

Specific part/body position or rotation

- Elbows flexed 90-degrees with the thumb up
- Shoulder, elbow, wrist and hand placed on the same horizontal plane
- Wrist true lateral
- Fingers can be flexed for support
- **Slight lateral rotation will achieve true lateral** position and superimpose the distal radius and ulna

Direction and point of entry of CR

- Perpendicular to the carpals

Fig. 37a. Position. Wrist – Lateral

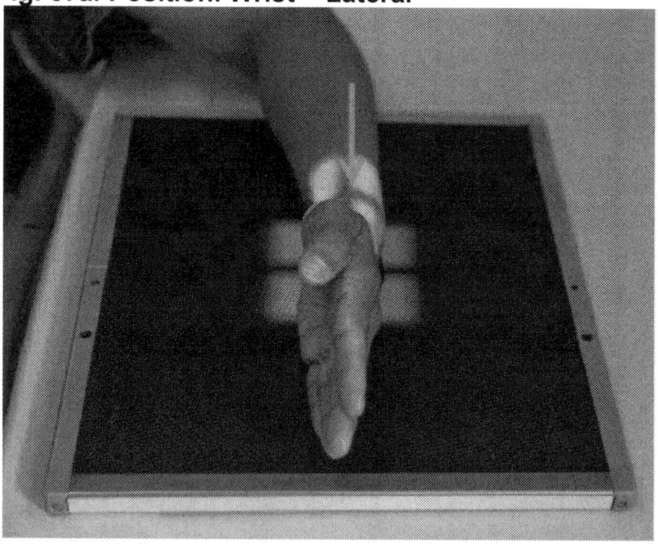

Collimation to include or structures demonstrated

- Carpals and 1-2 inches (2-5 cm) of the distal radius & ulna and the metacarpals

Image evaluation

- Soft tissue and bony trabeculae with the ulna head superimposed on distal radius
- Proximal 2nd through 5th metacarpals all superimposed
- Capital, lunate and distal radius demonstrated in straight line
- Scaphoid and trapezium seen anterior to the capitate and lunate

Fig. 37b. Radiograph. Wrist – Lateral

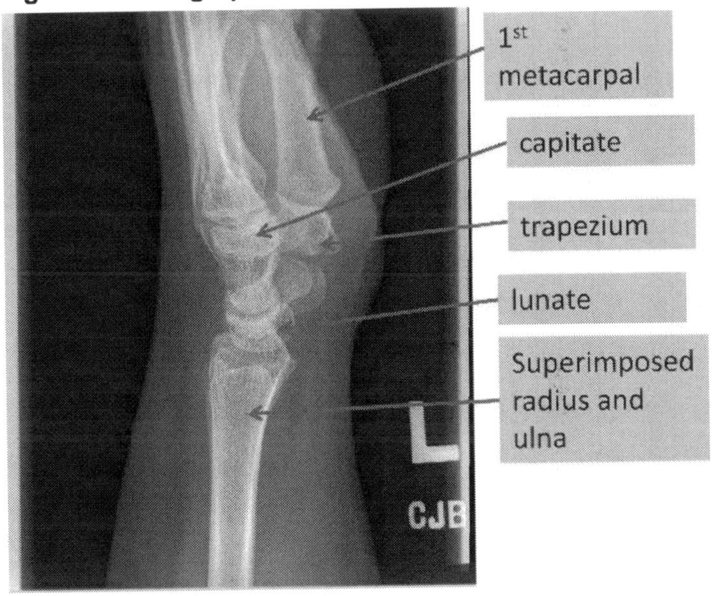

Wrist–Posteroanterior (PA) with Ulnar deviation

SID, Technical factors, Shielding

- 40 inches (100 cm). No Grid. 55 kVp @ 1.6 mAs. No AEC. Gonadal shielding

Patient/part position

- Seated, face turned away with side to the x-ray table to reduce radiation to gonads, eyes and thyroid

Specific part/body position- ulnar deviation

- Wrist PA with shoulder, elbow, wrist and hand on same horizontal plane
- Without moving forearm evert hand (turn to ulnar side)

Direction and point of entry of CR

- Perpendicular to the scaphoid or ¾inch (2 cm) distal and medial to radial styloid process

Fig.38a. Position. Wrist–Posteroanterior(PA) with Ulnar Deviation

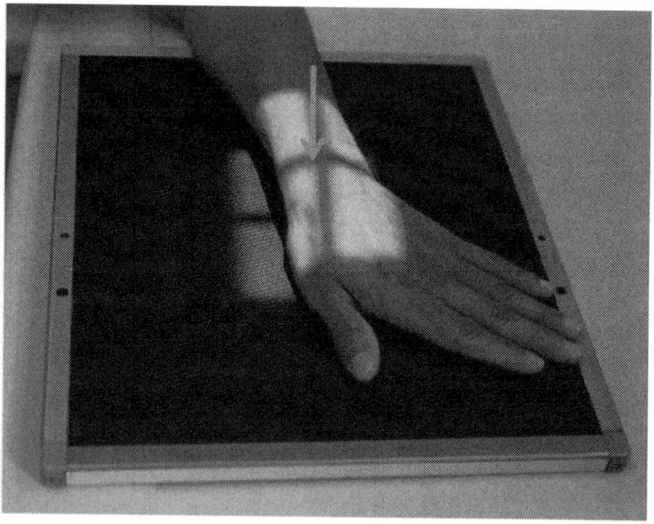

Collimation to include or structures demonstrated

- Carpals, 1inch (2.5cm) of the distal radius and ulna plus 1inch (2.5cm) of the metacarpals
- The scaphoid and the lateral carpals

Image evaluation

- Soft tissue and bony trabecular of the scaphoid
- Minimal superimposition of distal radioulnar joint

Notes

- This projection can be taken with or without tube angulation
- The scaphoid demonstrated without foreshortening with CR angulation of 10 to 15-degrees proximally–along forearm and toward elbow. The CR is directed perpendicular to the long axis of scaphoid.
- Scaphoid demonstrated with foreshortening if no tube angulation
- Too much angulation will result in elongation of the scaphoid.

Fig.38a. Position. Wrist–Posteroanterior(PA) with Ulnar Deviation

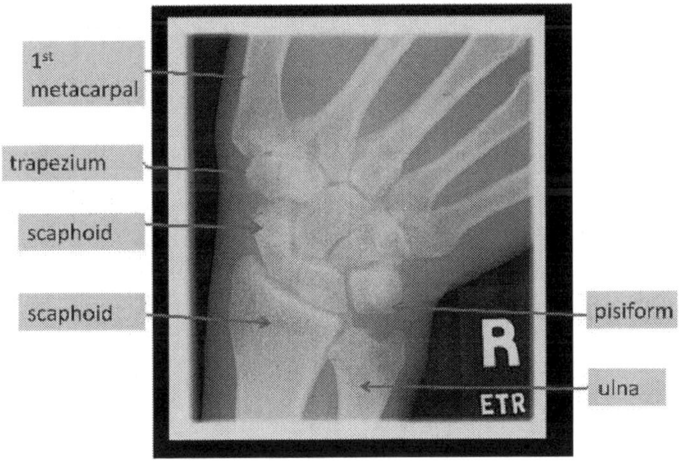

Wrist–Posteroanterior (PA) with Radial Deviation

SID, Technical factors, Shielding

- 40 inches (100 cm). No Grid. 55 kVp @ 1.6 mAs. No AEC. Gonadal shielding

Patient/part position

- Seated, face turned away with side to the x-ray table to reduce radiation to gonads, eyes and thyroid

Specific part/body position or rotation

- Elbows flexed 90-degrees with thumb up
- Shoulder, elbow, wrist and hand on same horizontal plane
- Without moving forearm, invert hand (turn medially to thumb, radial side)

Direction and point of entry of CR

- To mid carpals area

Fig. 39a. Position. Wrist – Posteroanterior (PA) with Radial Deviation

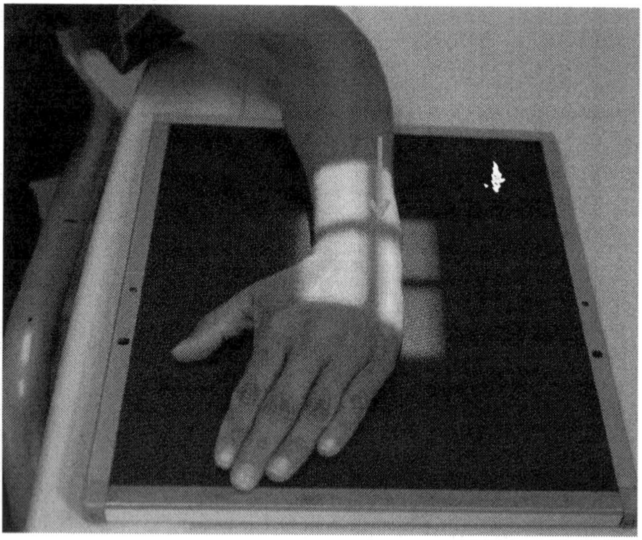

Collimation to include or structures demonstrated

- Carpals and 1inch (2.5cm) of the distal radius and ulna, plus 1inch (2.5cm) of the metacarpals with minimal superimposition of distal radioulnar joint

Image evaluation

- All trabeculae and soft tissues of the medial carpals plus medial interspaces open

Fig. 39b. Radiograph. Wrist – Posteroanterior (PA) with Radial Deviation

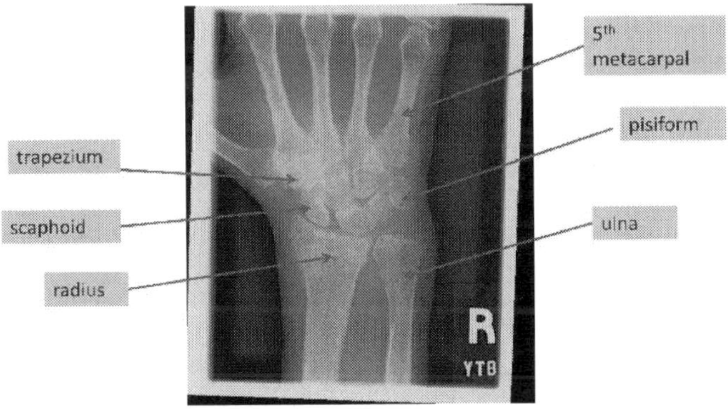

Wrist–Posteroanterior (PA) Scaphoid

Stecher method

SID, Technical factors, Shielding

- 40 inches (100 cm). No Grid. 55 kVp @ 1.6 mAs. No AEC. Gonadal shielding

Patient/part position

- Seated, face turned away with side to the x-ray table to reduce radiation to gonads, eyes and thyroid
- Wrist PA with shoulder, elbow, wrist and hand on the same horizontal plane

Specific part/body position or rotation (two options)

1. Place wrist on a 20-degree wedge sponge
2. Have patient clench fist (to achieve a 20-degree angle)

Direction and point of entry of CR

- Perpendicular to IR ¾inch (2 cm) distal and medial to radial styloid process

Fig. 40a. Position. Wrist – Posteroanterior (PA) Scaphoid Stecher method.

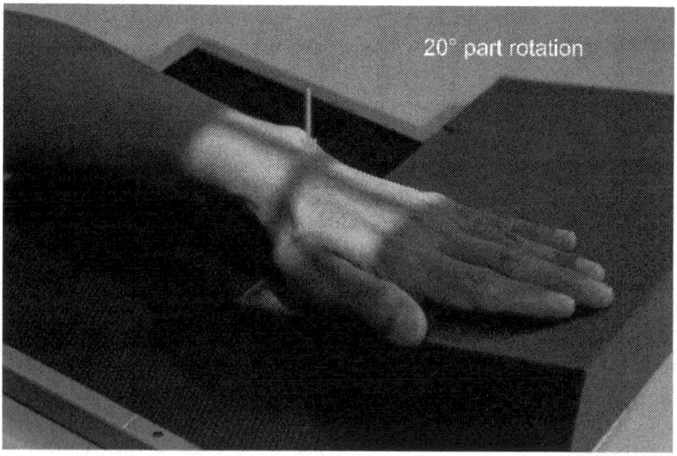

Collimation to include or structures demonstrated

- Carpals and 1inch (2.5cm) of the distal radius and ulna, plus 1inch (2.5cm) of the metacarpals

Image evaluation

- Soft tissue and bony trabecular of the lateral interspaces visible and open
- Demonstrates the scaphoid without foreshortening or superimposition
- Demonstrates minimal superimposition of distal radioulnar joint

Note

- A 20-degree tube angulation towards the elbow can be used instead of the using part angulation.

Fig. 40b. Radiograph. Wrist – Posteroanterior (PA) Scaphoid Stecher method.

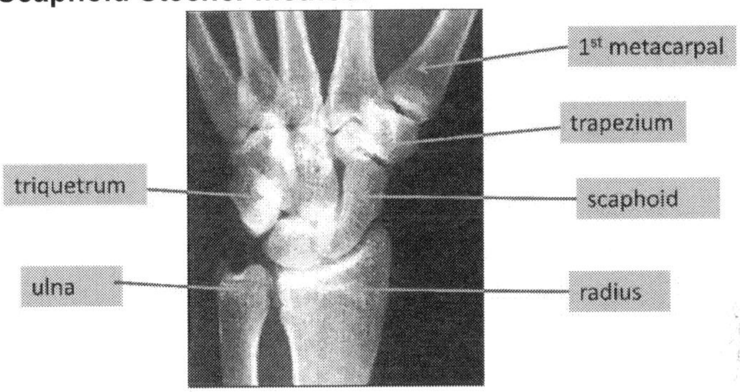

Wrist–Carpal Canal, Tangential Inferosuperior
Gaynor-Hart method

SID, Technical factors, Shielding

- 40 inches (100 cm). No Grid. 57 kVp @ 1.6 mAs. No AEC. Gonadal shielding

Patient/part position

- Patient seated at end of the x-ray table
- Hand pronated with wrist and forearm resting on IR

Specific part/body position or rotation

- Hyperextend wrist (dorsiflex) as far as possible to place long axis of metacarpals near vertical or 90-degrees to forearm
- Rotate hand and wrist 10-degrees laterally (to radial side) to prevent superimposition of pisiform and hamate

Direction and point of entry of CR

- Use 25-30degrees tube angulation to long axis of hand
- Increase angulation if patient cannot hyperextend wrist
- CR to a point 1 cm (2.5 cm) distal to base of 3rd metacarpal (on palm of hand)

Fig. 41a. Position. Wrist- Carpal Canal- Tangential Inferiosupeior (Gaynor-Hart Method)

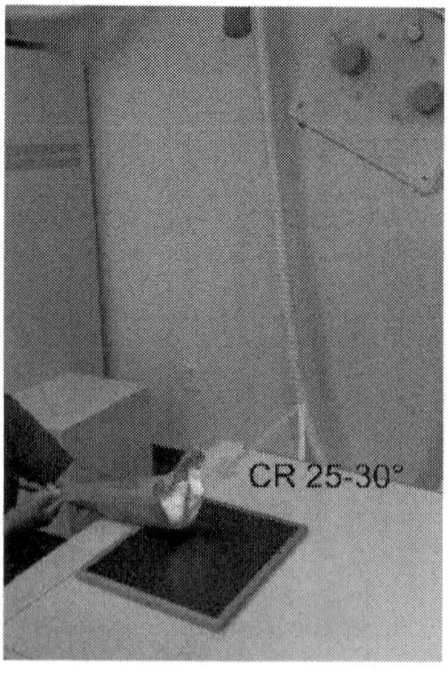

Collimation to include or structures demonstrated

- The carpals and superimposed metacarpals and radius & ulna

Image evaluation

- Soft tissue and bony trabeculae of the carpals in a tunnel-like arrangement
- Pisiform and hamulus of hamate separate and in profile without superimposition.

Note

- A narrow tunnel could indicate pinched nerves

Fig. 41b. Radiograph. Wrist- Carpal Canal- Tangential Inferiosupeior (Gaynor-Hart Method)

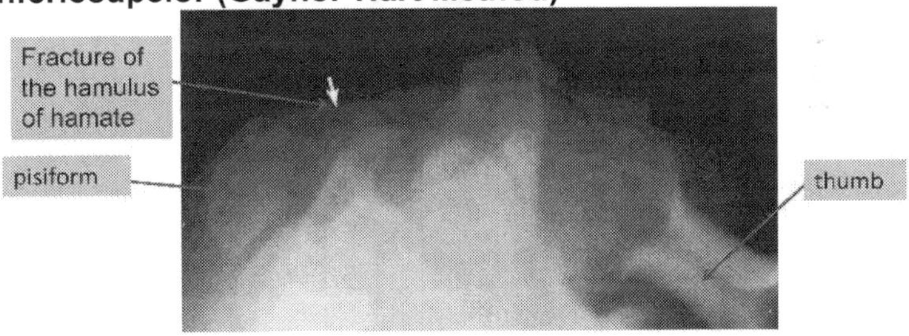

Forearm–Anteroposterior (AP) projection

SID, Technical factors, Shielding

- 40 inches (100 cm). No Grid. 55 kVp @ 2.3 mAs. No AEC. Gonadal shielding

Patient/part position

- Seated, face turned away with side to the x-ray table to reduce radiation to gonads, eyes and thyroid

Specific part/body position or rotation

- Shoulder, elbow, wrist and hand on same horizontal plane
- Elbows extended with hand supinated, thumb up
- Patient should lean laterally to place medial and lateral epicondyles parallel to IR and wrist true AP

Direction and point of entry of CR

- Perpendicular to the mid forearm

Fig. 42a. Position. Forearm – Anteroposterior (AP) projection

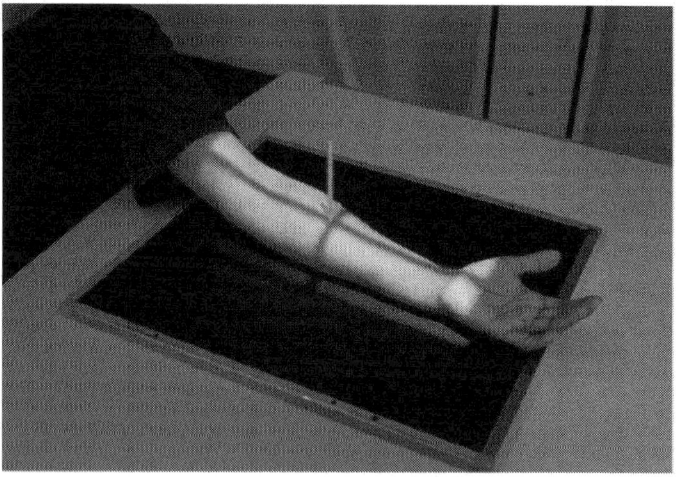

Collimation to include or structures demonstrated

- To include the radius, ulna plus carpals and ½ of metacarpals and 1-1 ½inches (2.5-3.8cm) of distal humerus

Image evaluation

- Soft tissue and bony trabecular with the shaft of the radius and ulna seen separated with the radial head, neck and tuberosity slightly superimposed over ulna

Fig. 42b. Radiograph. Forearm – Anteroposterior (AP) projection

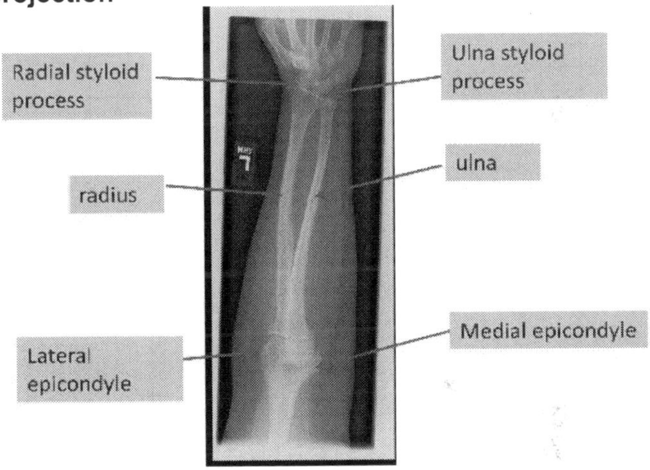

Forearm–Lateral

SID, Technical factors, Shielding

- 40 inches (100 cm). No Grid. 57 kVp @ 2.3 mAs. No AEC. Gonadal shielding

Patient/part position

- Seated, face turned away with side to the x-ray table to reduce radiation to gonads, eyes and thyroid

Specific part/body position

- Elbows flexed 90-degrees with hand true lateral, thumb up
- Shoulder, elbow, wrist and hand on same horizontal plane
- Support under hand and wrist if necessary, to keep part parallel to IR

Direction and point of entry of CR

- Perpendicular to the mid shaft.

Fig. 43a. Position. Forearm - Lateral

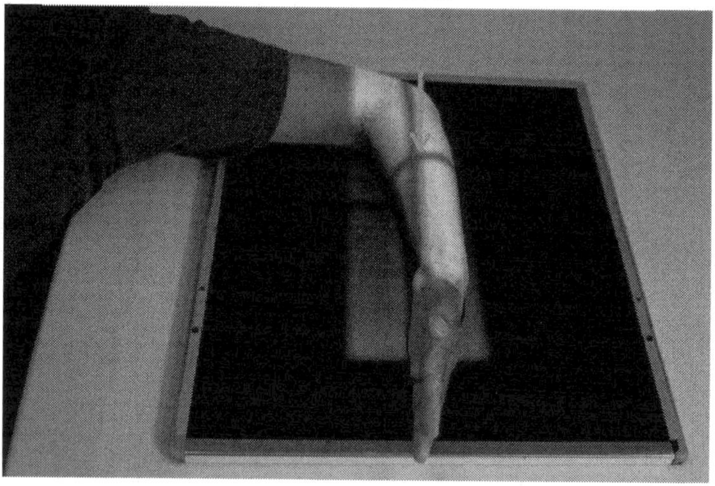

Collimation to include or structures demonstrated

- To include the radius ulna plus carpals and ½ of metacarpals and 1-1 ½inches (2.5-3.8 cm) of distal humerus

Image evaluation

- Soft tissue and bony trabecular with minimum superimposed proximal row of carpals & distal humerus
- Elbow at 90-degree with distal radius & ulna and humeral epicondyles superimposed
- Radial tuberosity seen anteriorly with radial head superimposed on coronoid process

Fig. 43b. Radiograph. Forearm - Lateral

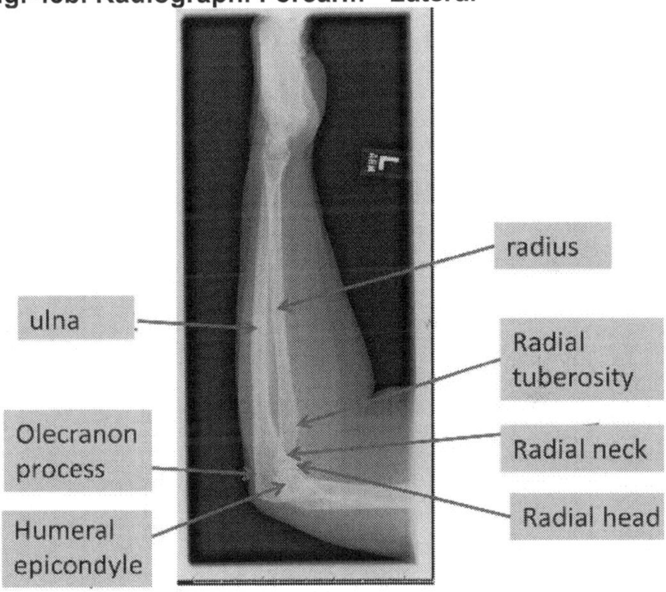

Elbow–Anteroposterior (AP)

SID, Technical factors, Shielding

- 40 inches (100 cm). No Grid. 60 kVp @ 2.3 mAs. No AEC. Gonadal shielding I

Patient/part position

- Seated, face turned away with side to the x-ray table to reduce radiation to gonads, eyes and thyroid

Specific part/body position or rotation

- Arm extended, hand supinated with forearm and humerus on the same plane
- Patient must lean laterally for true AP to place epicondyles parallel to IR

Direction and point of entry of CR

- Perpendicular to mid elbow joint ¾ inch (2cm) distal to midpoint of a line through epicondyles

Fig 44a. Position. Elbow – Anteroposterior (AP)

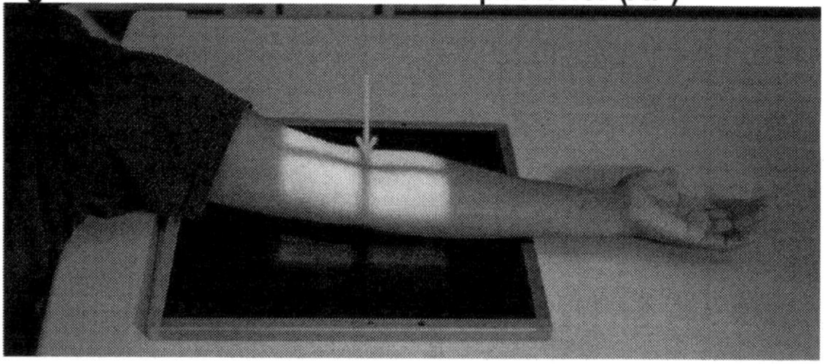

Collimation to include or structures demonstrated

- At least 4-5 inches (10-13cm) of distal humerus and proximal forearm

Image evaluation

- To include bone trabeculae and soft tissue with bilateral epicondyles seen in profile
- Radial head, neck and tubercles separated or slightly superimposed by ulna

Note:

- Ulna and humerus are the only bones articulating to form the elbow joint

Fig. 43b.Radiograph. Forearm - Lateral

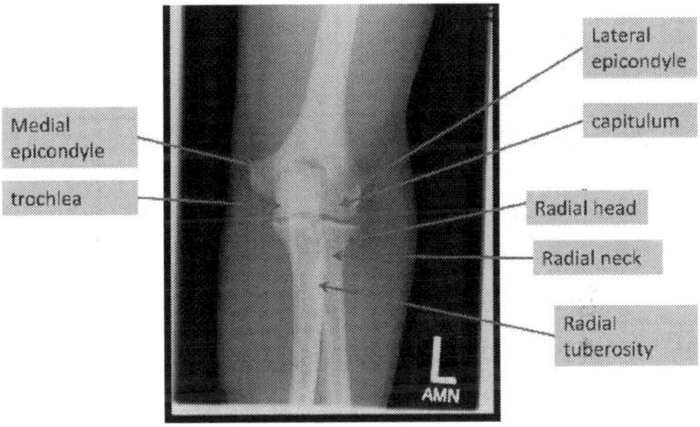

Elbow–Lateral

SID, Technical factors, Shielding

- 40 inches (100 cm). No Grid.62 kVp @ 2.3 mAs. No AEC. Gonadal shielding

Patient/part position

- Seated, face turned away with side to the x-ray table to reduce radiation to gonads, eyes and thyroid

Specific part/body position or rotation

- Elbows flexed 90-degrees with wrist true lateral and on same plane with shoulders

Direction and point of entry of CR

- 1½-inch (3.8 cm) medial to olecranon process

Fig. 45a. Position. Elbow – Lateral

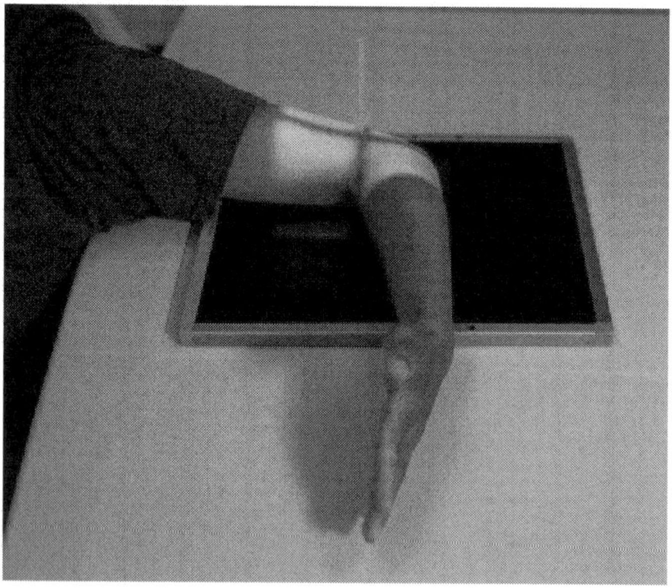

Collimation to include or structures demonstrated

- 1½-2 inches (2-5 cm) of distal humerus and proximal radius/ulna

Image evaluation

- Soft tissue and bony trabecular detail with 1/2 of the radial head superimposed on the coronoid process of the ulna
- The olecranon process in profile, with the epicondyles of humerus superimposed and radial tuberosity facing anteriorly

Notes

- To relax joint & visualize the three areas of fat pads the wrist, elbow and should must be on the same plane
- The anterior and supinator fat pads are seen on the lateral
- Posterior fat pad is seen only if there is a fracture

Fig. 43b. Radiograph. Forearm - Lateral

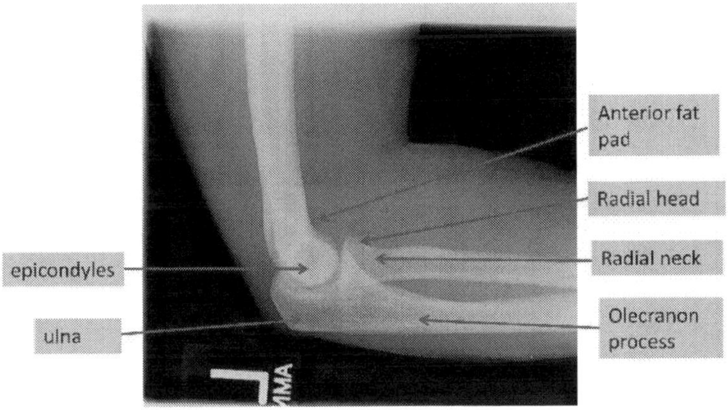

Elbow–Medial Oblique (internal rotation)

SID, Technical factors, Shielding

- 40 inches (100 cm). No Grid. 60kVp @ 2.3 mAs. No AEC. Gonadal shielding

Patient/part position

- Seated, face turned away with side to the x-ray table to reduce radiation to gonads, eyes and thyroid

Specific part/body position or rotation

- Arm extended with wrist, shoulder on same plane as elbow and hand pronated to place the epicondyles 45-degree to IR

Direction and point of entry of CR

- To elbow joint, ¾ inch (2 cm) distal to midpoint of line through epicondyles.

Fig. 46a. Position. Elbow - Medial Oblique (Internal Rotation)

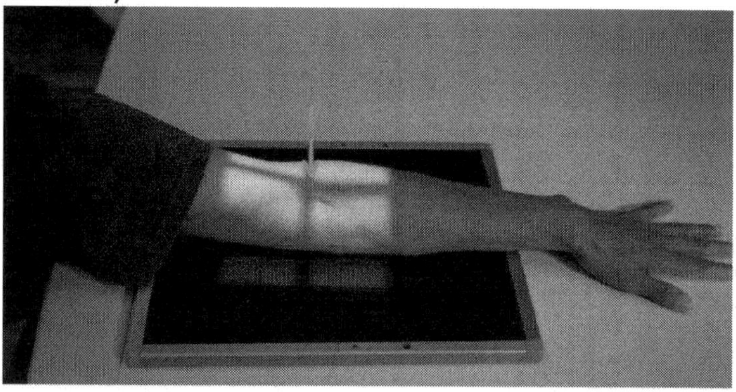

Collimation to include or structures demonstrated

- 1½ - 2 inches (2-5 cm) of distal humerus and proximal radius and ulna

Image evaluation

- Soft tissue and bony trabecular detail with the medial epicondyle, trochlea, radial head and neck superimposed on proximal ulna
- Coronoid process clearly seen and olecranon process in olecranon fossa

Fig. 46b. Radiograph. Elbow - Medial Oblique (Internal Rotation)

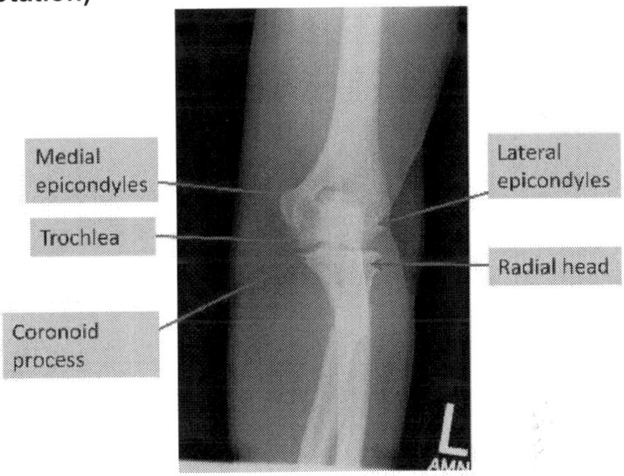

Elbow–Lateral Oblique (external rotation)

SID, Technical factors, Shielding

- 40 inches (100 cm). No Grid.62 kVp @ 2.3 mAs. No AEC. Gonadal shielding

Patient/part position

- Seated, face turned away with side to the x-ray table to reduce radiation to gonads, eyes and thyroid

Specific part/body position or rotation

- Arm extended with wrist, shoulder on same plane as elbow and hand
- Supinated hand and rotate laterally to place the epicondyles 45-degree to IR

Direction and point of entry of CR

- To the elbow joint, ¾-inch (2 cm) distal to midpoint of line through epicondyles.

Fig. 47a. Position. Elbow – Lateral Oblique (External Rotation)

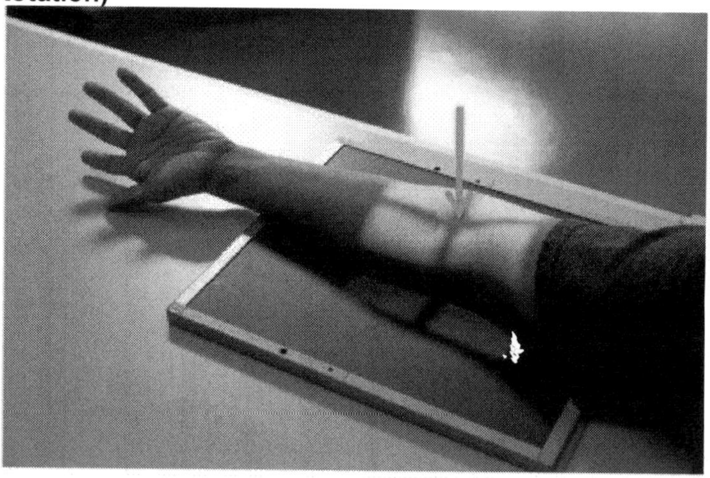

Collimation to include or structures demonstrated

- 1½ - 2 inches (2- 5 cm) of distal humerus plus proximal radius and ulna

Image evaluation

- Soft tissue and bony trabeculae detail with the radial head, neck & tuberosity free of superimposition and the lateral epicondyles clearly seen

Fig. 47b. Radiograph. Elbow – Lateral Oblique (External Rotation)

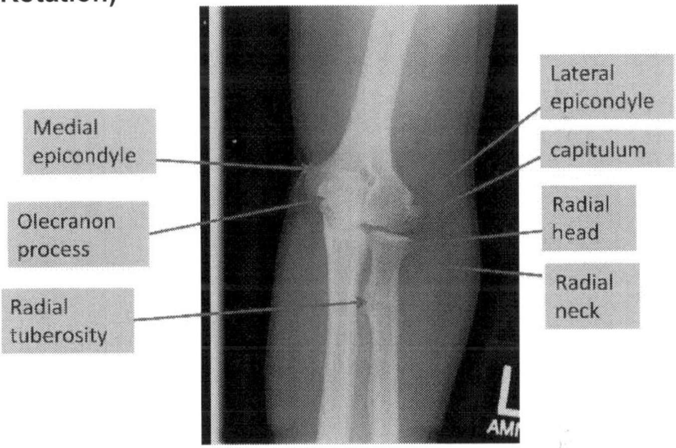

Elbow–Anteroposterior (AP) Partial Flexion
Part 1 of 2–Humerus parallel to the table-top

SID, Technical factors, Shielding

- 40 inches (100 cm). No Grid. 62kVp @ 2.3 mAs. No AEC. Gonadal shielding

Patient/part position

- Seated, face turned away with side to the x-ray table to reduce radiation to gonads, eyes and thyroid

Specific part/body position or rotation

- Two projections taken, one with forearm parallel to IR, the other with one with humerus parallel to IR

Direction and point of entry of CR

- Mid elbow joint (2cm) or ¾ inch distal to midpoint of line through epicondyles

Fig. 48a. Position. Elbow – Anteroposterior (AP) Partial Flexion, Humerus parallel to detector.

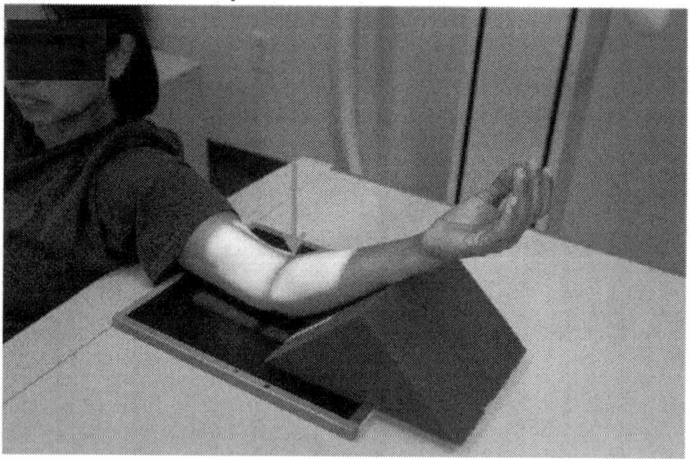

Collimation to include or structures demonstrated

- At least 4-5 inches (10-13 cm) of the distal humerus and proximal forearm

Image evaluation

- Bone trabeculae patterns and soft tissue
- With the humerus parallel to IR, the distal humerus is seen clearly
- Bilateral epicondyles seen in profile with the radial head, neck and tubercles separated or slightly superimposed by ulna

Note

- If elbow is flexed near 90-degree, use 10-15-degree tube angulation (to elbow joint)
- If flexion is more than 90-degree, this projection is not possible

Fig. 48b. Radiograph. Elbow – Anteroposterior (AP) Partial Flexion, Humerus parallel to detector.

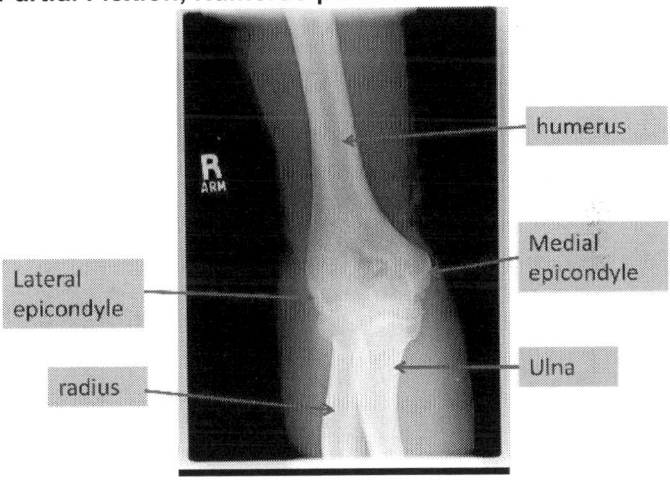

Elbow–Anteroposterior (AP) Partial Flexion

Part 2 of 2–Forearm parallel to the table-top

SID, Technical factors, Shielding

- 40 inches (100 cm). No Grid. 62kVp @ 2.3 mAs. No AEC. Gonadal shielding

Patient/part position

- Seated, face turned away with side to the x-ray table to reduce radiation to gonads, eyes and thyroid

Specific part/body position or rotation

- Two projections taken, one with forearm parallel to IR, the other with one with humerus parallel to IR

Direction and point of entry of CR

- Mid elbow joint (2cm) or ¾ inch distal to midpoint of line through epicondyles

Fig. 49a. Position. Elbow – Anteroposterior (AP) Partial Flexion, Forearm parallel to detector

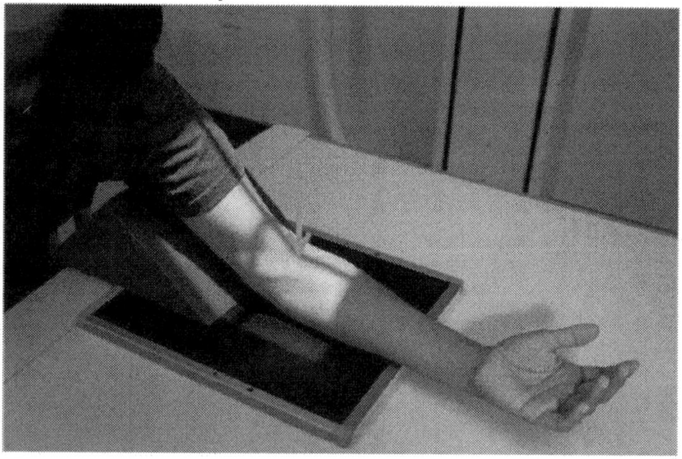

Collimation to include or structures demonstrated

- At least 4-5 inches (10-13 cm) of the distal humerus and proximal forearm

Image evaluation

- Bone trabeculae patterns and soft tissue
- With the forearm parallel to IR, the proximal forearm is seen clearly
- Bilateral epicondyles seen in profile with the radial head, neck and tubercles separated or slightly superimposed by ulna

Note

- If elbow is flexed near 90-degree, use 10-15-degree tube angulation (to elbow joint)
- If flexion is more than 90-degree, this projection is not possible

Fig. 49b. Radiograph. Elbow – Anteroposterior (AP) Partial Flexion, Forearm parallel to detector

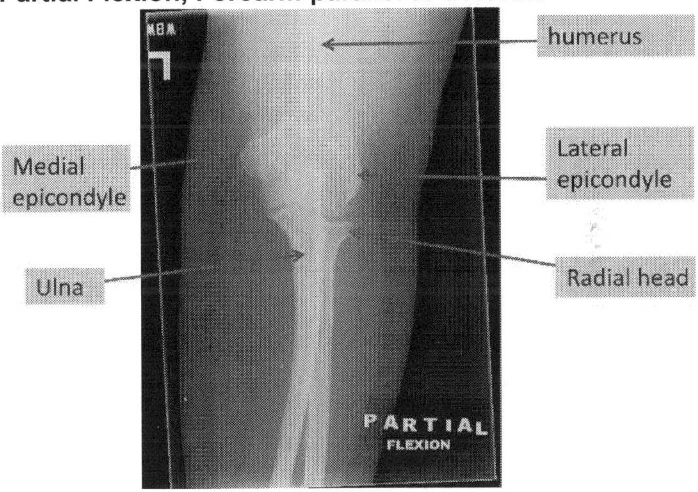

Elbow–Acute Flexion

SID, Technical factors, Shielding

- 40 inches (100 cm). No Grid. 62kVp @ 2.3 mAs. No AEC. Gonadal shielding

Patient/part position

- Seated, face turned away with side to the x-ray table to reduce radiation to gonads, eyes and thyroid

Specific part/body position or rotation

- The humerus placed to align with the long axis of IR
- Fingertips resting on the shoulder

Direction and point of entry of CR

To image the distal humerus

- CR perpendicular to IR and humerus, midpoint between epicondyles

To image the proximal forearm

- CR perpendicular to forearm (tube angulation may be necessary), 2 inches (5cm) proximal or superior to olecranon process

Fig. 50a. Position. Elbow – Acute Flexion

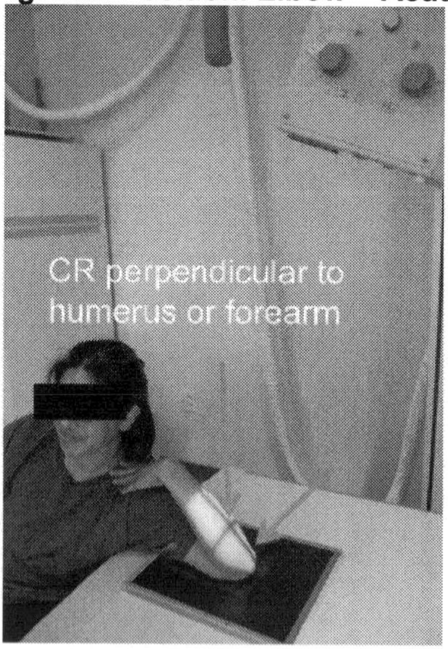

Collimation to include or structures demonstrated

- 2 inches (5 cm) of the proximal forearm and distal humerus

Image evaluation

- The soft tissue and bony trabeculae patterns
  Distal humerus
- Forearm and humerus superimposed. Olecranon process medial & lateral epicondyles in profile
  Proximal forearm
- Distal humerus superimposed on proximal ulna & radius

Note

- To visualize both distal humerus and proximal radius/ulna two projections are required *without moving patient.* One with the CR perpendicular to humerus the other with the CR perpendicular to forearm

Fig. 50b. Radiograph. Elbow – Acute Flexion

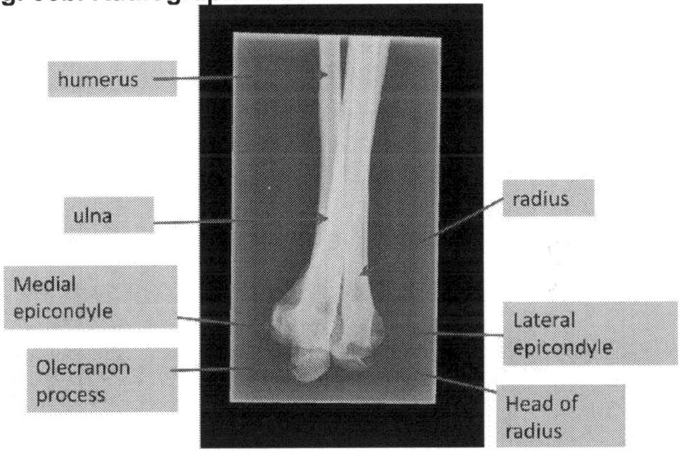

Elbow–Radial head Rotational Projections

Part1 of 4 –Hand supinated & elbow lateral

SID, Technical factors, Shielding

- 40 inches (100 cm). No Grid.62 kVp @ 2.3 mAs. No AEC. Gonadal shielding

Patient/part position

- Seated, face turned away with side to the x-ray table to reduce radiation to gonads, eyes and thyroid

Specific part/body position or rotation

- Elbow flexed 90-degrees with forearm and humerus on same plane

Direction and point of entry of CR

- Using a perpendicular beam the CR is directed to the radial head, 2.5cm or 1 inch distal to lateral epicondyle
- Hand supinated & externally rotated as far as possible–palm up
- Maximum external rotation of hand
- The thumb side of the hand should be up

Fig. 51a. Position. Radial Head Rotational Projections – Hand Supinated

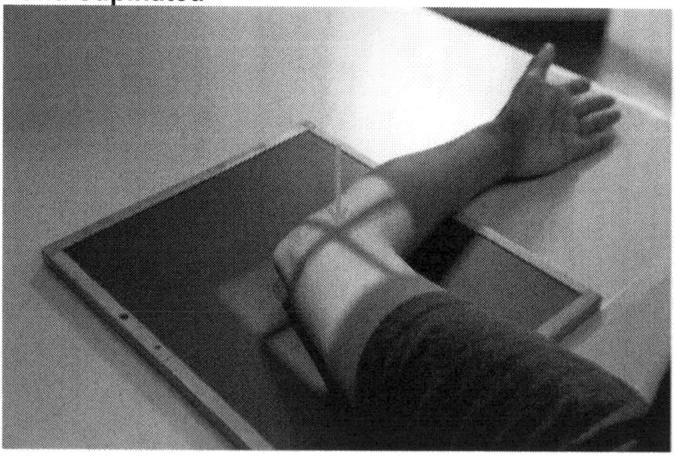

Collimation to include or structures demonstrated

- 2 inches (5cm) of proximal forearm and distal humerus

Image evaluation

- Bony trabeculae and soft tissue seen with the epicondyles superimposed with radial head partial superimposed on ulna
    - Radial tuberosity faces anterior on maximum external rotation
    - Radial tuberosity faces posterior on maximum internal rotation
    - Four images are taken–from maximum external rotation to maximum internal rotation to demonstrate the circumference of the radial head

Fig. 51b. Radiograph. Radial Head Rotational Projections – Hand Supinated

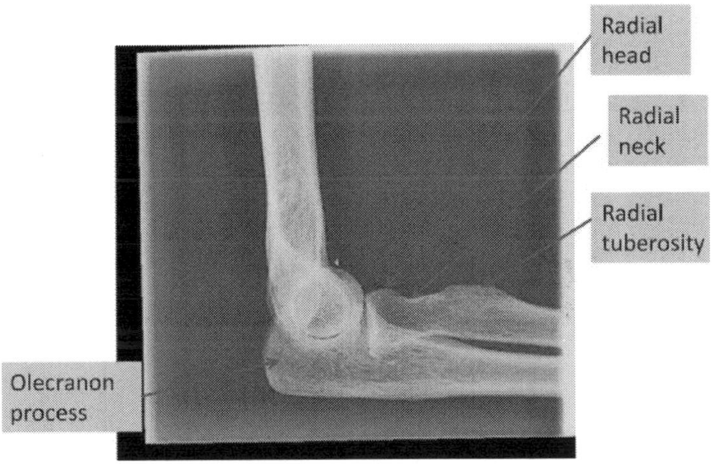

Elbow–Radial head Rotational Projections

Part 2 of 4–Hand lateral & elbow lateral

SID, Technical factors, Shielding

- 40 inches (100 cm). No Grid.62 kVp @ 2.3 mAs. No AEC. Gonadal shielding

Patient/part position

- Seated, face turned away with side to the x-ray table to reduce radiation to gonads, eyes and thyroid

Specific part/body position or rotation

- Elbow flexed 90-degrees with forearm and humerus on same plane
- Hand should be in the true lateral position

Direction and point of entry of CR

- Using a perpendicular beam, the CR is directed to the radial head, 2.5cm or 1 inch distal to lateral epicondyle

Fig. 51c. Position. Radial Head Rotational Projections – Hand Lateral

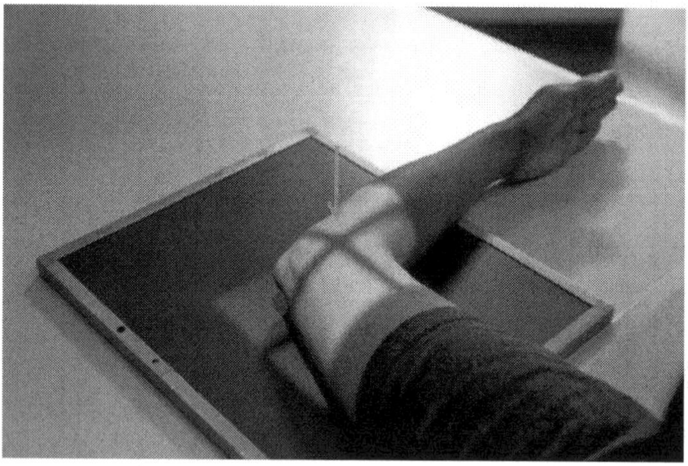

Collimation to include or structures demonstrated

- 2 inches (5cm) of proximal forearm and distal humerus

  Image evaluation

- Bony trabeculae and soft tissue seen with the epicondyles superimposed with radial head partial superimposed on ulna
  - Radial tuberosity faces anterior on maximum external rotation
  - Radial tuberosity faces posterior on maximum internal rotation
  - Four images are taken–from maximum external rotation to maximum internal rotation to demonstrate the circumference of the radial head

Fig. 51d. Radiograph. Radial Head Rotational Projections – Hand Lateral

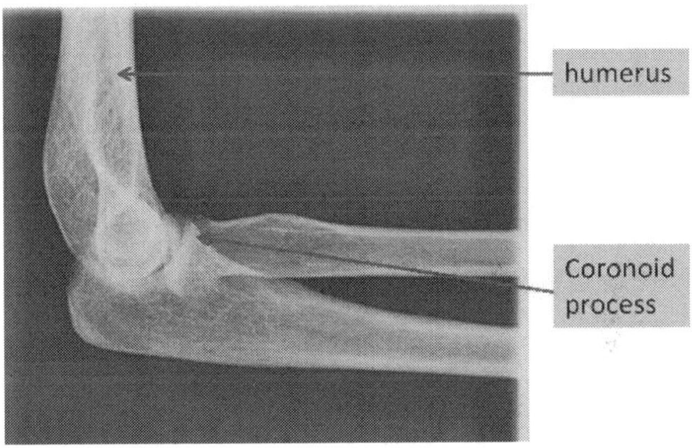

Elbow–Radial head Rotational Projections

Part 3 of 4–Hand pronated & elbow lateral

SID, Technical factors, Shielding

- 40 inches (100 cm). No Grid.62 kVp @ 2.3 mAs. No AEC. Gonadal shielding

Patient/part position

- Seated, face turned away with side to the x-ray table to reduce radiation to gonads, eyes and thyroid

Specific part/body position or rotation

- Elbow flexed 90-degrees with forearm and humerus on same plane
- Hand pronated with the palm flat on IR

Direction and point of entry of CR

- Using a perpendicular beam, the CR is directed to the radial head, 2.5cm or 1 inch distal to lateral epicondyle

Fig. 52a. Position. Radial Head Rotational Projections – Hand Pronated

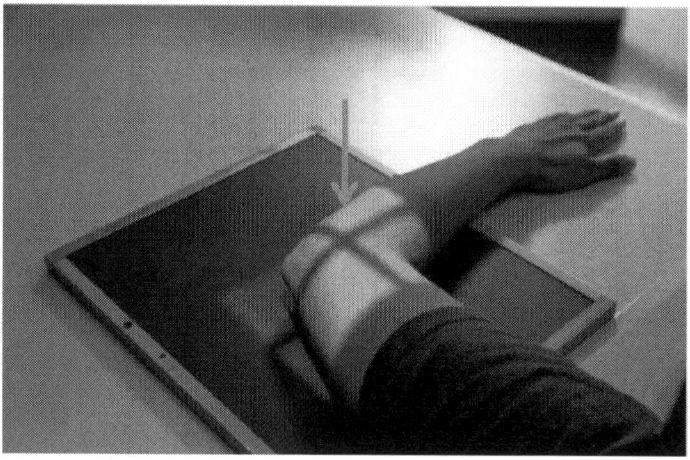

Collimation to include or structures demonstrated

- 2 inches (5cm) of proximal forearm and distal humerus

    Image evaluation

- Bony trabeculae and soft tissue seen with the epicondyles superimposed with radial head partial superimposed on ulna
    - Radial tuberosity faces anterior on maximum external rotation
    - Radial tuberosity faces posterior on maximum internal rotation
    - Four images are taken–from maximum external rotation to maximum internal rotation to demonstrate the circumference of the radial head

Fig. 52b. Radiograph. Radial Head Rotational Projections – Hand Pronated

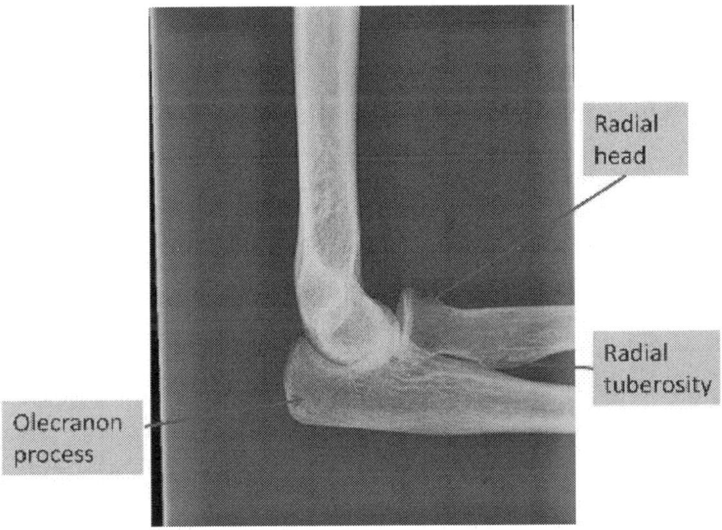

Elbow–Radial head Rotational Projections

Part 4 of 4–Hand supinated & elbow lateral

SID, Technical factors, Shielding

- 40 inches (100 cm). No Grid.62 kVp @ 2.3 mAs. No AEC. Gonadal shielding

Patient/part position

- Seated, face turned away with side to the x-ray table to reduce radiation to gonads, eyes and thyroid

Specific part/body position or rotation

- Elbow flexed 90-degrees with forearm and humerus on same plane
- Hand internally rotated with thumb down as far as possible

Direction and point of entry of CR

- Using a perpendicular beam, the CR is directed to the radial head, 2.5cm or 1 inch distal to lateral epicondyle

Fig. 52c. Position. Radial Head Rotational Projections – Hand Internally Rotated

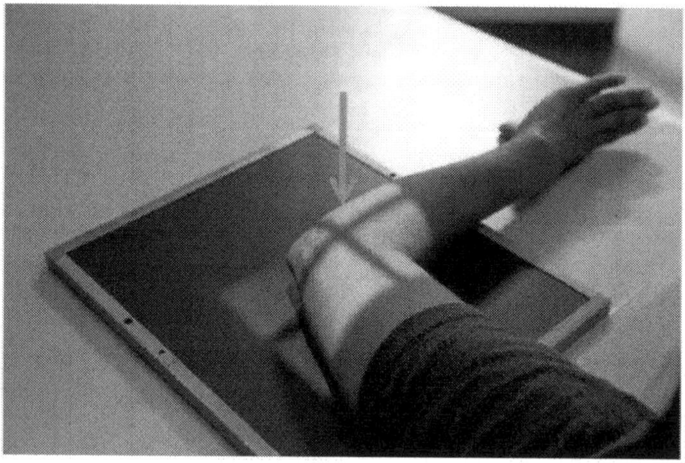

Collimation to include or structures demonstrated

- 2 inches (5cm) of proximal forearm and distal humerus
   Image evaluation
- Bony trabeculae and soft tissue seen with the epicondyles superimposed with radial head partial superimposed on ulna
   - Radial tuberosity faces anterior on maximum external rotation
   - Radial tuberosity faces posterior on maximum internal rotation
   - Four images are taken–from maximum external rotation to maximum internal rotation to demonstrate the circumference of the radial head

Fig. 52d. Radiograph. Radial Head Rotational Projections – Hand Internally Rotated

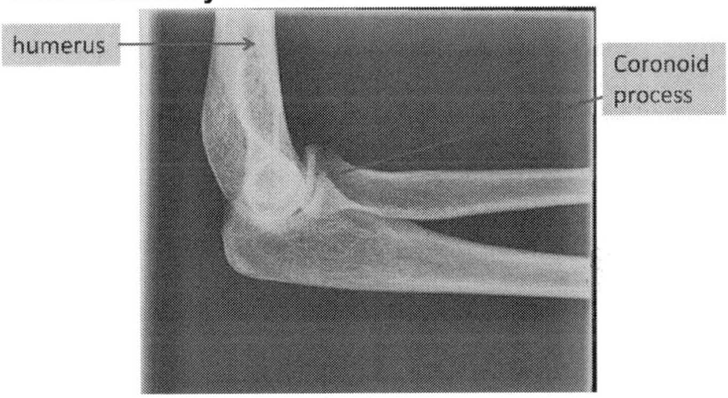

Elbow–Radial Head Projection

Part 1 of 2 of the trauma (Coyle method) of imaging the elbow–Greenspan & Normal position

SID, Technical factors, Shielding

- 40 inches (100 cm). No Grid. 62kVp @ 2.3 mAs. No AEC. Gonadal shielding

Patient/part position

- Seated, face turned away with side to the x-ray table to reduce radiation to gonads, eyes and thyroid

Specific part/body position or rotation

- Elbow flexed 90-degrees with forearm and humerus on same plane and hand pronated

Direction and point of entry of CR

- CR is directed 45-degrees to shoulder passing through the radial head

Fig. 53a. Position. Elbow – Radial Head Projection

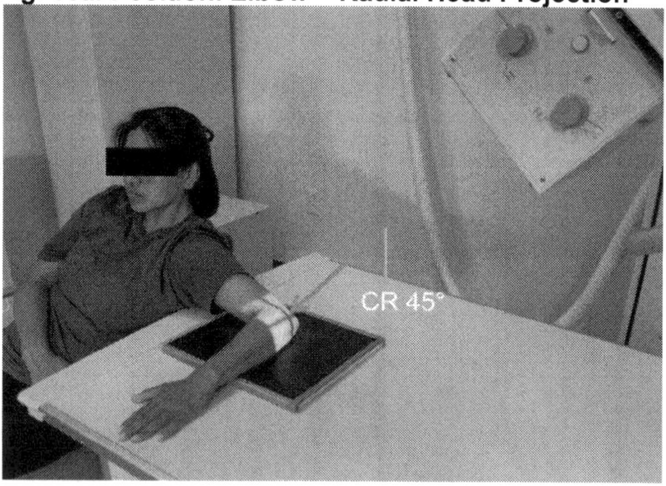

Collimation to include or structures demonstrated

- 2 inches (5 cm) of the proximal forearm & distal humerus

Image evaluation

- Include bony trabecular and soft tissue with the joint space between radial head and capitulum open
- Radial head partly superimpose on coronoid
- Radial neck and tuberosity in profile and free of superimposition
- Distal humerus distorted

Fig. 53b. Radiograph. Elbow – Radial Head Projection

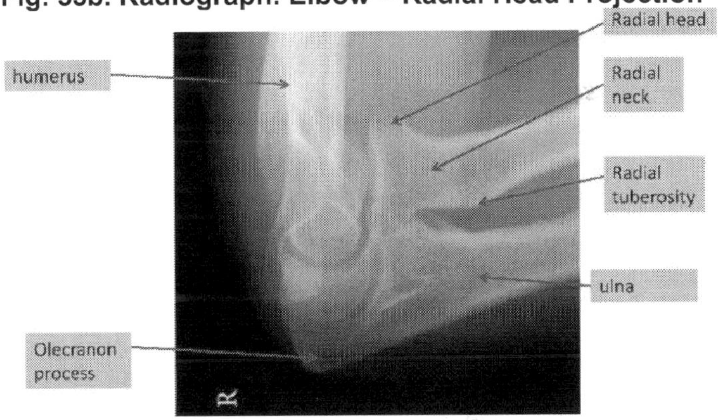

Elbow–Coronoid Process Projection

Part 2 of 2 of the trauma (Coyle method) of imaging the elbow

SID, Technical factors, Shielding

- 40 inches (100 cm). No Grid. 62kVp @ 2.3 mAs. No AEC. Gonadal shielding

Patient/part position

- Seated, face turned away with side to the x-ray table to reduce radiation to gonads, eyes and thyroid

Specific part/body position or rotation

- Elbow flexed 80-degrees from extended position (more flexion will obscure coronoid) with forearm and humerus on same plane and hand pronated

Direction and point of entry of CR

- CR is directed 45-degrees away from the shoulder passing through the radial head

Fig. 54a. Position. Elbow- Coronoid Process

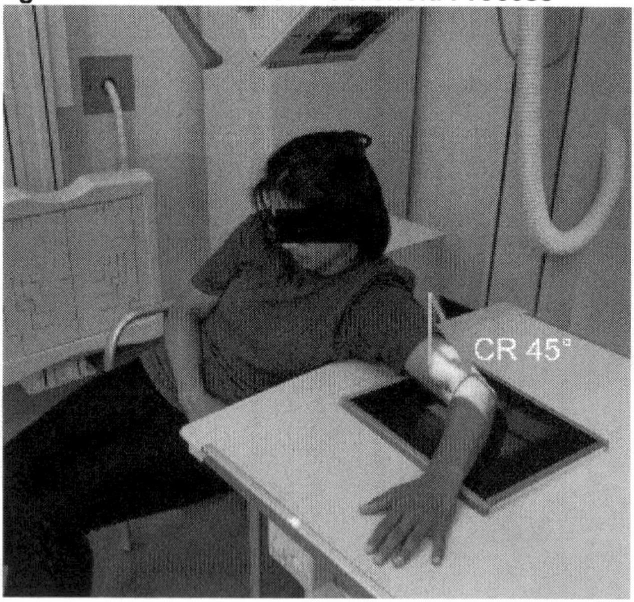

Collimation to include or structures demonstrated

- 2 inches (5 cm) of the proximal forearm & distal humerus

Image evaluation

- Include bony trabecular and soft tissue with the distal coronoid process elongated but seen in profile
- Open joint space between coronoid process and trochlear
- Radial head and neck superimposed by ulna

Fig. 54b. Radiograph. Elbow- Coronoid Process

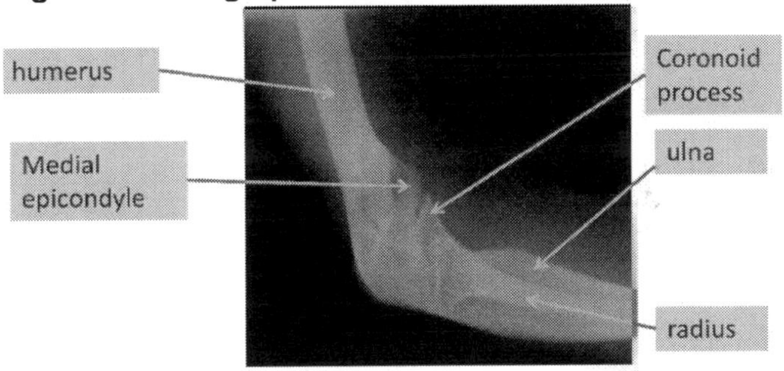

Humerus–Anteroposterior (AP)

SID, Technical factors, Shielding

- 40 inches (100 cm). Grid. 65-70kVp @ 3.2 mAs or AEC. Gonadal shielding

Patient/part position

- Patient supine or erect facing the CR

Specific part/body position or rotation

- Rotate body to affected side with arm abducted
- Extend the arm and forearm with hand supinated

Direction and point of entry of CR

- Perpendicular to mid humeral shaft

Fig.55a. Position. Humerus – Anteroposterior (AP)

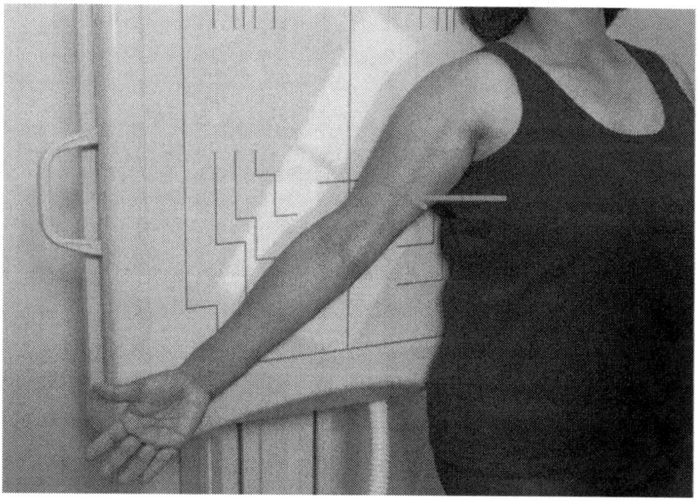

Collimation to include or structures demonstrated

- The shoulder and elbow joints, plus 1 inch (2.5 cm) of proximal forearm)

Breathing instructions

- Image taken with arrested respiration

Image evaluation

- Bony trabeculae and soft tissue with the greater tubercle is seen in profile on the laterally aspect of humerus
- Minimal superimposition of humeral head on glenoid cavity
- Medial and lateral epicondyles seen in profile

Notes

- Do not manipulate arm in cases of suspected fracture.
- To minimize the anode heel effect and allows uniform exposure, the humeral head is placed to the cathode side of the tube

Fig.55b. Radiograph. Humerus – Anteroposterior (AP)

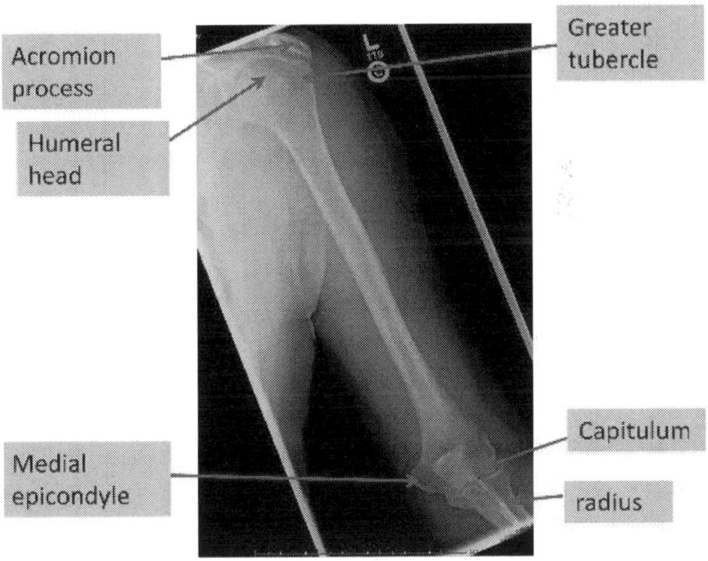

Humerus–Lateral (mediolateral)

SID, Technical factors, Shielding

- 40 inches (100 cm). Grid. 65-70kVp @ 3.2 mAs or AEC. Gonadal shielding

Patient/part position

- Patient supine or erect

Specific part/body position or rotation

- Patient starts PA then rotate affected side to the IR with the elbow flexed 90-degrees to place the epicondyles perpendicular to the IR

Direction and point of entry of CR

- Perpendicular to mid humeral shaft

Fig. 56a. Position. Humerus – Lateral (Mediolateral, patient PA)

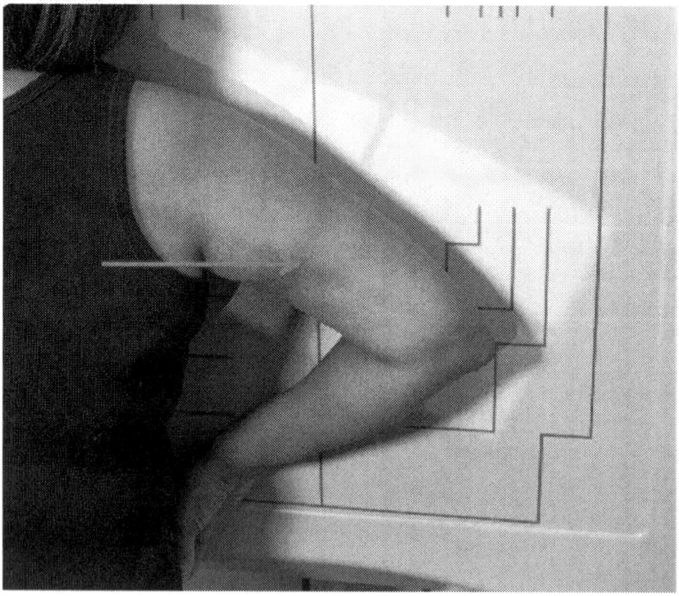

Collimation to include or structures demonstrated

- The shoulder and elbow joints plus 1 inch (2.5 cm) of proximal forearm

Breathing instructions

- Image taken with arrested respiration

Image evaluation

- Bony trabeculae and soft tissue with the epicondyles superimposed
- Lesser tubercle in profile medially

Notes:

- To minimize the anode heel effect and allows uniform exposure, the humeral head is placed to the cathode side of the tube
- Do not manipulate arm if suspected fracture.
- Imaging can be performed mediolateral or lateromedial

Fig. 56b. Radiograph. Humerus – Lateral (Mediolateral, patient PA)

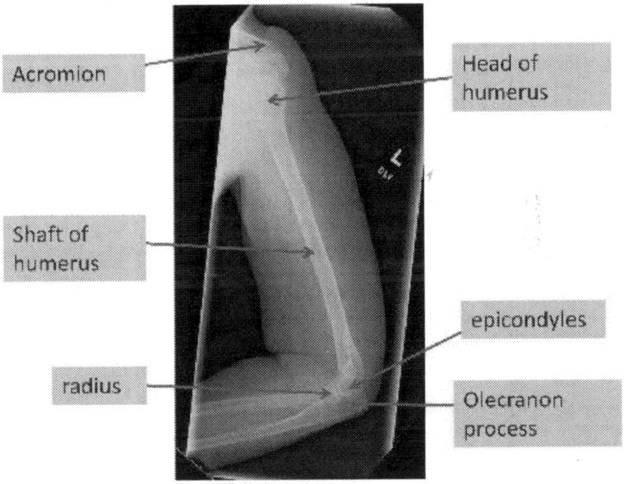

Humerus–Lateral (lateromedial)

SID, Technical factors, Shielding

- 40 inches (100 cm). Grid. 65-70kVp @ 3.2 mAs or AEC. Gonadal shielding

Patient/part position

- Patient supine or erect

Specific part/body position or rotation

- Patient starts AP then rotated to affected side
- Internally rotate the arm to place the epicondyles perpendicular to the IR
- Keep elbows partially flexed

Direction and point of entry of CR

- Perpendicular to mid humeral shaft

Fig. 57a. Position. Humerus – Lateral (Mediolateral, patient AP)

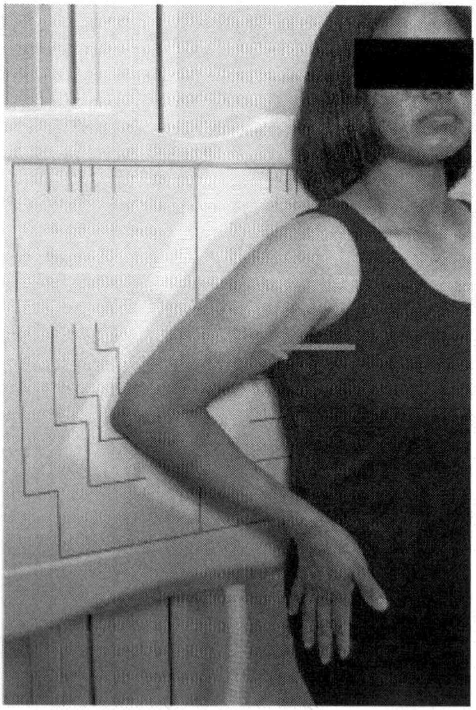

Collimation to include or structures demonstrated

- The shoulder and elbow joints plus 1 inch (2.5 cm) of proximal forearm)

Breathing instructions

- Image taken with arrested respiration

Image evaluation

- Bony trabeculae and soft tissue with the epicondyles superimposed with the lesser tubercle in profile medially.

Notes:

- To minimize the anode heel effect and allows uniform exposure, the humeral head is placed to the cathode side of the tube
- No manipulation of the arm in cases of suspected fracture
- Imaging can be performed mediolateral or lateromedial

Fig. 57b. Radiograph. Humerus – Lateral (Mediolateral, patient AP)

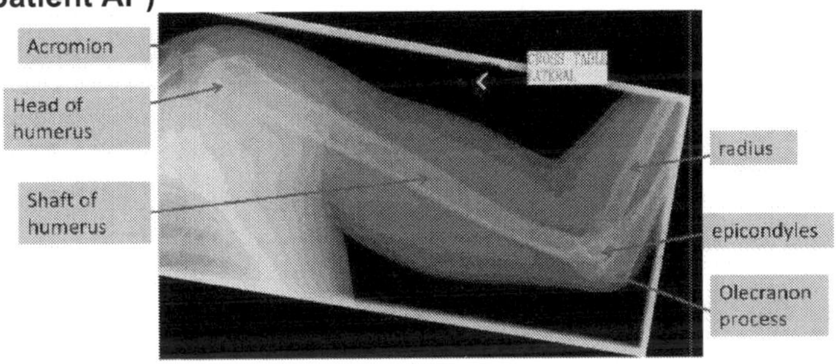

Shoulder Girdle

- Bones of the shoulder girdle –Clavicle and scapula

- Bones of the shoulder Joint –Humerus, scapula, clavicle
    - Clavicle:
        - laterally it articulates with acromion of scapula- Acromioclavicular joint
        - Medially it articulates with sternal manubrium & 1st costal cartilage- Sternoclavicular joint.
    - Scapula: humeral head articulates within glenoid fossa of scapula-Scapulohumeral joint (Glenohumeral joint)

External rotation

- Position of hand –Supinated
- Interepicondylar line position in relationship to the IR
    - Parallel to IR
- Location of lesser and greater tubercle
    - Lesser seen anteriorly; Greater seen laterally in profile

Internal rotation

- Position of hand–Back of hand against the hip
- Interepicondylar line position in relationship to the IR
    - Perpendicular to IR
- Location of lesser and greater tubercle
    - Lesser medially in profile; Greater anterior & medial

Neutral rotation

- Position of hand –Palm faces inward against thigh
- Interepicondylar line position in relationship to the IR
    - –45° to IR
- Location of lesser and greater tubercle
    - –Lesser anterior & medial; Greater anterior and lateral

Anatomy of the Shoulder

Fig. 58a. AP scapula

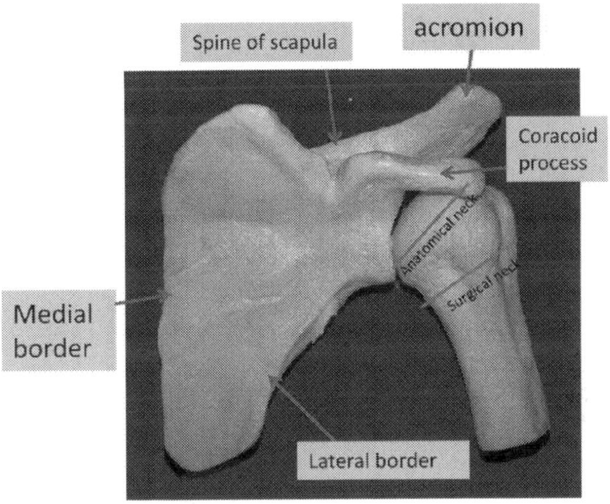

Fig. 58b. Lateral scapula

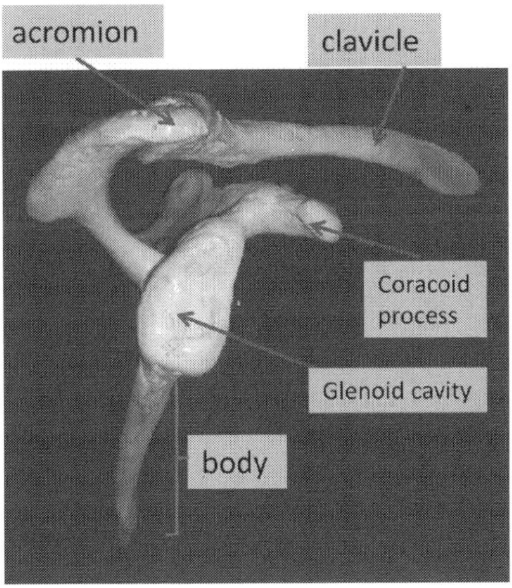

Shoulder–Anteroposterior (AP) projection, External Rotation

For non-trauma imaging only

SID, Technical factors, Shielding

- 40 inches (100 cm). Grid. 70kVp @ 5 mAs or AEC. Gonadal shielding

Patient/part position

- Patient imaged erect or supine

Specific part/body position or rotation

- Rotate affected part slightly to the rest shoulder on IR, and abduct arm
- Externally rotate arm to supinated hand with epicondyles parallel to the IR

Direction and point of entry of CR

- To a point 1-inch (2.5 cm) inferior to coracoid process.

Fig. 59a. Position. Shoulder -Anteroposterior (AP) projection external rotation

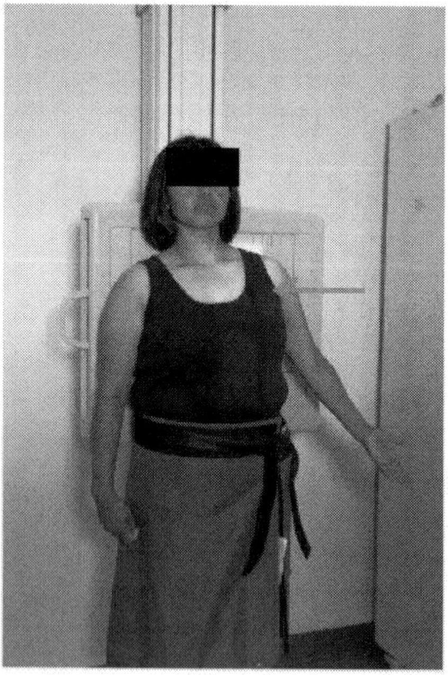

Collimation to include or structures demonstrated

- At least 2/3 of clavicle medially; 1/3 of proximal humerus inferiorly; humeral head superiorly & laterally

Breathing instructions

- Image on suspend respiration

Image evaluation

- Soft tissue and bony trabeculae with the greater tubercle seen in profile on lateral aspect of humerus
- Lesser tubercle superimposed on humeral head
- Slight overlap of humeral head on glenoid cavity

Note

- The coracoid process is ¾ in (2 cm) inferior to most lateral portion of clavicle

Fig. 59b. Radiograph. Shoulder -Anteroposterior (AP) projection external rotation

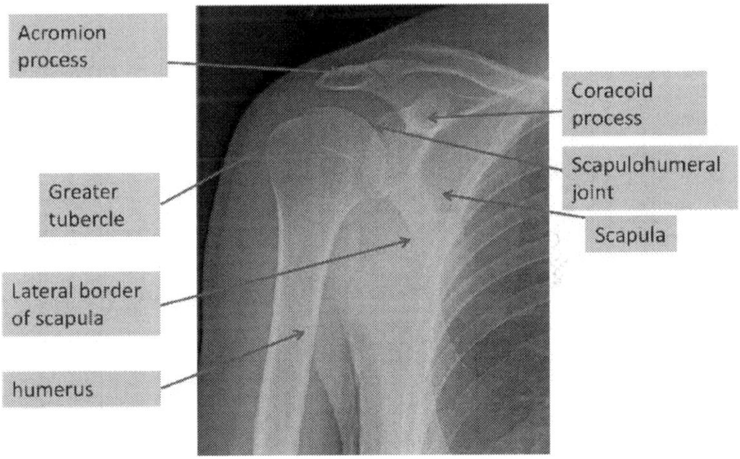

Shoulder–Anteroposterior projection, Internal Rotation

For non-trauma imaging only

SID, Technical factors, Shielding

- 40 inches (100 cm). Grid. 70kVp @ 5 mAs or AEC. Gonadal shielding

Patient/part position

- Patient imaged erect or supine

Specific part/body position or rotation

- Rotate affected part slightly to the rest shoulder on IR, and abduct arm
- Internally rotate arm, to pronate hand with epicondyles perpendicular to the IR

Direction and point of entry of CR

- To a point 1-inch (2.5 cm) inferior to coracoid process

Fig. 60a. Position. Shoulder – Anteroposterior projection, Internal Rotation

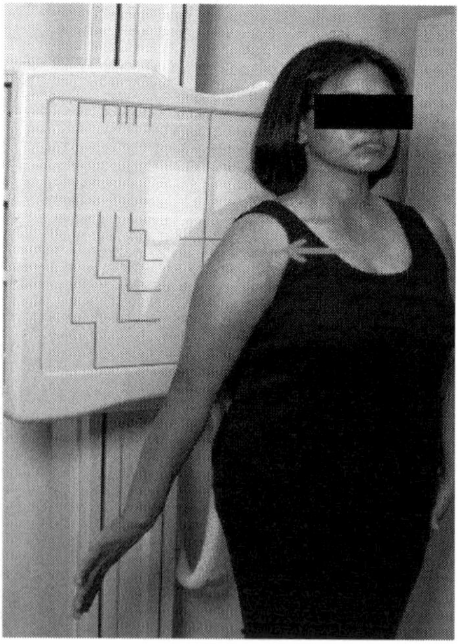

Collimation to include or structures demonstrated

- At least 2/3 of clavicle medially; 1/3 of proximal humerus inferiorly; humeral head superiorly & laterally.

Breathing instructions

- Suspend respiration

Image evaluation

- Soft tissue and bony trabeculae with the lesser tubercle seen in profile on medial aspect of humerus
- The greater tubercle superimposed on humeral head
- More overlap of humeral head on glenoid cavity than seen on the external rotation

Note

- The coracoid process is ¾ in (2 cm) inferior to most lateral portion of clavicle

Fig. 60b. Radiograph. Shoulder – Anteroposterior projection, Internal Rotation

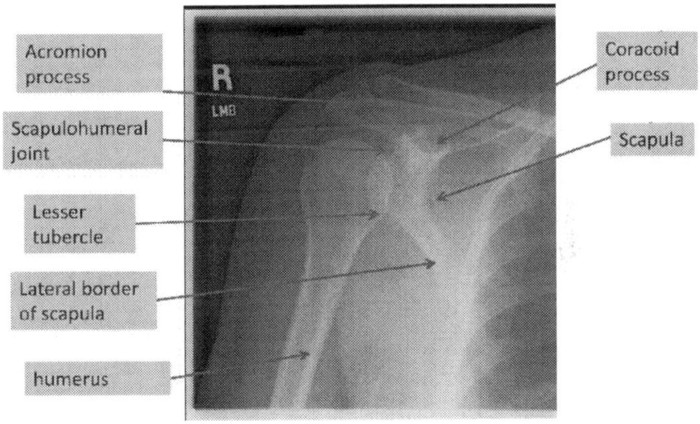

Shoulder–Anteroposterior projection, Neutral Rotation

For trauma imaging

SID, Technical factors, Shielding

- 40 inches (100 cm). Grid. 70kVp @ 5 mAs or AEC. Gonadal shielding

Patient/part position

- Patient imaged erect or supine

Specific part/body position or rotation

- The arm should be imaged as is. DO NOT manipulate the arm of the trauma patient

Direction and point of entry of CR

- To a point 1-inch (2.5 cm) inferior to coracoid process.

Fig.61a. Position. Shoulder – Anteroposterior projection, Neutral Rotation

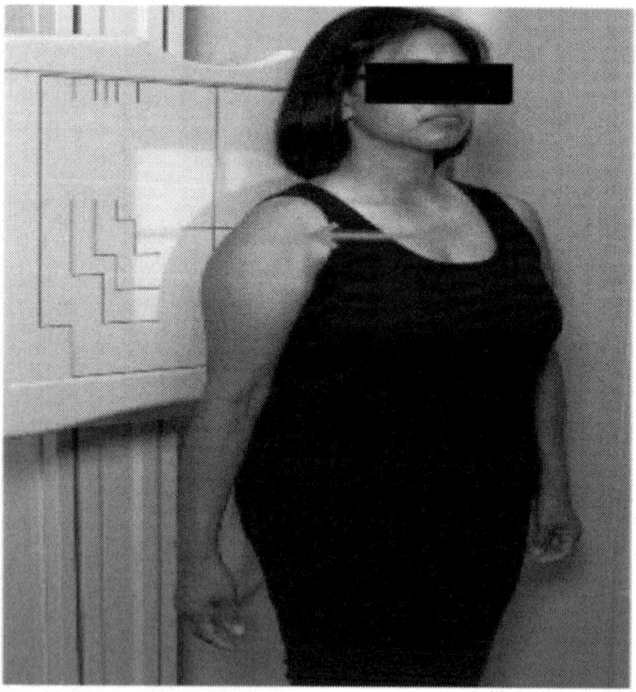

Collimation to include or structures demonstrated

- At least 2/3 of clavicle medially; 1/3 of proximal humerus inferiorly; humeral head superiorly & laterally

Breathing instructions

- Image on suspend respiration

Image evaluation

- Soft tissue and bony trabeculae with the MSP & epicondyles typically imaged 45-degrees to the IR when the arm is neutral
- The greater and lesser tubercle will be superimposed on humeral head with the greater tubercle more lateral

Note

- The coracoid process is ¾ in (2 cm) inferior to most lateral portion of clavicle

Fig.61b. Radiograph. Shoulder – Anteroposterior projection, Neutral Rotation

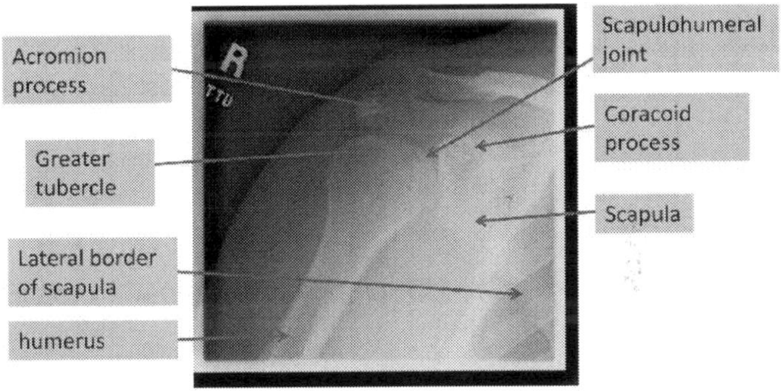

Shoulder–Transthoracic Lateral projection

For trauma imaging, Lawrence method

SID, Technical factors, Shielding

- 40 inches (100 cm). Grid. 80kVp @ 5 mAs or AEC. Gonadal shielding

Patient/part position

- The preferred position is erect however the patient can be supine
- Lateral (affected side) resting on the IR with MSP parallel to IR

Specific part/body position or rotation

- Affected arm kept in neutral position with no manipulation, or allowed it to drop if possible
- Elevate unaffected arm (raised over the patient's head) to elevate the unaffected shoulder and prevent superimposition of both shoulders

Direction and point of entry of CR

- Directed perpendicular to IR through thorax to surgical neck of the humerus

Fig. 62a. Position. Shoulder – Transthoracic Lateral projection

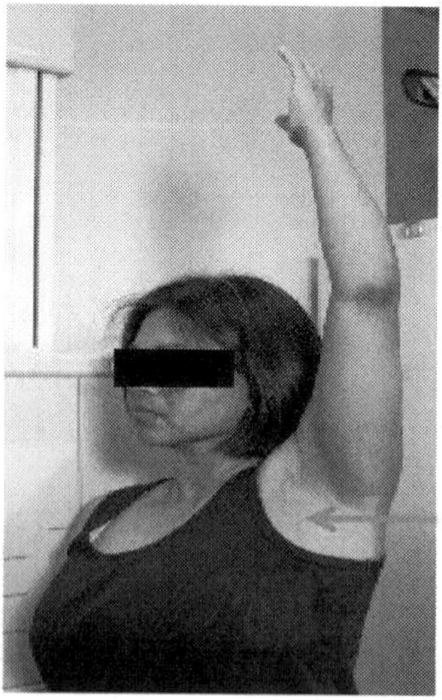

Collimation to include or structures demonstrated

- The glenohumeral joint and entire humeral head plus 1-/3 of the humeral shaft

Breathing instructions–two options

- Breathing technique can be used to blur out ribs and lungs. The exposure is taken with slow breathing using a long exposure time of 2-3 seconds
- Full arrested inspiration used to improve contrast and decrease exposure necessary to penetrate body.

Image evaluation

- Soft tissue and bony trabecular detail the glenohumeral joint and proximal humerus visualized through the thorax
- The unaffected humerus free of superimposition by affected humerus
- Humerus visualized anterior to the thoracic spine
- Blurred ribs and lung markings if using breathing technique

Note

- If patient cannot drop affected shoulder to prevent superimposition of shoulders 10–15° cephalic tube angulation needed

Fig. 62b. Radiograph. Shoulder – Transthoracic Lateral projection

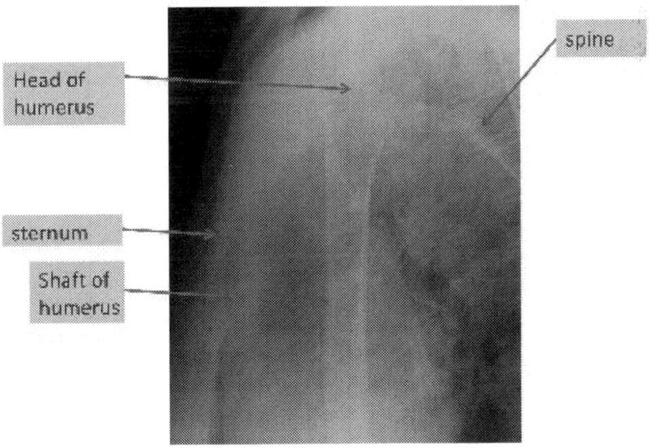

Shoulder–Superoinferior Axial projection

For non-trauma imaging

SID, Technical factors, Shielding

- 40 inches (100 cm). Grid. 80kVp @ 5 mAs. No AEC. Gonadal shielding

Patient/part position

- Patient seated at end of x-ray table
- Head rotated/tilted away from affected side

Specific part/body position or rotation

- Lean patient laterally with arm abducted
- Flex elbow 90° and place hand prone

Direction and point of entry of CR

- CR is directly vertical using 5 –15° tube angulation laterally through the acromioclavicular joint or axilla
- Less abduction of arm will require more lateral angulation

Fig. 63a. Position. Shoulder- Superoinferior Axial projection

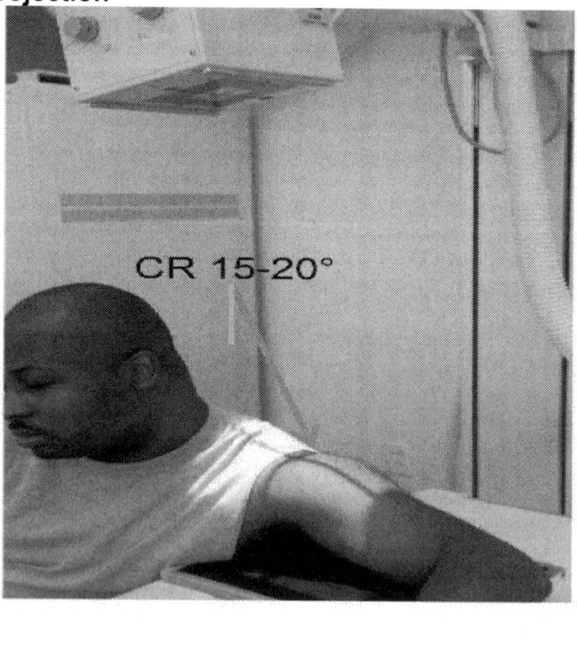

Collimation to include or structures demonstrated

- The proximal 1/3 of the humerus plus lateral 1/3 of clavicle

Breathing instructions

- Exposure on suspend respiration

Image evaluation

- Bony trabeculae and soft tissue showing the relationship of proximal humerus in glenoid cavity
- The coracoid process above clavicle
- Lesser tubercle in profile
- Spine of scapula seen on edge below the scapulohumeral joint
- Superior and inferior borders of glenoid cavity directly superimposed

Fig. 63b. Radiograph. Shoulder- Superoinferior Axial projection

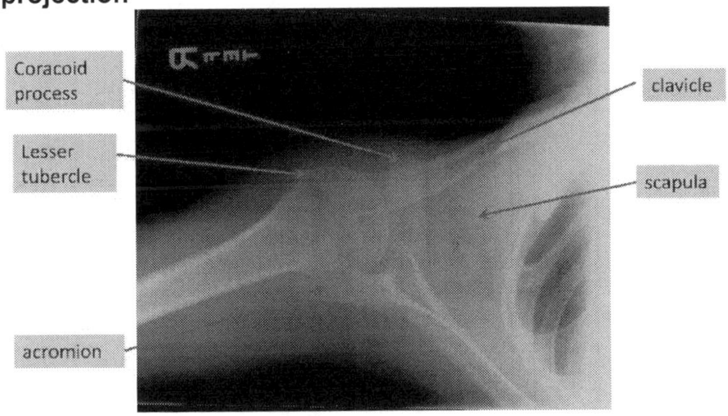

Shoulder–Inferosuperior Axial projection

For non-trauma imaging, Lawrence method

SID, Technical factors, Shielding

- 40 inches (100 cm). Grid. 80kVp @ 5 mAs. No AEC. Gonadal shielding

Patient/part position

- Patient is supine with upper torso on a raised support
- Head rotated away from affected side

Specific part/body position or rotation

- The arm is extended and abducted 90-degree with thumb down and arm in external rotation
- Support the IR vertically against the patient's shoulder as close to the neck as possible

Direction and point of entry of CR

- The CR is directed horizontal and medially 10-30 degrees
- Decrease tube angulation if the arm is abducted less than 90

Fig. 64a. Position. Shoulder- Inferosuperior Axial projection

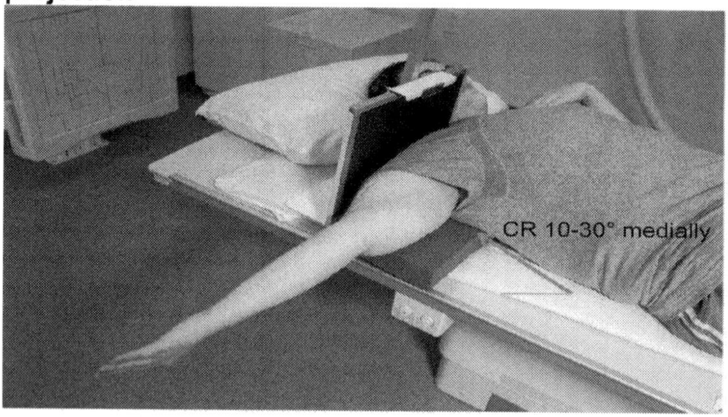

Collimation to include or structures demonstrated

- The proximal 1/3 of the humerus plus lateral 1/3 of clavicle

Breathing instructions

- Exposure on suspend respiration

Image evaluation

- Bony trabeculae and soft tissue showing the relationship of proximal humerus in glenoid cavity
- AC joint, acromion and lateral clavicle seen through the humeral head
- The coracoid process and lesser tubercle seen in profile
- Superior and inferior borders of glenoid cavity directly superimposed

Fig. 64b. Radiograph. Shoulder- Inferosuperior Axial projection

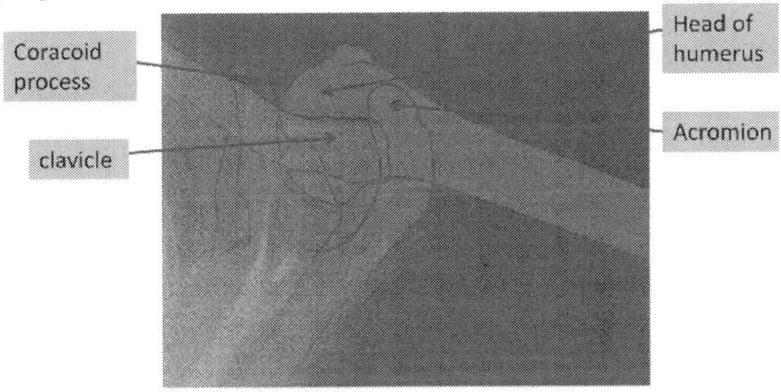

Shoulder– Anterior Oblique position, RAO & LAO, Scapular Y projection

For trauma imaging

SID, Technical factors, Shielding

- 40 inches (100 cm). Grid. 80kVp @ 5 mAs or AEC. Gonadal shielding

Patient/part position

- Patient erect or supine
- The erect is more comfortable for the trauma patient

Specific part/body position or rotation for the RAO or LAO

- Patient facing the x-ray tube with affected side touching the IR and body rotated with MCP forming an angle of 45-60 degree to IR
- Slightly abduct the arm without manipulation to avoid superimposition of humerus on ribs
- Palpate for the scapular borders to position the medial and lateral borders superimposed

Direction and point of entry of CR

- To the scapulohumeral joint or 2-2 ½ inches (5-6 cm) below top of shoulder

Fig. 65a. Position. Shoulder – Oblique, Scapular Y projection. Anterior Oblique position, RAO or LAO

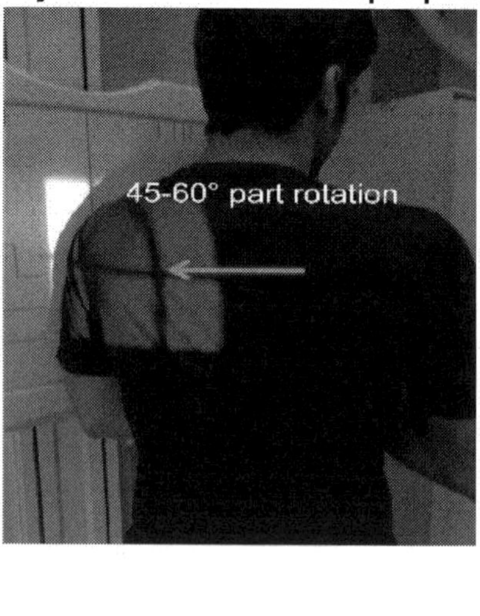

Collimation to include or structures demonstrated

- The humeral head superimposed in the glenoid cavity
- The acromion and coracoid process appearing as the letter **Y** with the acromion projected laterally and the coracoid medially

Breathing instructions

- Imaging on arrested respiration

Image evaluation

- Sharp bony trabecular and soft tissue detail of a true lateral scapula with the medial and lateral borders of the scapula superimposed
- The scapula body clear of the ribs

Notes

- With anterior dislocation–humeral head projects inferior to coracoid
- With posterior dislocation–humeral head projects inferior to acromion
- If the thicker (lateral border) of the scapula is seen on the outside this indicates too little rotation

Fig. 65b. Radiograph. Shoulder – Oblique, Scapular Y projection. Anterior Oblique position, RAO or LAO

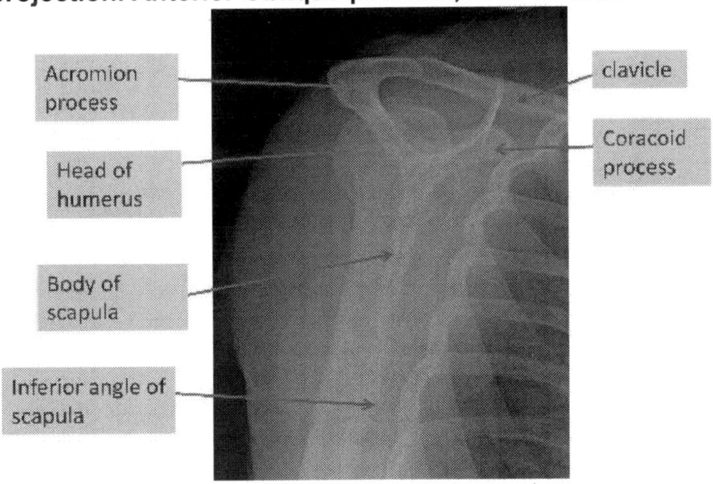

Shoulder–Posterior Oblique position, RPO & LPO, Scapular Y projection

For trauma imaging

SID, Technical factors, Shielding

- 40 inches (100 cm). Grid. 80kVp @ 5 mAs or AEC. Gonadal shielding

Patient/part position

- Patient erect or supine. The erect is more comfortable for the trauma patient

Specific part/body position or rotation for the RPO or LPO

- Patient's back to the x-ray tube with the affected side away from the IR and body rotated with MCP forming an angle of 45-60° to IR
- Slightly abduct the arm without manipulation to avoid superimposition of humerus on ribs
- Palpate and position the medial and lateral scapula borders superimposed

Direction and point of entry of CR

- To the scapulohumeral joint or 2-2 ½ inches (5-6 cm) below top of shoulder

Fig. 65c. Position. Shoulder – Oblique, Scapular Y projection. Posterior Oblique position, RPO or LPO

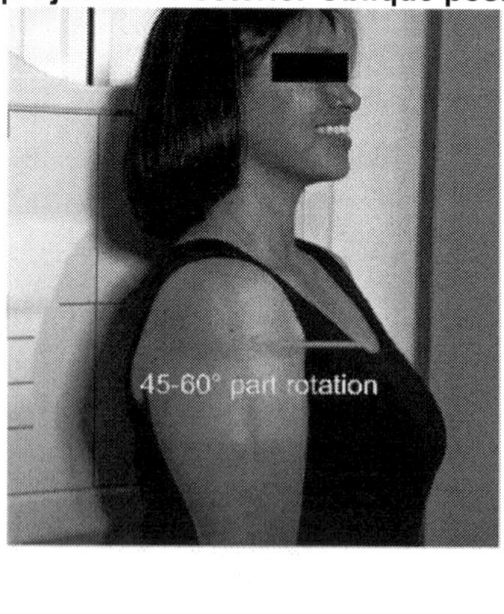

Collimation to include or structures demonstrated

- The humeral head superimposed in the glenoid cavity
- The acromion and coracoid process appearing as the letter **Y** with the acromion projected laterally and the coracoid medially

Breathing instructions

- Imaging on arrested respiration

Image evaluation

- Sharp bony trabecular and soft tissue detail of a true lateral scapula with the medial and lateral borders of the scapula superimposed
- The scapula body clear of the ribs

Notes:

- The radiograph is the same as the RAO or LAO with slight magnification because of the OID
- With anterior dislocation–humeral head seen inferior to coracoid
- With posterior dislocation–humeral head seen inferior to acromion

Fig. 65d. Radiograph. Shoulder – Oblique, Scapular Y projection. Posterior Oblique position, RPO or LPO

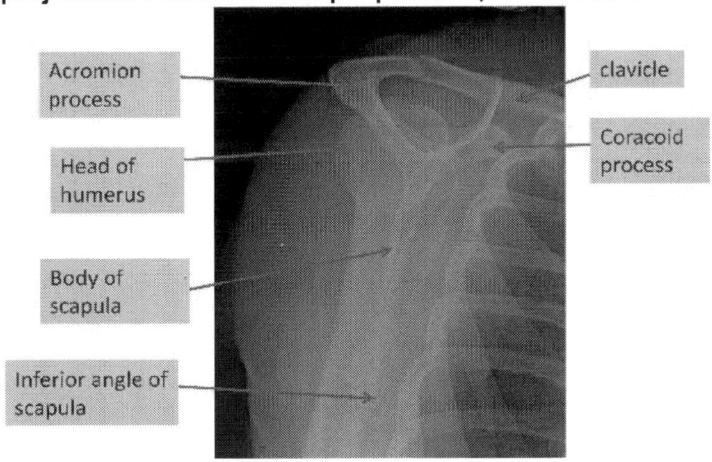

Shoulder–Posterior Oblique, LPO or RPO position with internal rotation

Non-trauma imaging, Grashey method

SID, Technical factors, Shielding

- 40 inches (100 cm). Grid. 70kVp @ 5 mAs or AEC. Gonadal shielding

Patient/part position

- Patient erect or supine

Specific part/body position or rotation

- Patient is rotated 45° to affected side to place the body of scapula against IR. Rounded shoulders requires more rotation
- The arm is abducted slightly with arm neutral rotation or placed with palm on stomach

Direction and point of entry of CR

- To the scapulohumeral joint, 2-inch (5 cm) inferior & medial to superolateral border of shoulder

Fig. 66a. Position. Shoulder- Posterior Oblique, LPO or RPO position with Internal Rotation.

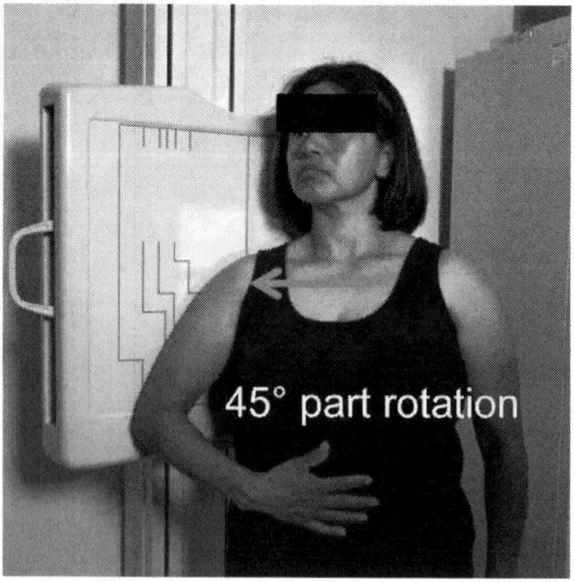

Collimation to include or structures demonstrated

- At least 2/3 of clavicle medially, 1/3 of proximal humerus and humeral head

Breathing instructions

- Imaging on suspend respiration

Image evaluation

- Soft tissue and bony trabecular with the glenoid cavity in profile without humeral head superimposition

Fig. 66b. Radiograph. Shoulder- Posterior Oblique, LPO or RPO position with Internal Rotation.

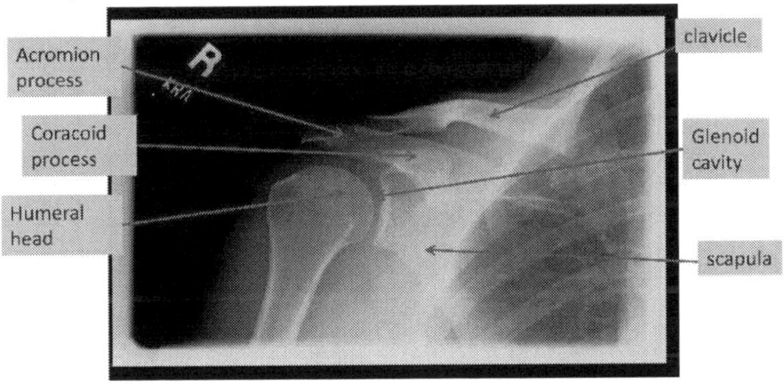

Clavicle–Anteroposterior (AP) projection or Posteroanterior (PA)

SID, Technical factors, Shielding

- 40 inches (100 cm). Grid. 70kVp @ 10 mAs or AEC. Gonadal shielding

Patient/part position

- Supine or erect in true AP position

Specific part/body position or rotation position

- Chin raised and arm at sides

Direction and point of entry of CR

- Using a perpendicular CR to the mid clavicle

Fig. 67a. Position. Clavicle – Anteroposterior (AP) proejction

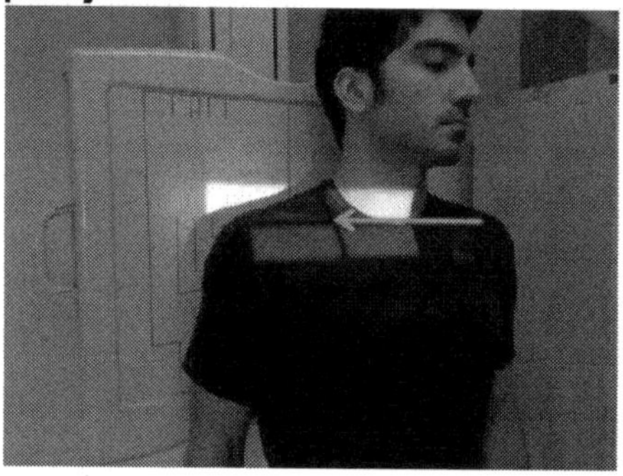

Fig. 67b. Position. Clavicle – Posteroanterior (PA) proejction

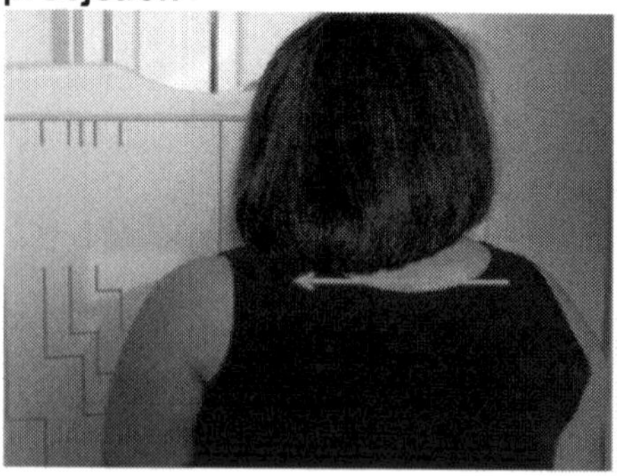

Collimation to include or structures demonstrated

- The entire clavicle including medial and lateral ends plus the acromioclavicular and sternoclavicular joints

Breathing instructions

- Image on arrested inspiration to place the clavicles higher

Image evaluation

- Sharp bony trabecular, soft tissue detail with the medial half of clavicle superimposed over thorax.

Note: The PA projection places the clavicle closer to IR but is difficult for patients with injuries

Fig. 67c. Radiograph. Clavicle – Anteroposterior (AP) or Posteroanterior proejction

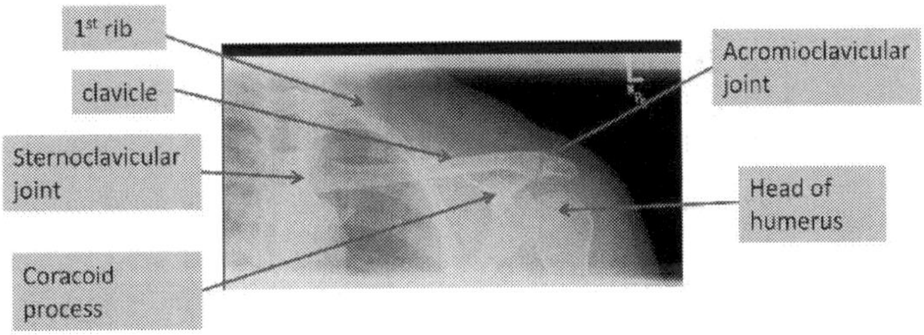

Clavicle–Anteroposterior (AP) projection or Axial Posteroanterior (PA)

SID, Technical factors, Shielding

- 40 inches (100 cm). Grid. 70kVp @ 10 mAs or AEC. Gonadal shielding

Patient/part position

- Supine or erect in true AP position

Specific part/body position or rotation

- Chin raised with arm at sides

Direction and point of entry of CR, AP axial

- Center to mid clavicle using 15-30 degrees cephalic tube angulation

Direction and point of entry of CR, PA axial

- Center to mid clavicle using 15-20 degrees caudal tube angulation

Fig. 68a. Position. Clavicle – Anteroposterior (AP) Axial projection

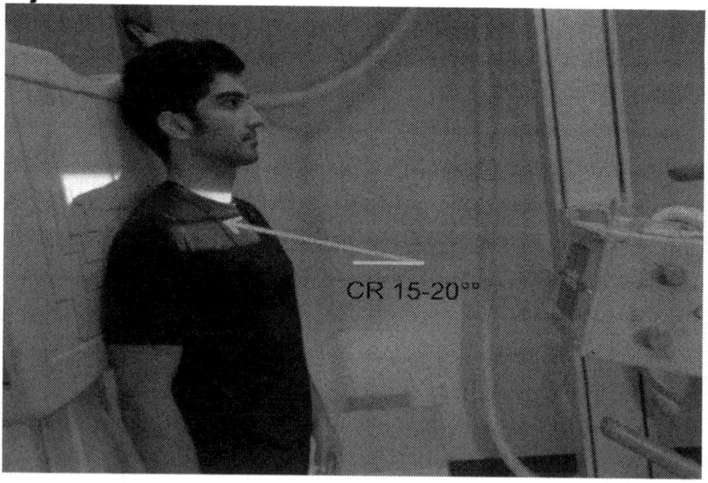

Collimation to include or structures demonstrated

- To include medial and lateral ends of the clavicle plus the AC and SC joints

Breathing instructions

- Image on arrested inspiration to place the clavicles higher

Image evaluation

- Sharp bony trabecular and soft tissue detail with most of clavicle projected above thorax
- The most medial end will superimpose the 1st or 2nd rib

Notes

- Thinner patients need more angulation
- Increase angulation up to 45 degrees for children
- Decrease angulation if the patient is imaged standing using the Lordotic position
- The PA projection places the clavicle closer to IR but is difficult for patients with injuries

Fig. 68b. Radiograph. Clavicle – Anteroposterior (AP) Axial projection

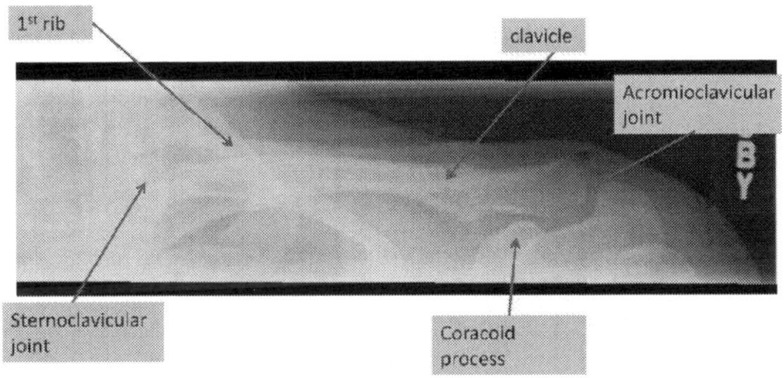

Acromioclavicular (AC) Joint–Anteroposterior (AP) projection

Part1 of 2—Imaging without weights

SID, Technical factors, Shielding

- 72-inch SID (183 cm). Grid. 75kVp @ 20mAs or AEC. Gonadal shielding

Patient/part position

- Patient erect either standing or seated

Specific part/body position or rotation

- Both shoulders should rest against the IR with body weight equally distributed on both feet

Direction and point of entry of CR & SID

- Horizontal to midline 1-inch (2.5 cm) above jugular notch

Fig. 69a. Position. Acromioclavicular (AC) joint – Anteroposterior (AP) projections, without weights.

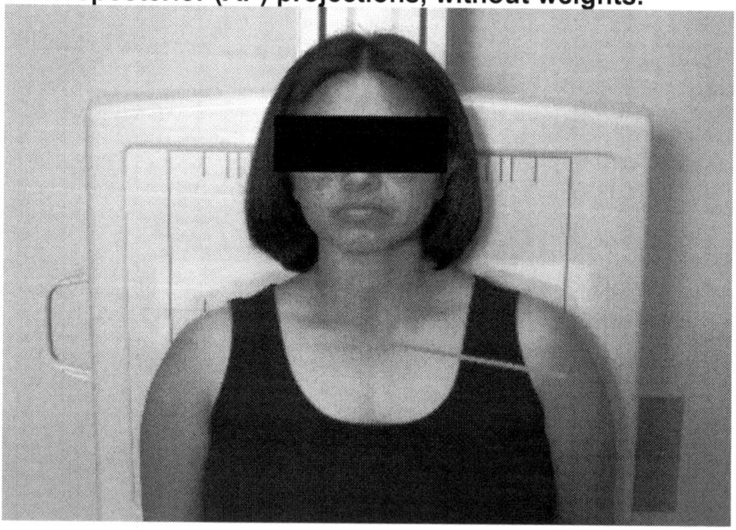

Collimation to include or structures demonstrated

- Include the upper borders of both shoulder with AC joints

Breathing instructions

- Arrested expiration to relax shoulders

Image evaluation

- Sharp bony trabecular and soft tissue detail with both AC joints, entire clavicle and SC joints
- AC joints on same horizontal plane with symmetric SC joint

Notes

- The projection must be taken erect because dislocation will reduce itself in the recumbent position
- Comparison radiographs, bilateral with and without weights of both sides always taken
- If both shoulders cannot fit on single IR, separate exposures taken but the patient should not move between exposures
- Longer SID needed because of increased OID
- Patient must be able to hold weights
- Equal weights average 5-10 lbs. (2.3-4.5 kg) recommended

Fig. 69b. Radiograph. Acromioclavicular (AC) joint – Anteroposterior (AP) projections, without weights.

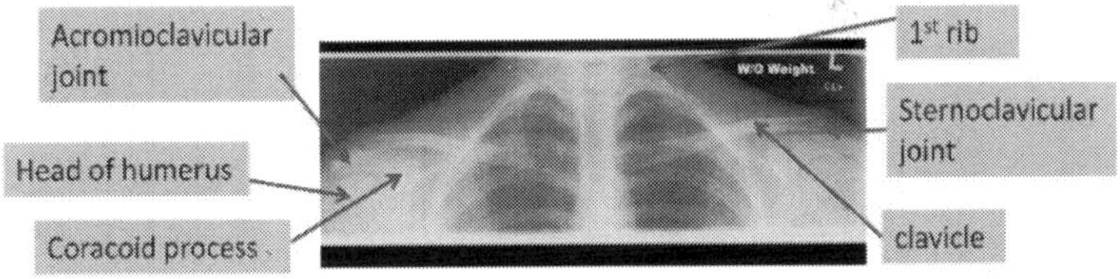

Acromioclavicular (AC) Joint–Anteroposterior (AP) projection

Part 2 of 2—Imaging with weights

SID, Technical factors, Shielding

- 72-inch SID (183 cm). Grid. 75kVp @ 20mAs or AEC. Gonadal shielding

Patient/part position

- Patient erect either standing or seated

Specific part/body position or rotation

- Both shoulders should rest against the IR with body weight equally distributed on both feet
- Just before the exposure the patient is given equal weights (5-10 lbs. average
- Weights should be strapped to wrist **not** held in the hands to allow gravity to pull the arm and shoulder down

Direction and point of entry of CR & SID

- Horizontal to midline 1-inch (2.5 cm) above jugular notch

Fig. 69c. Position. Acromioclavicular (AC) joint – Anteroposterior (AP) projections, with weights.

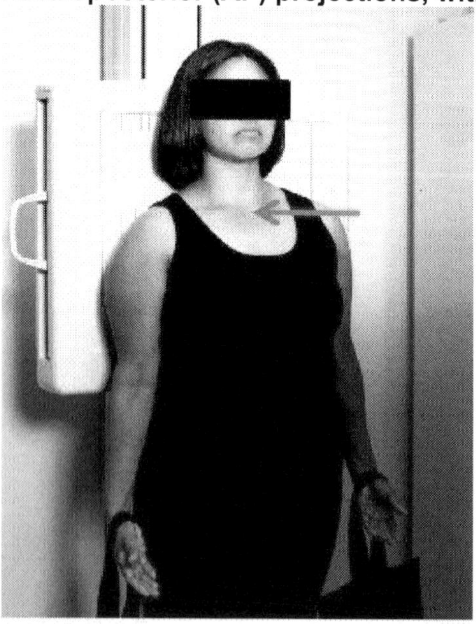

Collimation to include or structures demonstrated

- Include the upper borders of both shoulder with AC joints
  Breathing instructions
- Arrested expiration to relax shoulders
  Image evaluation
- Sharp bony trabecular and soft tissue detail with both AC joint
- Entire clavicle and SC joint
- AC joints on same horizontal plane and symmetric SC joint
  Notes:
- The projection must be taken erect because dislocation will reduce itself in the recumbent position
- Comparison radiographs, bilateral with and without weights, of both sides always taken
- If both shoulders cannot fit on a single IR, separate exposures taken but the patient should not move between exposures
- Longer SID needed because of increased OID
- Patient must be able to hold weights equal weights. Average 5-10 lbs. (2.3-4.5 kg) recommended
- Weights held in hands will contract instead of relaxing the shoulders

Fig. 69d.Radiograph. Acromioclavicular (AC) joint – Anteroposterior (AP) projections, with weights.

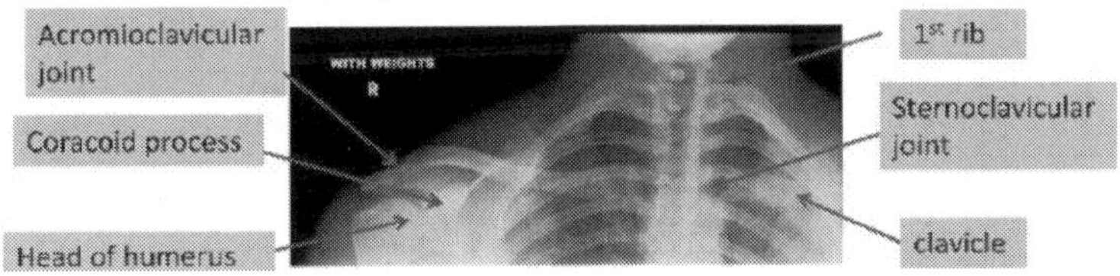

Scapula–Anteroposterior (AP)

SID, Technical factors, Shielding

- 40 inches (100 cm). Grid. 80kVp @ 5 mAs or AEC. Gonadal shielding

Patient/part position and reason

- Patient erect or supine

Specific part/body position or rotation

- To allow separation of the scapula from the thorax DO NOT rotate patient to the affected side
- Abducted arm 90º with long axis of body, flex elbow 90º and supinate hand to remove scapula from under thorax

Direction and point of entry of CR

- CR is directed perpendicular to the IR to the mid scapula 2 inches (5cm) inferior to coracoid process or at the level of axilla 2 inches (5cm) medial from lateral border of patient

Fig. 70a. Position. Scapula – Anteroposterior (AP)

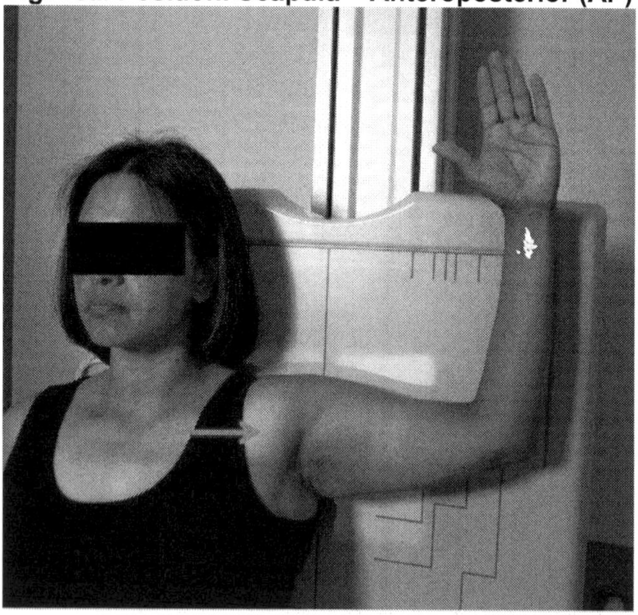

Collimation to include or structures demonstrated

- To include head of humerus, medial & lateral borders of scapula and ¾ of clavicle

Breathing instructions

- Normal breathing to blur out lung markings

Image evaluation

- Sharp bony trabecular and soft tissue detail with the lateral scapula free of superimposition & medial scapula seen through thorax

Fig. 70b. Radiograph. Scapula – Anteroposterior (AP)

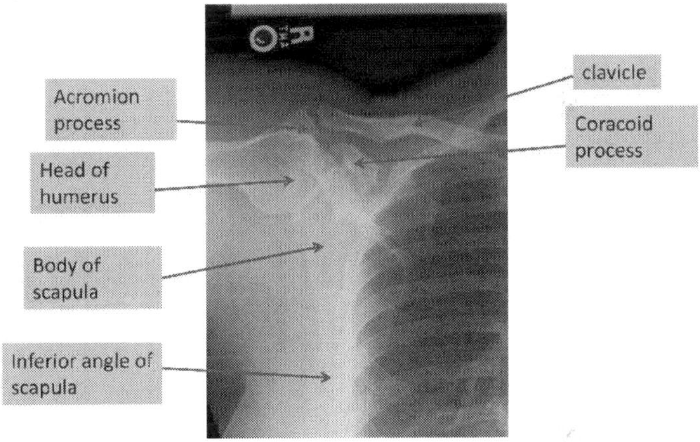

Scapula–Lateral, LAO or RAO positions

To demonstrate the scapula body

Note

- In trauma cases the patient can be imaged using the reverse, LPO or RPO positions

SID, Technical factors, Shielding

- 40 inches (100 cm). Grid. 80kVp @ 5 mAs or AEC. Gonadal shielding

Patient/part position

- Patient erect or recumbent back to the x-ray tube, LAO or RAO

Specific part/body position or rotation

- Rotate patient 45-60 degrees with the affected side to the IR
- Less rotation if arm is placed up or across anterior chest
- Raise affected arm and place hand on upper thorax, unaffected shoulder or forehead to avoid superimposing humerus on scapula

Direction and point of entry of CR

- CR to midvertebral border (medial) of scapula

Fig. 71a. & Fig 71b. Position. Scapula – Lateral, LAO & LPO

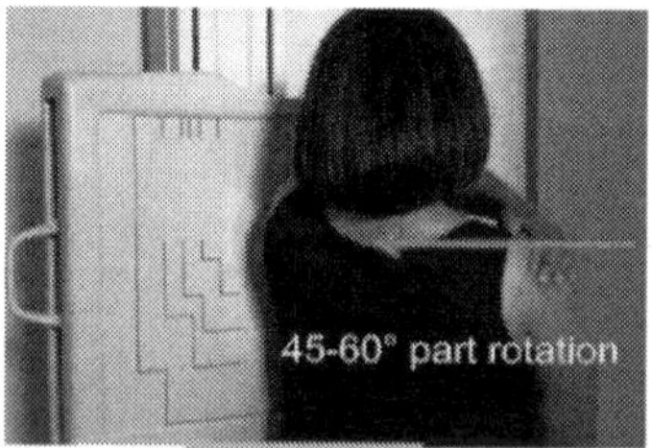

Fig 71a LAO

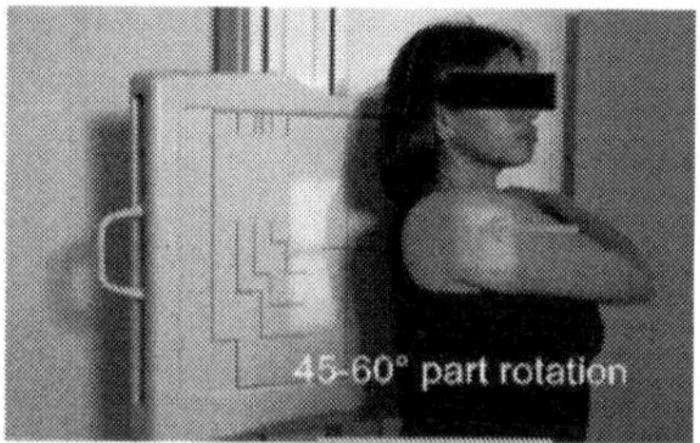

Fig 71b

Collimation to include or structures demonstrated

- The entire scapula
  Breathing instructions
- Arrested respiration
  Image evaluation
- Sharp bony trabecular and soft tissue detail with the medial and lateral borders of scapula superimposed.
- Body of the scapula visualized free of superimposition of ribs and humerus

Fig. 71c. Radiograph. Scapula – Lateral, LAO & LPO

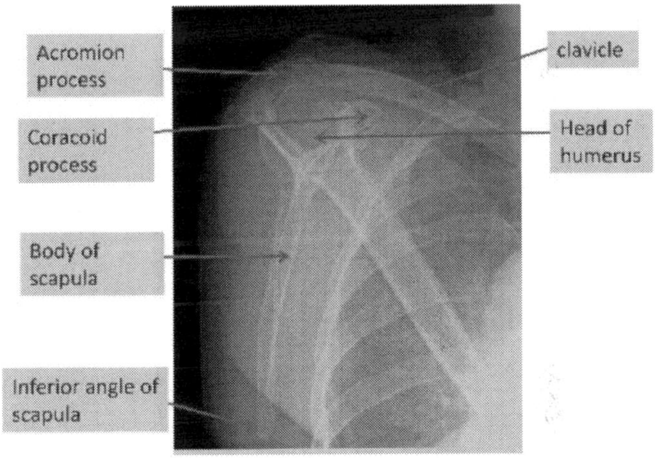

Scapula–Lateral, LAO or RAO positions
To demonstrate the acromion and coracoid process

Note

- In trauma cases the patient can be imaged using the reverse, LPO or RPO positions

SID, Technical factors, Shielding

- 40 inches (100 cm). Grid. 80kVp @ 5 mAs or AEC. Gonadal shielding

Patient/part position

- Patient erect or recumbent, prone—LAO or RAO

Specific part/body position or rotation

- Rotate patient 45-60° with affected side to the IR

To demonstrate the acromion & coracoid process

- Place arm down–by side, on chest or behind back

To demonstrate the scapulo-humeral joint or anterior or posterior dislocation

- Keep arm down to allow humerus to superimposed on wing of scapula as in "Y" projection

Direction and point of entry of CR

- CR to the lateral border of scapula

Fig. 72a. & Fig. 72b. Position. Scapula – Lateral, LAO & LPO

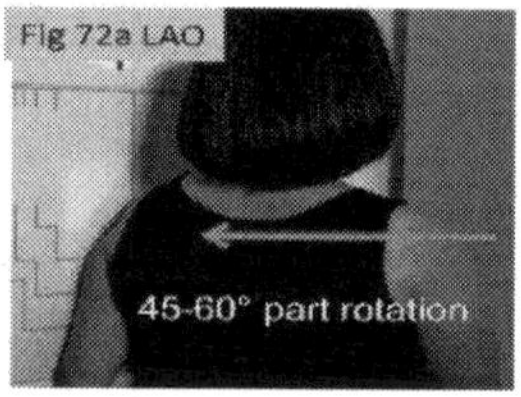

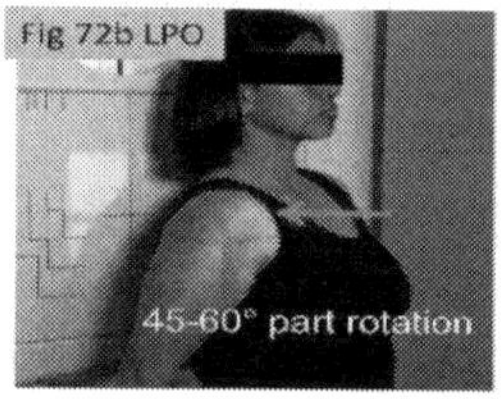

Collimation to include or structures demonstrated

- Entire scapula

Breathing instructions

- Arrested respiration

Image evaluation

- Sharp bony trabecular, soft tissue detail with the medial and lateral borders of scapula superimposed.
- Entire scapula visualized free of superimposition of ribs

Fig. 72c. Radiograph. Scapula – Lateral, LAO & LPO

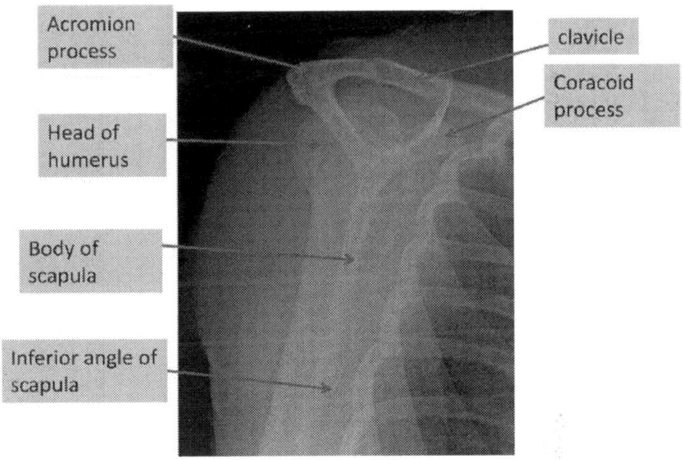

Lower Extremity Imaging

Grid use

- A grid/Bucky will improve image contrast and should be used when imaging parts greater than 10 cm/4 inches thick or when using kVp in excess of 80

Breathing instructions

- Not necessary however a child or anxious adult is more likely to keep still when told to stop breathing.

External preparations

- Remove anything metallic from the area of interest

Radiation protection

- Gonad and thyroid shielding should be provided to all patients, especially to children and females of child bearing age
- Always shield if gonads lie within 5cm or 2 in of the collimated field or primary beam
- Gonad shielding always be wrap around shielding to protect against back scatter

Bones of the Lower Extremity

Number of bones on each side of the body

Foot – 26 bones (including the tarsals

- 14 phalanges articulate proximally with the metacarpals (**metatarsophalangeal joints**) and distally with the second row of the phalanges of each toe (**interphalangeal joints**)
    - The great toe has 2 phalanges–proximal and distal
    - The other toes have 3 phalanges – proximal, middle and distal
- 5 metacarpals named 1-5
    - The metacarpals articulate with the phalanges proximally, and the with the tarsals distally
- 7 tarsals

- Calcaneus (Os calcis), Talus, Navicular, Cuboid, Medial Cuneiform, Intermediate Cuneiform, Lateral Cuneiform.
- **Articulations** –Intermetatarsal joints, tarsometatarsal joint, calcaneocuboid, cuneocuboid, intercuneiform, cuboidonavicular, navicularcuneiform, subtalar, talocalcaneal, talocalcaneonavicular

Sesamoid Bones–2 bones

- Located inferior to the 1st metatarsal

Leg–2 bones

- Tibia – on the medial side.
  - Tibia articulates with the talus–tibiotalar joint and with the fibula –tibiofibular joint
- Fibula–on the lateral side
  - The fibula articulates with proximally with the tibia – proximal tibiofibular joint) and distally with the fibula – distal tibiofibular joint and with the talus–talofibular

Patella–1 bone

- The patella articulates with the femur–Patellofemoral joint

Thigh–1 bone

- **Femur**–1
- The femur articulates with the tibial distally – femorotibial joint(knee joint) and proximally in the acetabulum of the pelvis

Toes–Anteroposterior (AP) dorsoplantar

SID, Technical factors, Shielding

- 40 inches (100 cm). No Grid. 50kVp @ 1.3 mAs. No AEC.

Gonadal shielding

Patient/part position

- Patient supine or seated on x-ray table with knees flexed

Specific part/body position or rotation

- Sole of foot rests flat on the x-ray table

Direction and point of entry of CR

- Great toe–CR to metatarsophalangeal (MTP) joint.
- Other toes–CR to proximal interphalangeal (PIP) joint

Fig. 73a. Position. Great Toe – Anteroposterior AP

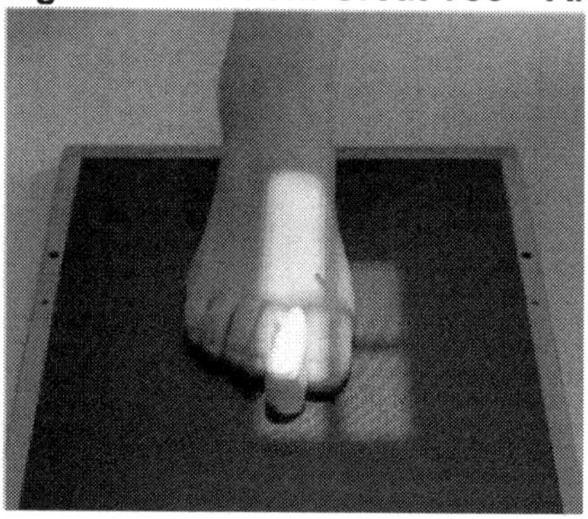

Fig. 73c. Position. 2nd Toe – Anteroposterior AP

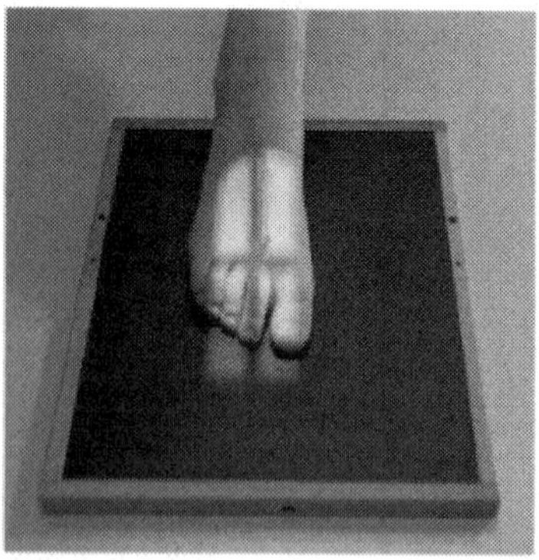

Collimation to include or structures demonstrated

- The toe of interest plus adjacent digit and distal metatarsal

Image evaluation

- Sharp bony trabecular and soft tissue detail with separated digits
- No overlap of soft tissue with metatarsal equal concavity both sides

Notes

- Increase concavity implies that the part is rotated away from IR
- Department routines can vary–to include all toes versus single toe

Fig. 73b. Radiograph. Great Toe – Anteroposterior(AP) & Fig. 73d. Radiograph. 2nd Toe – Anteroposterior (AP)

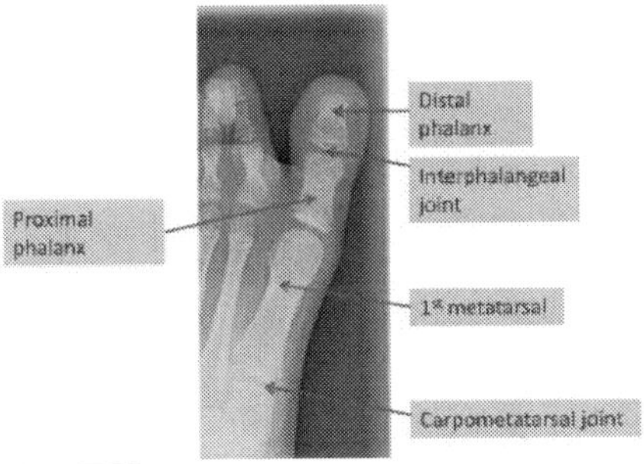

Fig. 72b

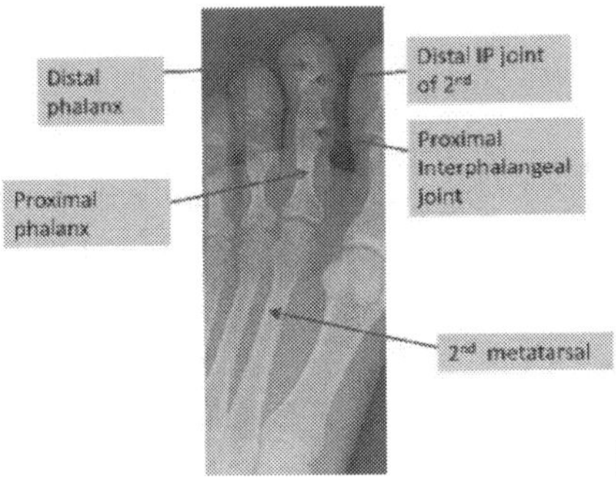

Fig. 73d

Toes –AP Oblique

SID, Technical factors, Shielding

- 40 inches (100 cm). No Grid. 50kVp @ 1.3 mAs. No AEC. Gonadal shielding

Patient/part position

- Patient supine or seated on x-ray table with knees flexed and sole of foot 30-45 degree to IR

Specific part/body position or rotation

- Use tape/ gauze to separate the toes
- For 1st & 2nd toes, rotate foot medially to reduce OID
- For 4th & 5th toes rotate foot laterally to reduce OID
- The 3rd toe can be rotated in any direction

Direction and point of entry of Central Ray/SID

- Great toe–perpendicular CR to MTP joint
- Other toes–perpendicular CR to PIP joint

Fig. 74a. Position. Great Toe – AP Oblique, & Fig. 74c. Position. 2nd Toe – AP Oblique

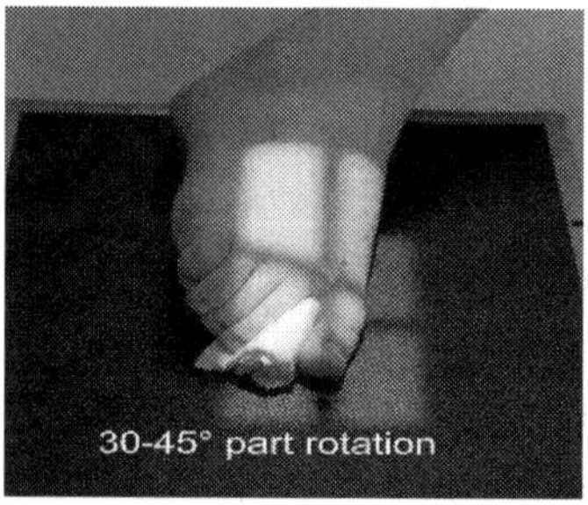

Fig. 74a

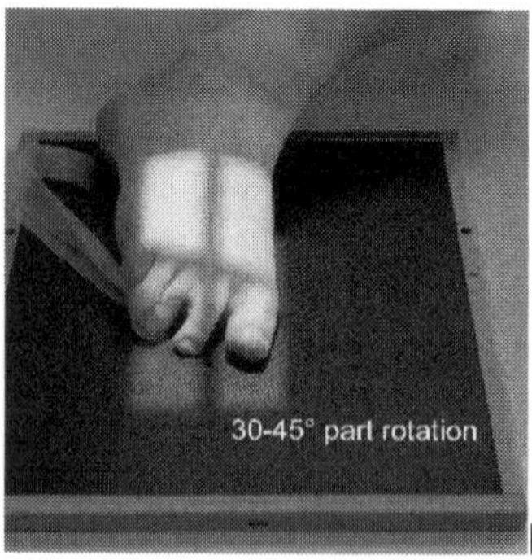

Fig.74c

Collimation to include or structures demonstrated

- Soft tissue and bony margins of toe of interest plus adjacent digit and distal metatarsal

Image evaluation

- Sharp bony trabecular and soft tissue detail with increased concavity on one side of shaft.

Fig. 74b . Radiograph. Great Toe – AP Oblique, & Fig. 74d. Radiograph. 2nd Toe – AP Oblique

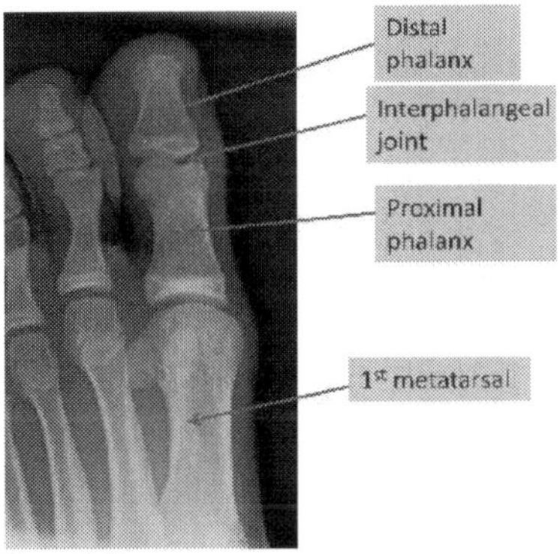

Fig. 74b

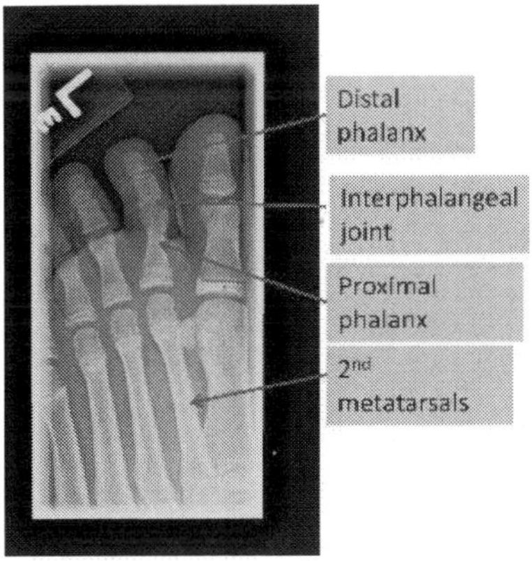

Fig.74d

Toes–Mediolateral or Lateromedial

SID, Technical factors, Shielding

- 40 inches (100 cm). No Grid. 50kVp @ 1.3 mAs. No AEC.

Gonadal shielding

Patient/part position

- Patient supine or seated on x-ray table with knees flexed

Specific part/body position or rotation

- Rotate foot medially for toes 1 & 2 (lateromedial projection).
- Rotate laterally for 4 & 5 (Mediolateral projection)
- The 3rd toe can be rotated in any direction
- Use tape/gauze to separate toe of interest

Direction and point of entry of Central Ray/SID

- Great toe–perpendicular CR to MTP joint
- Other toes–perpendicular CR to PIP joint

Fig. 75a. Position. Great Toe – Mediolateral & Fig. 75c. Position. 2nd Toe–. Mediolateral

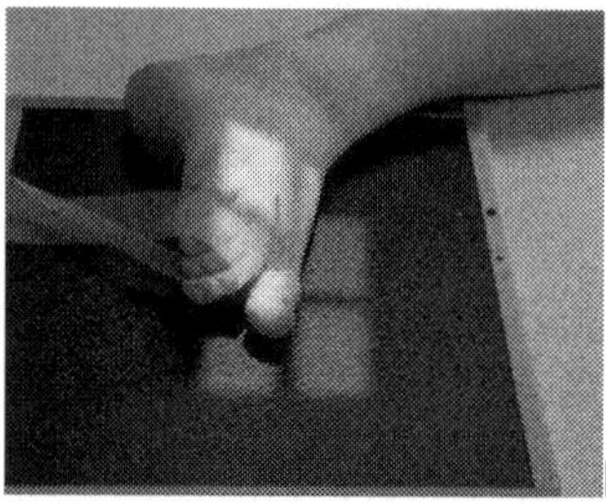

Fig. 75a

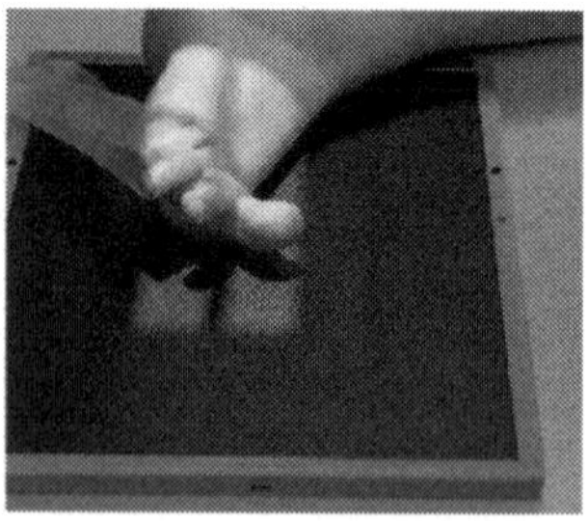

Fig.75c

Collimation to include or structures demonstrated

- Soft tissue margins of toe of interest plus distal metatarsal

Image evaluation

- Sharp bony trabecular and soft tissue detail
- The lateral digit free of superimposition by other digits, if possible. Increase concavity of anterior surface of distal phalanx & posterior surface of proximal phalanx.

Fig. 75b. Radiograph. Great Toe– Mediolateral & Fig. 75d. Radiograph. 2nd Toe– Mediolateral

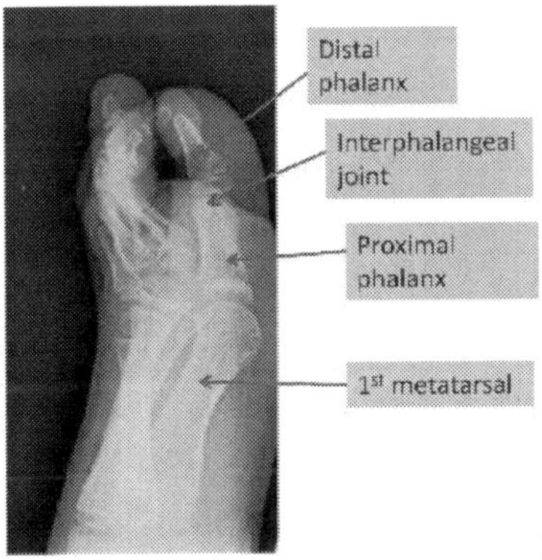

Fig 75b

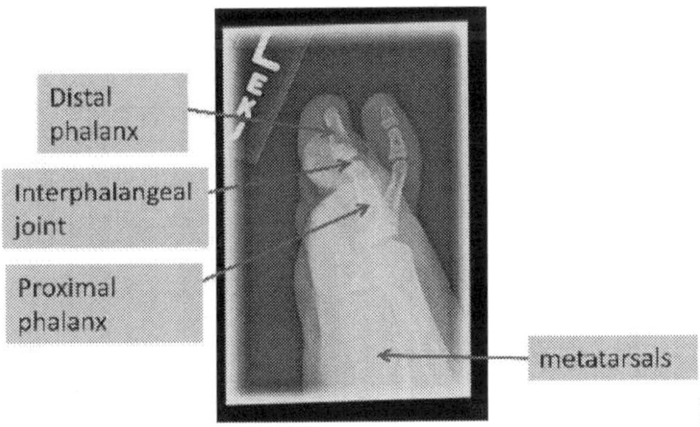

Fig. 75d

Sesamoid bones–Tangential projection

Lewis & Holly methods

SID, Technical factors, Shielding

- 40 inches (100 cm). No Grid. 52kVp @ 1.3 mAs. No AEC.

Gonadal shielding

Patient/part position

- Patient supine or prone on the x-ray table

Specific part/body position or rotation

PRONE (Lewis method)

- Patient kneeling or sitting with legs parallel to the tabletop.

Foot dorsiflexed with plantar surfaces of toes on tabletop. Pad under knee for comfort.

SUPINE (Holly method). This result in increased OID)

- Patient seated. A gauze bandage used to hold toes in flexed position.
- Medial border of foot vertical & plantar surface at angle of 75-degrees with IR.

Direction and point of entry of Central Ray/SID

- CR perpendicular to IR. Tangential to posterior aspect of first MTP joint

Fig. 76a & 76b. Position. Sesamoid Bones– Tangential projection

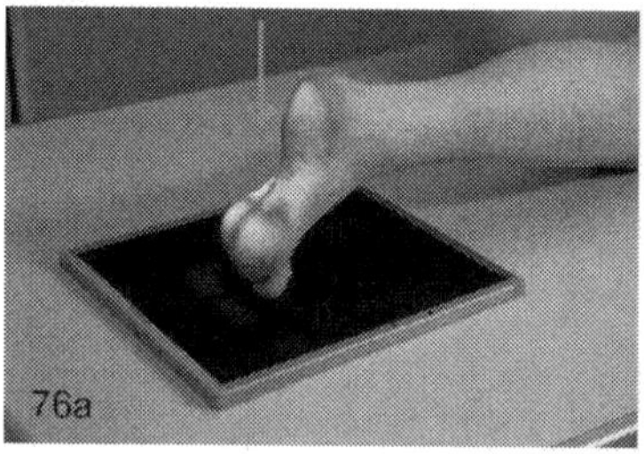

Fig. 76a. Prone

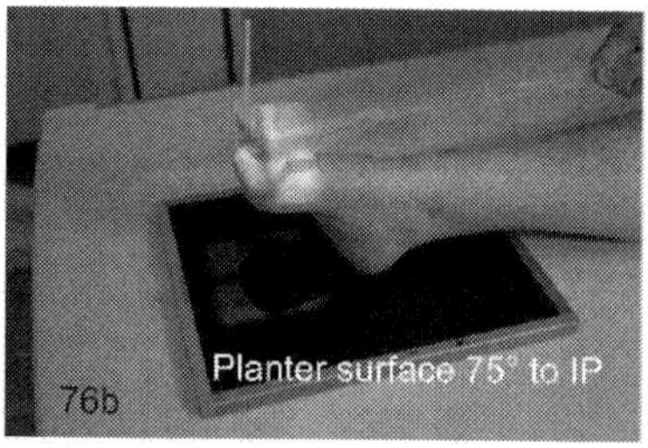

Fig. 76b. Supine

Collimation to include or structures demonstrated

- Must include the sesamoid

Image evaluation

- Sharp bony trabecular and soft tissue detail

Note: In addition to the tangential, a lateral of first digit in dorsiflexion can be taken

Fig. 76c. Radiograph. Sesamoid Bones– Tangential projection

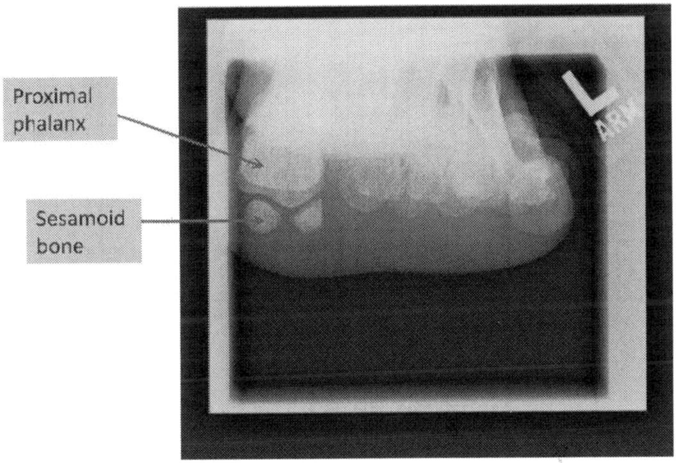

Foot–Anteroposterior (AP) Axial

SID, Technical factors, Shielding

- 40 inches (100 cm). No Grid. 55kVp @ 1.3 mAs. No AEC.

Gonadal shielding

Patient/part position and reason

- Patient seated or supine with knees flexed and planter surface on IR

Direction and point of entry of Central Ray/SID

- CR to the base of 3rd metatarsal using 10 degrees tube angulation to the heel (posteriorly) placing the CR perpendicular to metatarsals.

Fig. 77a. Position. Foot– Anteroposterior (AP) Axial

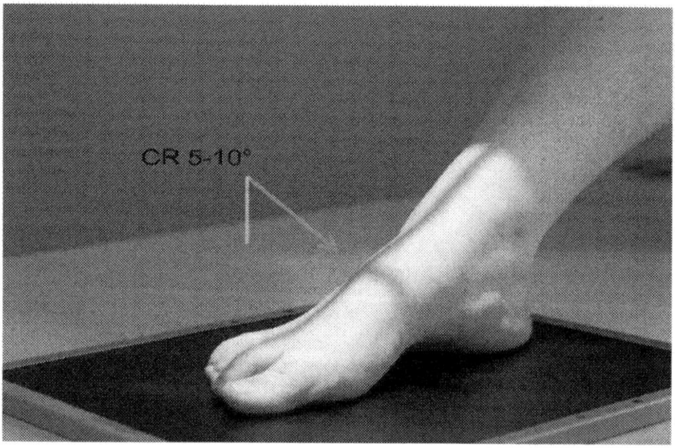

Collimation to include or structures demonstrated

- All phalanges, metatarsals and tarsals

Image evaluation

- Sharp bony trabecular and soft tissue detail with equal distance between 2nd -5th metatarsal
- Base of 1st through 2nd metatarsal separated
- Bases of 2nd through 5th metatarsal overlapped
- Joint space seen between 1 through 2 cuneiforms.

Fig. 77b. Position. Foot– Anteroposterior (AP) Axial

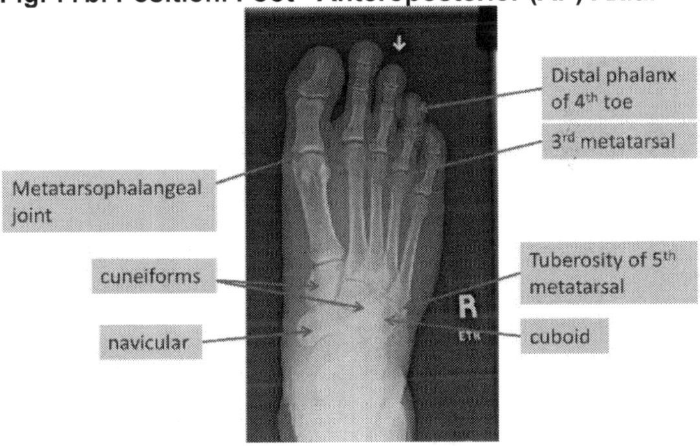

Foot–Medial Oblique (medial rotation)

SID, Technical factors, Shielding

- 40 inches (100 cm). No Grid. 55kVp @ 1.3 mAs. No AEC.

Gonadal shielding

Patient/part position

- Patient seated or supine with knees flexed. affected side

Specific part/body position or rotation

- Keeping the medial edge of foot on IR, rotate the sole of the foot away from the IR to form an angle of 30 to 45 degrees to the IR.

Direction and point of entry of Central Ray/SID

- CR directed to the base of the 3rd metatarsal.

Fig. 78a. Position. Foot – Medial Oblique (medial rotation)

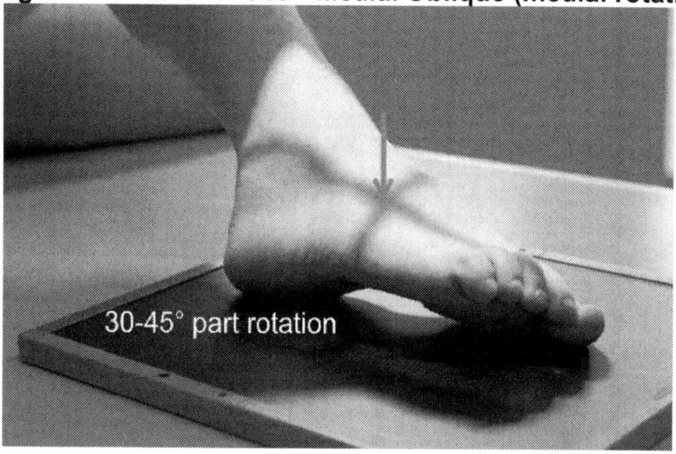

Collimation to include or structures demonstrated

- All phalanges, metatarsals and tarsals

Image evaluation

- Sharp bony trabecular and soft tissue detail seen with all sides of the cuboid joint
- The bases of the 2nd -5th metatarsals superimposed and with tarsals and proximal metatarsals shafts free of superimposition

Fig. 78b. Radiograph. Foot – Medial Oblique (medial rotation)

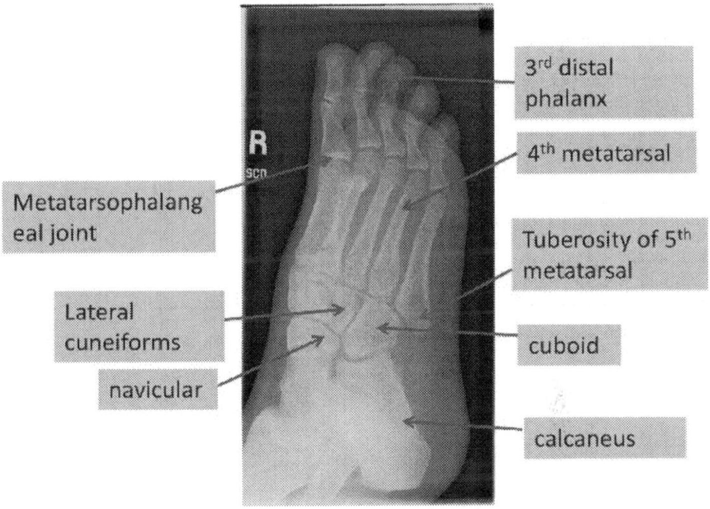

Foot–Lateral (mediolateral and lateromedial)

SID, Technical factors, Shielding

- 40 inches (100 cm). No Grid. 57kVp @1.6 mAs. No AEC.

Gonadal shielding

Patient/part position

- Patient recumbent with foot dorsiflexed.

Specific part/body position or rotation

- Either the lateral or the medial side of foot resting on the IR. The plantar surface should be perpendicular to the IR. Elevate the knee to keep foot in position.

Direction and point of entry of CR

- CR directed to the base of the3rd metatarsal

Fig. 79a. Position. Foot– Lateral (lateromedial)

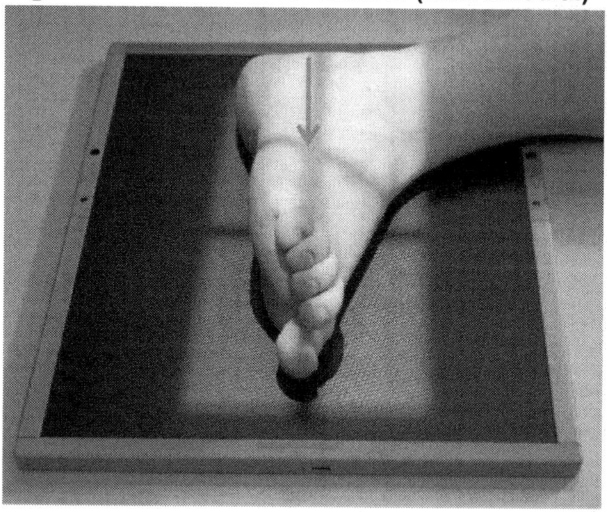

Collimation to include or structures demonstrated

- All phalanges, metatarsals and tarsals

Image evaluation

- Sharp bony trabecular and soft tissue detail with the metatarsal nearly superimposed on the posterior portion of the tibia.

Note

- The mediolateral is more comfortable for patient **but** the lateromedial gives a truer lateral.

Fig. 79b. Radiograph. Foot– Lateral (lateromedial)

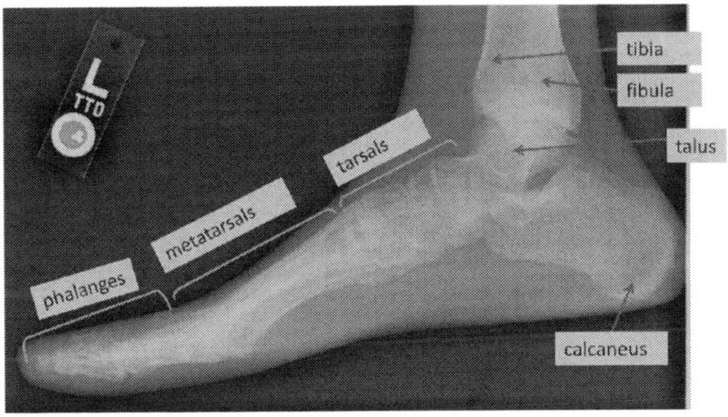

Foot–Lateral, Weight Bearing

SID, Technical factors, Shielding

- 40 inches (100 cm). No Grid. 57kVp @ 1.6 mAs. No AEC. Gonadal shielding

Patient/part position

- Patient standing usually imaged bilateral

Specific part/body position or rotation

- Patient stands with the medial or lateral side of the foot close to the IR

Direction and point of entry of CR

- CR just above base of 3rd metatarsal

Fig. 80a. Position. Foot– Lateral, Weight Bearing

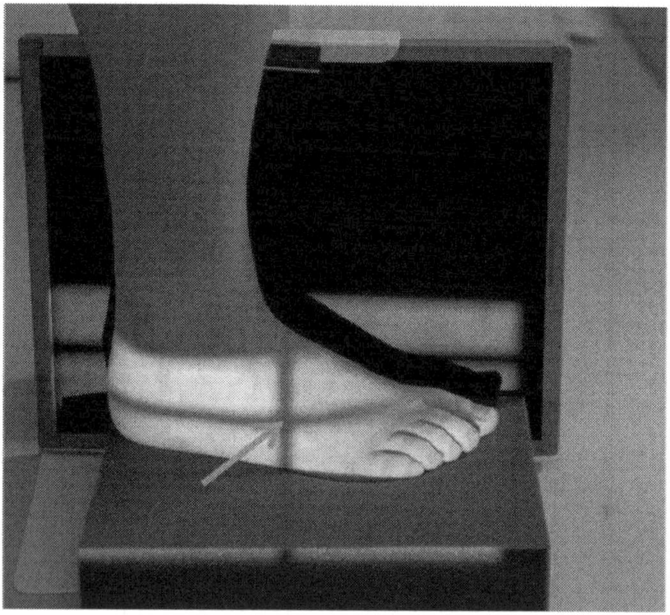

Collimation to include or structures demonstrated

- All phalanges, metatarsals and tarsals

Image evaluation

- Sharp bony trabecular and soft tissue detail with the metatarsal nearly superimposed on the posterior portion of the tibia

Note: To permit accurate evaluation of the tarsals and metatarsals, an additional projection used is the AP axial. Patient stands on the IR with weight equally distributed on feet. Image using 15-degree tube angulation to tarsals.

Fig. 80b. Radiograph. Foot– Lateral, Weight Bearing

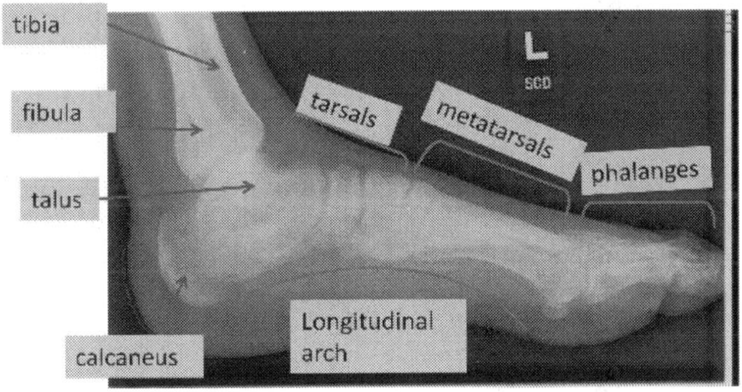

Calcaneus—Axial

(plantodorsal or dorsoplantar)

SID, Technical factors, Shielding

- 40 inches (100 cm). No Grid. 60kVp @ 2.3 mAs. No AEC.

Gonadal shielding

Patient/part position

- Patient prone or seated with the long axis of leg parallel to long axis of table (if seated)

Specific part/body position or rotation

- The IR placed under the ankle of the seated patient and against the plantar surface of foot for the prone patient.

Direction and point of entry of CR

- Plantodorsal, patient supine: CR directed to midpoint of IR using 40 –degree tube angulation with the central ray entering at the base of the 3rd metatarsal. Dorsoplantar, patient prone: CR enters the dorsal surface from the ankle and emerges on plantar surface (at level of base of 3rd metatarsal

Fig. 81a. Position. Calcaneus–Axial (plantodorsal) & Fig. 81b. Calcaneus –Axial (dorsoplantar)

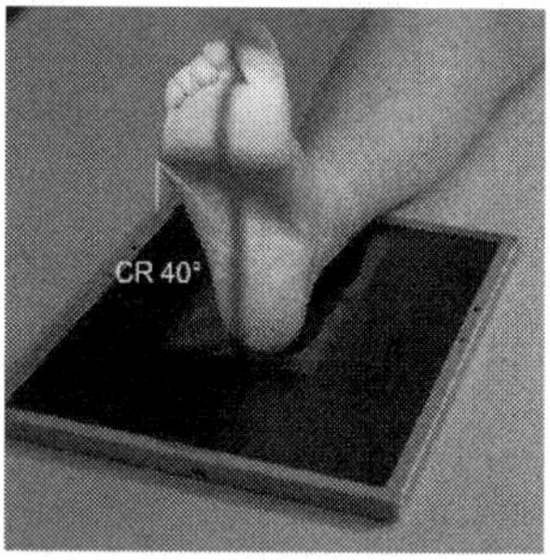

Fig. 81a.Patient Supine

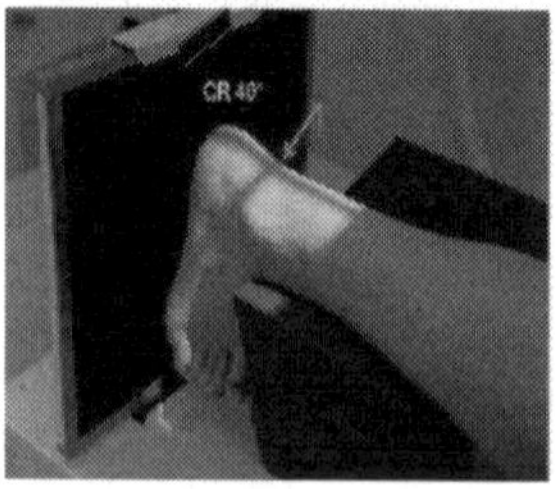

Fig. 81b. Patient Prone

Collimation to include or structures demonstrated

- Entire calcaneus from tuberosity to talocalcaneal joint

Image evaluation

- Soft tissue and bone trabeculae with details with the sustentaculum tali seen medially & the trochlear process (peroneal trochlea) seen laterally
- The talocalcaneal or subtalar joint clearly seen.

Note

- The calcaneus has 3 articular surfaces: anterior, middle & posterior.

Fig. 81c. Radiograph. Calcaneus–Axial (plantodorsal or dorsoplantar)

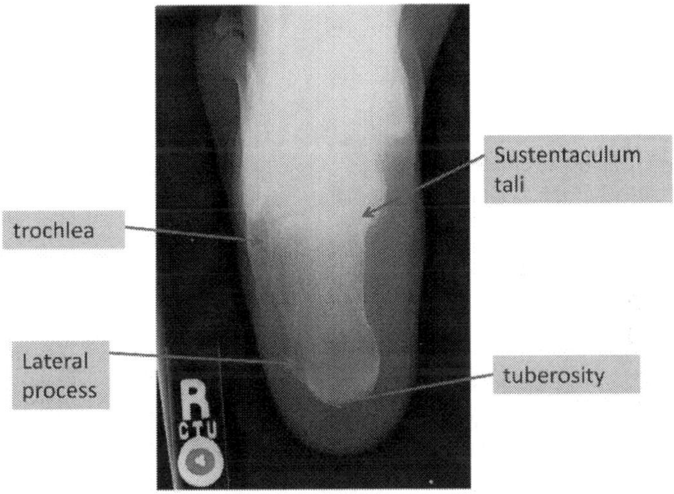

Calcaneus–Lateral

(mediolateral or lateromedial) Os Calcis

SID, Technical factors, Shielding

- 40 inches (100 cm). No Grid. 62kVp @ 2.3 mAs. No AEC.

Gonadal shielding

Patient/part position

- Patient recumbent with either lateral or medial side of foot closest to IR. The mediolateral is more comfortable for patient but the lateromedial give a truer lateral.
- Foot dorsiflexed

Specific part/body position or rotation–mediolateral

- The plantar surface should form an angle of 90-degrees with the IR
- Elevate the knee to keep foot in position

Direction and point of entry of CR

- Center 1–1 ½ (3-4 cm) distal to medial malleolus

Fig. 82a. Position. Calcaneus – Lateral (mediolateral)

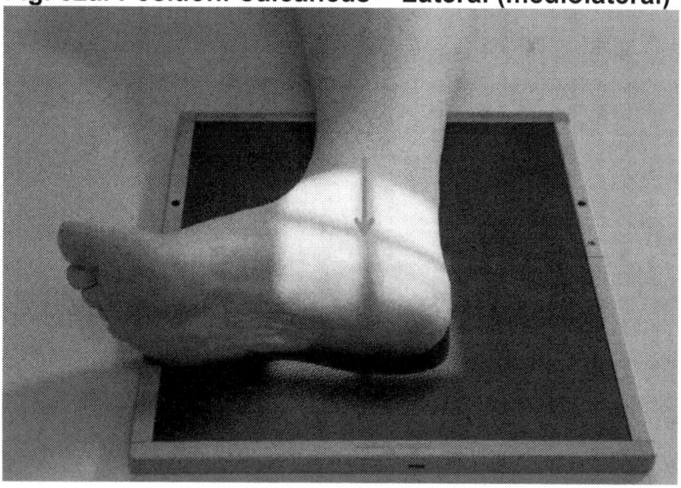

Collimation to include or structures demonstrated

- The entire calcaneus plus proximal metatarsals and the ankle joint

Image evaluation

- Include soft tissue and bony trabecular detail of calcaneus
- Open talocalcaneal joint (subtalar), calcaneocuboid joint and talonavicular joint with the fibula superimposed on the posterior portion of the tibia.

Fig. 82b. Radiograph. Calcaneus – Lateral (mediolateral or lateromedial)

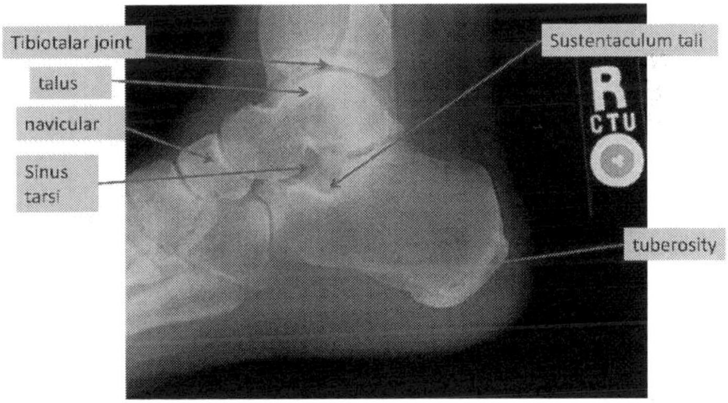

Ankle–Anteroposterior (AP) projection

SID, Technical factors, Shielding

- 40 inches (100 cm). No Grid. 60kVp @ 2.3 mAs. No AEC.

Gonadal shielding

Patient/part position

- Patient seated; legs parallel to the long axis of table

Specific part/body position or rotation

- Foot dorsi-flexed with the plantar surface to form a 90° angle with lower leg. No rotation of leg. (medial malleolus should be higher than lateral when positioning)

Direction and point of entry of CR

- Perpendicular to ankle joint

Fig. 83a. Position. Ankle – Anteroposterior (AP) projection

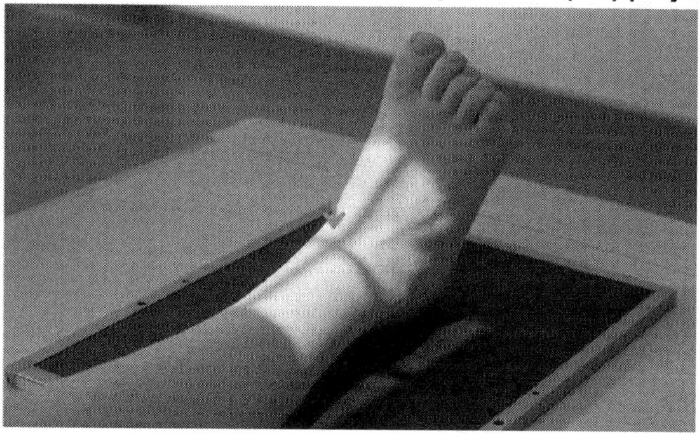

Collimation to include or structures demonstrated

- Distal tibial and fibular, talus, medial and lateral malleoli, the talus and proximal metatarsals.

Image evaluation

- Include soft tissue and bony trabecular detail of the ankle joint
- The distal tibia & fibula will be slightly superimposed
- The medial mortise open and lateral mortise closed.

Fig. 83b. Radiograph. Ankle – Anteroposterior (AP) projection

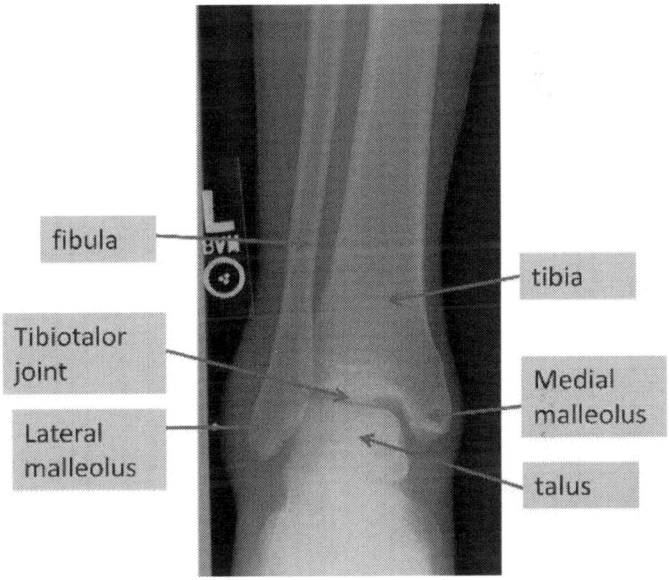

Ankle–Oblique, Mortise 15-20 degree (medial rotation)

SID, Technical factors, Shielding

- 40 inches (100 cm). No Grid. 60kVp @ 2.3 mAs. No AEC. Gonadal shielding

Patient/part position

- Patient seated; legs parallel to the long axis of table

Specific part/body position or rotation

- Do not dorsiflex foot. Plantar flexion will show tuberosity of 5th metatarsal.
- Internally rotate leg and foot 15-20 degrees to place intermalleolar plane parallel with IR

Direction and point of entry of CR

- Perpendicular midway between the malleoli

Fig. 84a. Position. Ankle – Oblique, Mortise 15-20° medial rotation

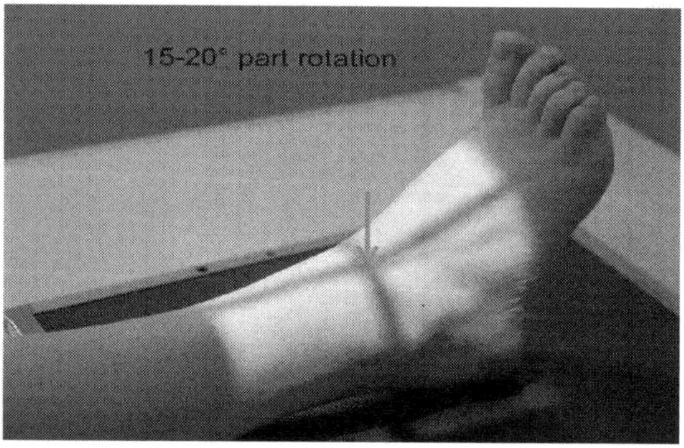

Collimation to include or structures demonstrated

- Distal tibial and fibular, talus, medial and lateral malleoli, the talus and proximal metatarsals.

Image evaluation

- Soft tissue and bone trabeculae with details. The three sides of the mortise joint should be visualized
- Talofibular joint space open.

Fig. 84b. Radiograph. Ankle – Oblique, Mortise 15-20° medial rotation

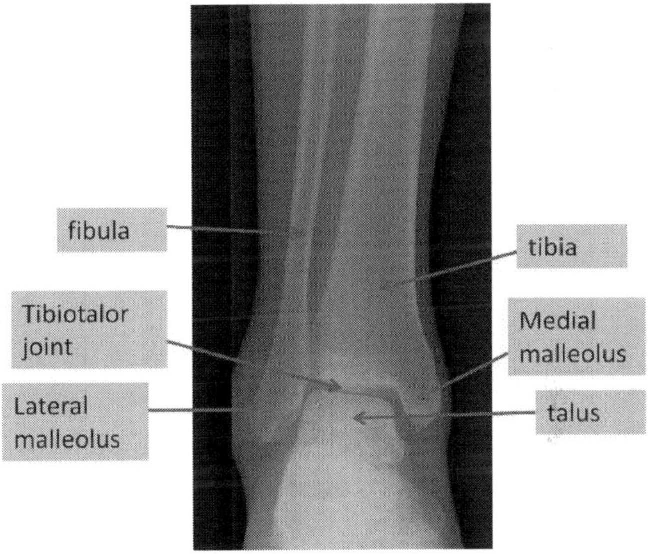

Ankle–Oblique, 45 degree (medial rotation)

SID, Technical factors, Shielding

- 40 inches (100 cm). No Grid. 60kVp @ 2.3 mAs. No AEC.

Gonadal shielding

Patient/part position

- Patient seated; legs parallel to the long axis of table

Specific part/body position or rotation

- Foot dorsi-flexed with the plantar surface to form a 90° angle with lower leg.
- Internally rotate leg and foot 45° (medial malleolus should be higher than lateral when positioning)

Direction and point of entry of CR

- Perpendicular midway between the malleoli

Fig. 85a. Position. Ankle–Oblique, 45° medial rotation

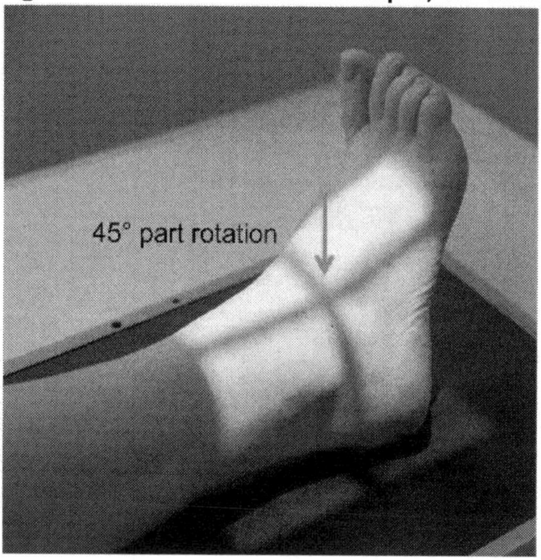

Collimation to include or structures demonstrated

- Distal tibial and fibular, talus, medial and lateral malleoli, the talus and proximal metatarsals.

Image evaluation

- Include soft tissue and bony trabecular detail of the ankle joint with the distal tibiofibular joint open

Fig. 85b. Radiograph. Ankle–Oblique, 45º medial rotation

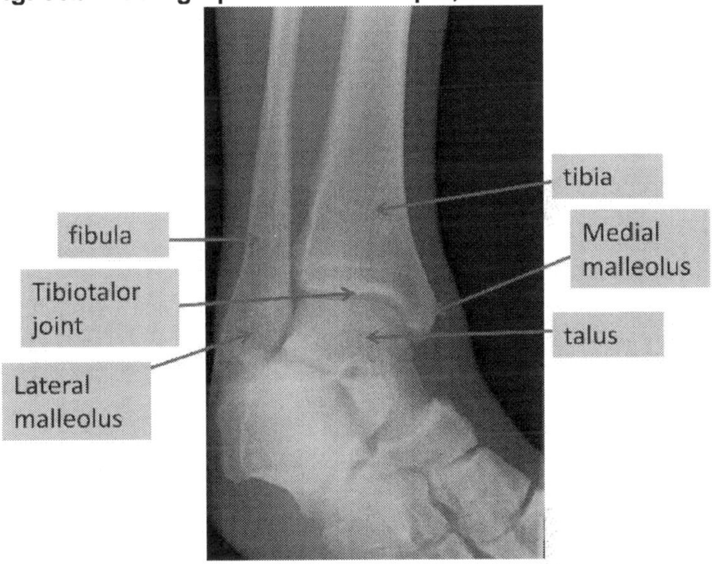

Ankle–Lateral
(mediolateral or lateromedial) projection

SID, Technical factors, Shielding

- 40 inches (100 cm). No Grid. 62kVp @ 2.3 mAs. No AEC. Gonadal shielding

Patient/part position

- Patient recumbent with either lateral or medial side of foot resting on IR.

Specific part/body position or rotation

- Foot dorsiflexed to prevent lateral rotation
- The plantar surface should form an angle of 90-degrees with the IR
- Elevate the knee to keep foot in position

Direction and point of entry of CR

- Centering to medial malleolus or ½ inch (1cm) superior to the lateral malleolus

Fig. 86a. Position. Ankle – Lateral (mediolateral)

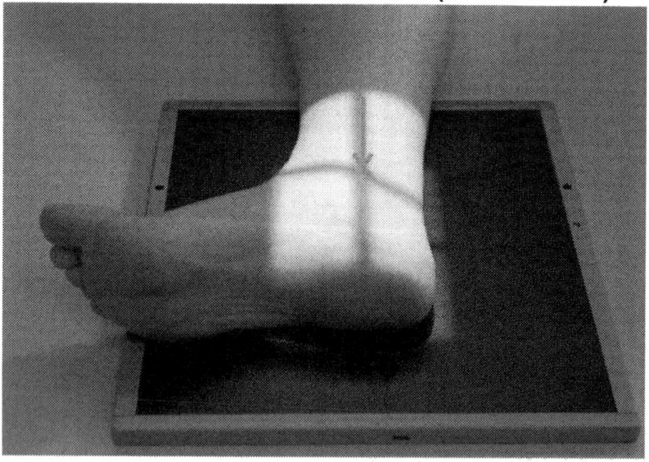

Collimation to include or structures demonstrated

- Distal 1/3 of tibial, calcaneus, talus, navicular, cuboid and proximal metatarsals including tuberosity of 5th

Image evaluation

- Soft tissue and bone trabeculae with details. Tibula superimposed on posterior half of the tibia
- Tibiotalar joint well visualized

Note

- The mediolateral is more comfortable for patient but the lateromedial give a truer lateral.

Fig. 86b. Radiograph. Ankle – Lateral (mediolateral or lateromedial)

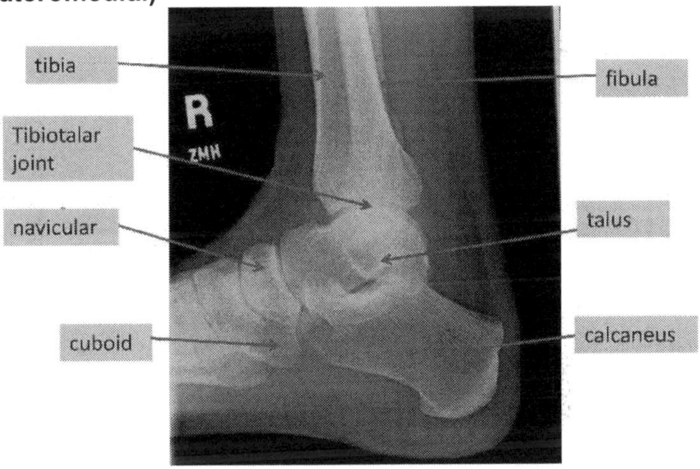

Ankle–AP Stress/subtalar projection

SID, Technical factors, Shielding

- 40 inches (100 cm). No Grid. 62kVp @ 2.3 mAs. No AEC. Gonadal shielding

Patient/part position

- Patient seated; legs extended parallel to the long axis of table

Specific part/body position or rotation

- Foot dorsiflexed
- Without moving or rotating the lower leg from the supine position, the foot is forcibly turned medially(inverted)

Direction and point of entry of CR

- Perpendicular, midway between the malleoli

Fig. 87a. Position. Ankle- AP Stress/Subtalar projection

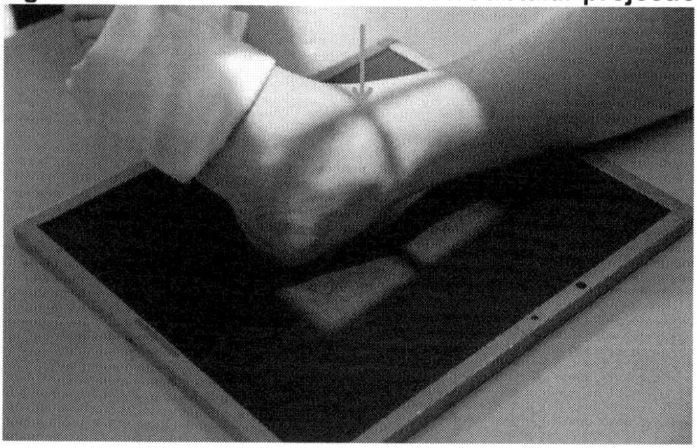

Collimation to include or structures demonstrated

- Distal tibial and fibular, talus, medial and lateral malleoli, the talus and proximal metatarsals.

Image evaluation

- Appearance will vary depending on injury
- Ruptured ligament is demonstrated by widening of the joint space on the side of the injury

Notes:

- A physician or other health clinical must be present to turn and hold the foot and ankle in stress positions
- Local anesthetic often used
- Straps may be used to maintain the position during exposure.
- Additional imaging often taken with the foot turned laterally (eversion)

Fig. 87b. Radiograph. Ankle- AP Stress/Subtalar projection

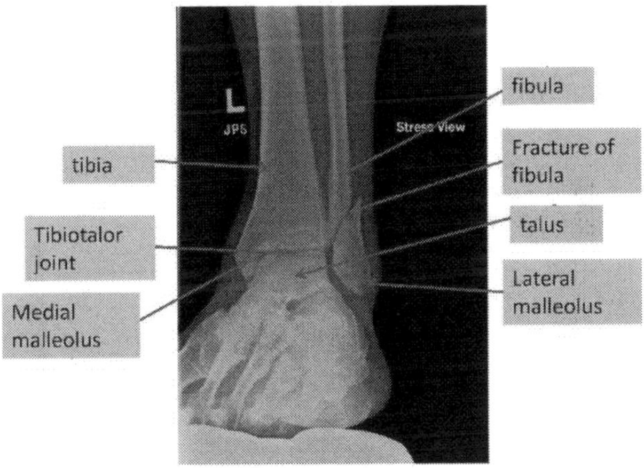

Tibia & Fibula–Anteroposterior (AP) projection

SID, Technical factors, Shielding

- 40 inches (100 cm). No Grid. 60kVp @ 2.3 mAs. No AEC. Gonadal shielding

Patient/part position

- Long axis parallel to IR (or diagonal to long axis of IR to image both joints on a single IR)

Specific part/body position or rotation

- Foot extended with dorsiflexion. Plantar surface perpendicular to IR

Direction and point of entry of CR

- Perpendicular to mid shaft

Fig. 88a. Position. Tibia & Fibula- Anteroposterior (AP) projection

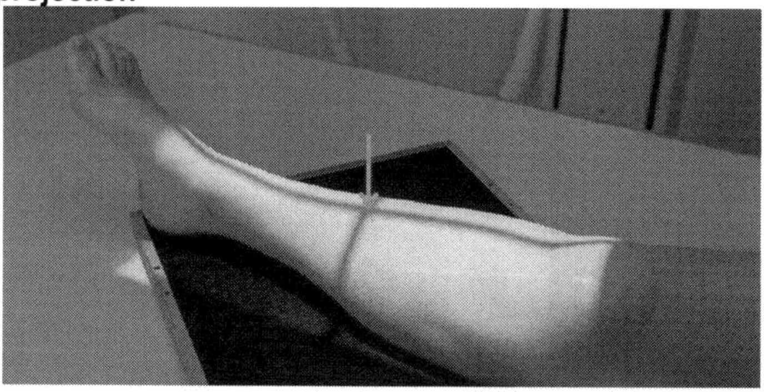

Collimation to include or structures demonstrated

- Image must include complete tibia and fibula and at least 1 inch (2.5 cm) of the distal femur plus the proximal talus

Image evaluation

- Anode heel effect used to ensure high contrast visualization of both joints with soft tissue and bone trabeculae details
- Symmetrical condyles

Fig. 88b. Radiograph. Tibia & Fibula- Anteroposterior (AP) projection

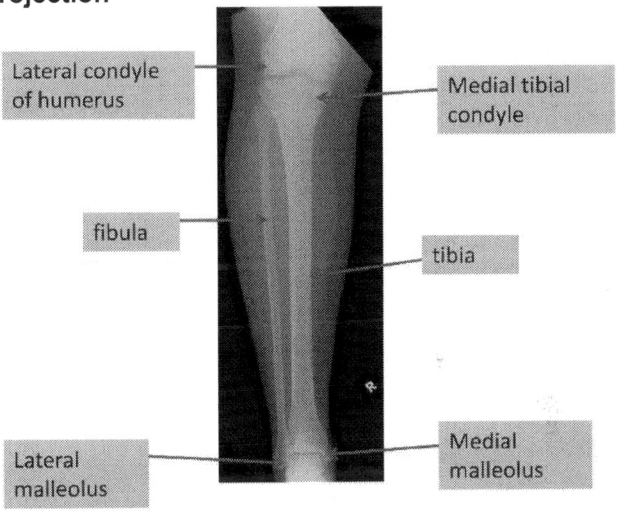

Tibia & Fibula–Lateral projection

SID, Technical factors, Shielding

- 40 inches (100 cm). No Grid. 60kVp @ 2.3 mAs. No AEC. Gonadal shielding

Patient/part position

- Parallel to long axis of IR (or diagonal to long axis of IR to image both joints on a single IR)

Specific part/body position or rotation

- Patient on affected side, knees slightly flexed, patella perpendicular, foot dorsiflexed

Direction and point of entry of CR

- Perpendicular to mid shaft

Fig. 89a. Position. Tibia & Fibula- Lateral projection

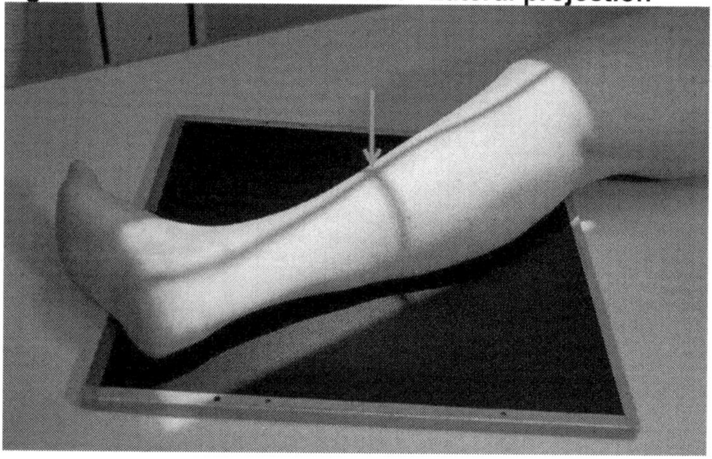

Collimation to include or structures demonstrated

- Complete tibia & fibula plus 1 inch (2.5 cm) of the distal femur and the proximal talus

Image evaluation

- Anode heel effect used to ensure high contrast visualization of both joints with soft tissue and bone trabeculae details
- Condyles will not project superimposed due to divergent rays

Fig. 89b. Radiograph. Tibia & Fibula- Lateral projection

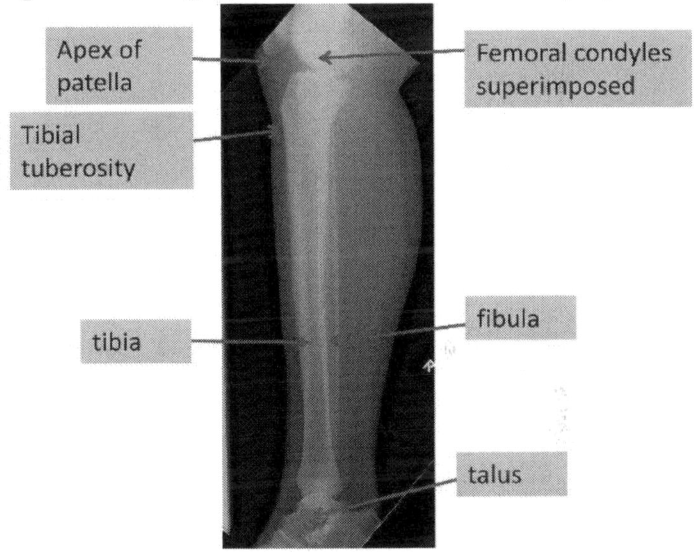

Knee–Anteroposterior (AP) projection

SID, Technical factors, Shielding

- 40 inches (100 cm). Grid. 70kVp @ 3.2 mAs or AEC.

Gonadal shielding

Patient/part position

- AP supine, no rotation

Specific part/body position or rotation

- Leg extended, centered to table/grid

Direction and point of entry of CR

- Perpendicular or angled to pass directly ½ inch (1.3 cm) below patella apex through the knee joint. Tube angulation depends on ASIS distance to tabletop.
- Less than (<)19cm =3°-5°caudal; 19-24cm perpendicular; greater than (>)24cm=3°-5° cephalic

Fig. 90a. Position. Knee– Anteroposterior (AP) projection

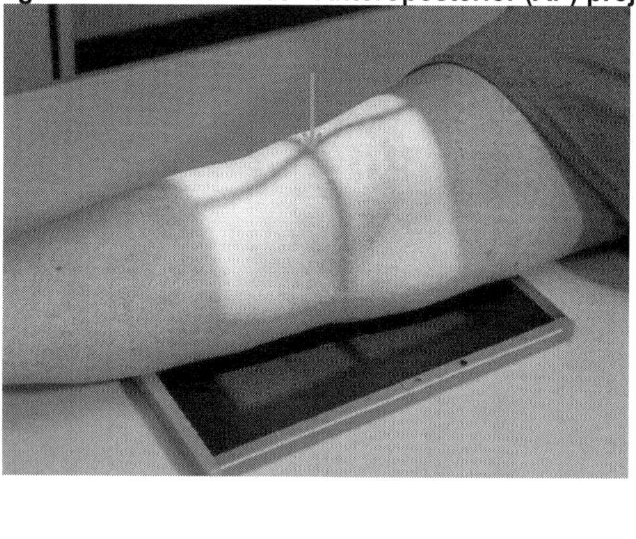

Collimation to include or structures demonstrated

- The knee joint plus 2 inches (5cm) of distal femur and proximal tibia/fibula

Image evaluation

- Include soft tissue and bony trabecular detail of knee
- Condyles should be symmetrical with open joint space
- Patella superimposed on femur

Fig. 90b. Radiograph. Knee– Anteroposterior (AP) projection

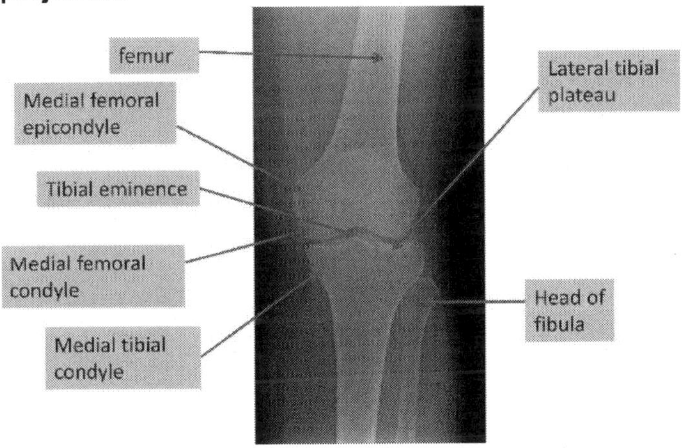

Knee–Lateral (mediolateral) projection

SID, Technical factors, Shielding

- 40 inches (100 cm). Grid. 70kVp @ 3.2 mAs or AEC.

Gonadal shielding

Patient/part position

- Recumbent and lateral on affected side

Specific part/body position or rotation

- Patella true lateral and perpendicular to tabletop. Knee flexed 20°-30° to relax muscles & shows maximum joint volume

Direction and point of entry of CR

- ½ inch (1.3 cm) below epicondyle or on condyle
- 5°-7° cephalic angulation to superimpose condyles and avoid superimposition on joint space by magnified medial femoral condyle

Fig.91a. Position. Knee-Lateral (mediolateral) projection

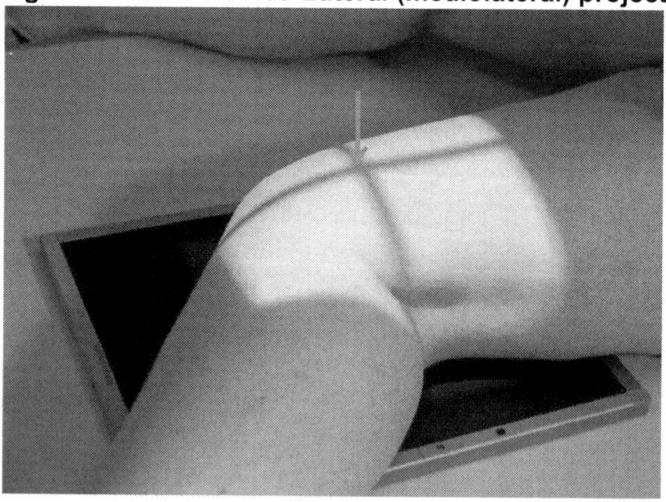

Collimation to include or structures demonstrated

- The knee joint plus 2 inches (5cm) of distal femur and proximal tibia/fibula

Image evaluation

- Include soft tissue and bony trabecular detail of knee
- Patella in profile
- Open patellofemoral joint
- Fibular head slightly superimposed on tibia.

Fig.91b. Radiograph. Knee-Lateral (mediolateral) projection

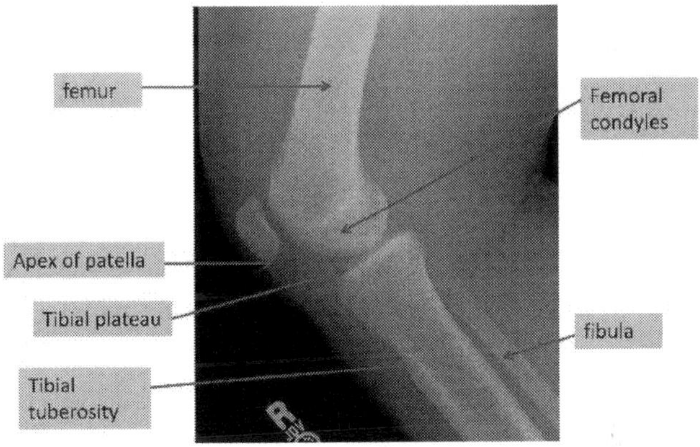

Knee–Anteroposterior (AP) Oblique projection, medial/internal rotation

SID, Technical factors, Shielding

- 40 inches (100 cm). Grid. 70kVp @ 3.2 mAs or AEC.

Gonadal shielding

Patient/part position

- Supine

Specific part/body position or rotation

- Elevate opposite and rotate patient's leg 45° medially and internally

Direction and point of entry of CR

- Perpendicular or angled to pass directly ½ inch (1.3 cm) below patella apex through the knee joint. Tube angulation depends on ASIS distance to tabletop.
- Less than (<)19cm =3°-5°caudal; 19-24cm perpendicular; greater than (>)24cm=3°-5° cephalic

Fig. 92a. Position. Knee- Anteroposterior (AP) Oblique projection, medial/internal rotation

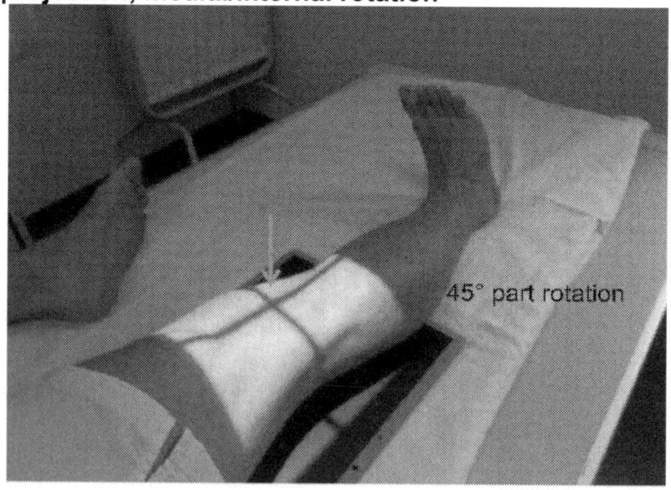

Collimation to include or structures demonstrated

- The knee joint plus 2 inches (5cm) of distal femur and proximal tibia/fibula

Image evaluation

- Proximal Tibiofibular articulation demonstrated.

Fig. 92b. Radiograph. Knee- Anteroposterior (AP) Oblique projection, medial/internal rotation

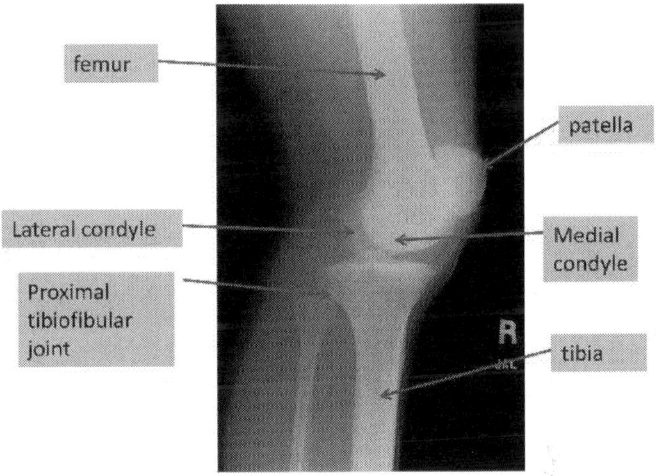

Knee– Anteroposterior (AP) Oblique projection, lateral/external rotation

SID, Technical factors, Shielding

- 40 inches (100 cm). Grid. 70kVp @ 3.2 mAs or AEC. Gonadal shielding

Patient/part position

- Supine

Specific part/body position or rotation

- Elevate opposite hip and rotate patient's leg 45° lateral & external

Direction and point of entry of CR

- Perpendicular or angled to pass directly ½ inch (1.3 cm) below patella apex through the knee joint. Tube angulation depends on ASIS distance to tabletop.
- Less than (<)19cm =3°-5°caudal; 19-24cm perpendicular; greater than (>)24cm=3°-5° cephalic

Fig. 93a. Position. Knee- Anteroposterior (AP) Oblique projection, lateral/external rotation

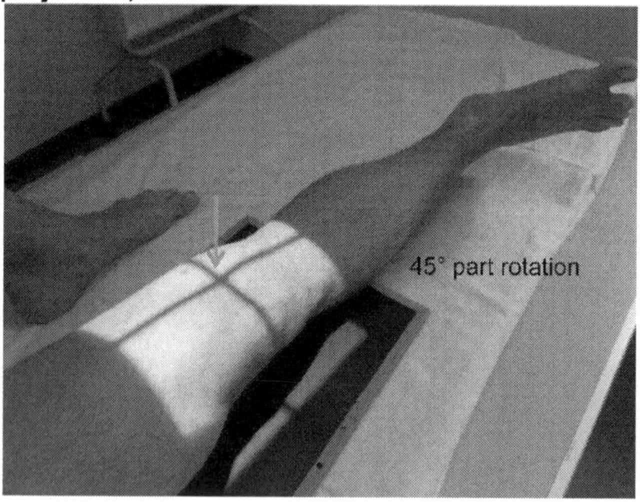

Collimation to include or structures demonstrated

- The knee joint plus 2 inches (5cm) of distal femur and proximal tibia/fibula

Image evaluation

- Tibia/fibula superimposed

Fig. 93b. Radiograph. Knee- Anteroposterior (AP) Oblique projection, lateral/external rotation

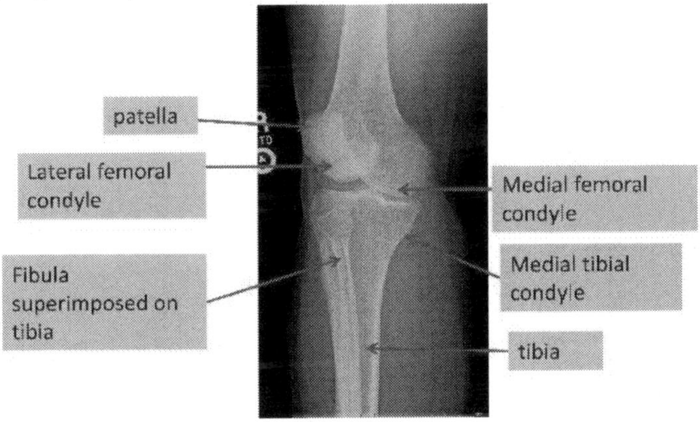

Knee–Posteroanterior (PA) Axial intercondylar fossa projection

Holmblad method

SID, Technical factors, Shielding

- 40 inches (100 cm). Grid. 70kVp @ 3.2 mAs or AEC.

Gonadal shielding

Patient/part position

- Kneeling with affected knee centered to Bucky.

Specific part/body position or rotation

- Lean patient forward to form an angle of 20 degrees between the elevated femur and the horizontal.
- Keep tibia/fibula parallel with tabletop

Direction and point of entry of CR

- Perpendicular to interpopoliteal surface. CR exits at patella apex

Fig. 94a. Position. Knee-Posteroanterior (PA) Axial Intercondylar Fossa Projection. Holmblad method

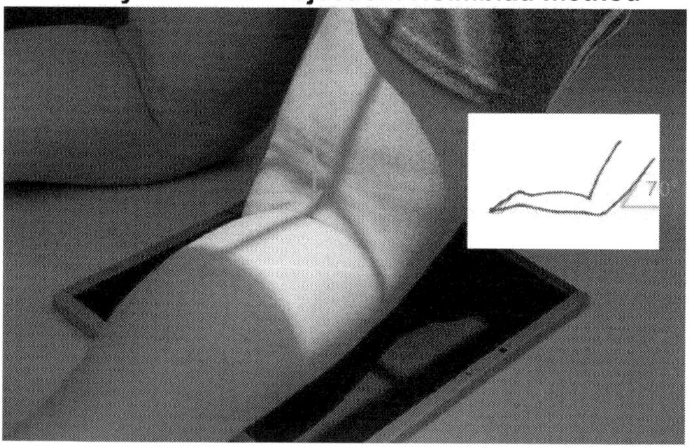

Collimation to include or structures demonstrated

- The knee joint plus 2 inches (5cm) of distal femur and proximal tibia/fibula

Image evaluation

- Intercondyloid fossa of femur, medial and lateral intercondylar tubercles of the intercondylar eminence in profile.
- Apex of patella should not superimpose in fossa
- Condyles symmetrical–fossa open and in center of collimated image.
- In all the intercondylar projections the central ray is directed 90-degree to the tib/fib

Fig. 94b. Radiograph. Knee-Posteroanterior (PA) Axial Intercondylar Fossa Projection. Holmblad method

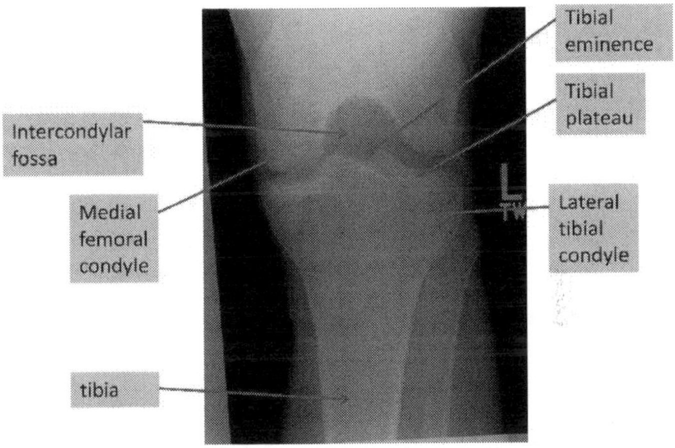

Knee–Posteroanterior (PA) axial, superoinferior intercondylar fossa projection
Camp-Coventry method

SID, Technical factors, Shielding

- 40 inches (100 cm). Grid. 70kVp @ 3.2 mAs or AEC.

Gonadal shielding

Patient/part position

- Prone

Specific part/body position or rotation

- Flex knee 40º–50º and rest foot on support.

Direction and point of entry of CR

- 40 inches (100cm) perpendicular to the long axis of tibia-fibula
- Therefore 40º caudal when knee is flexed 40º or 50ºcaudal if knee is flexed 50º

Fig. 95a. Position. Knee-Posteroanterior (PA) Axial Intercondylar Fossa Projection. Comp-Coventry method

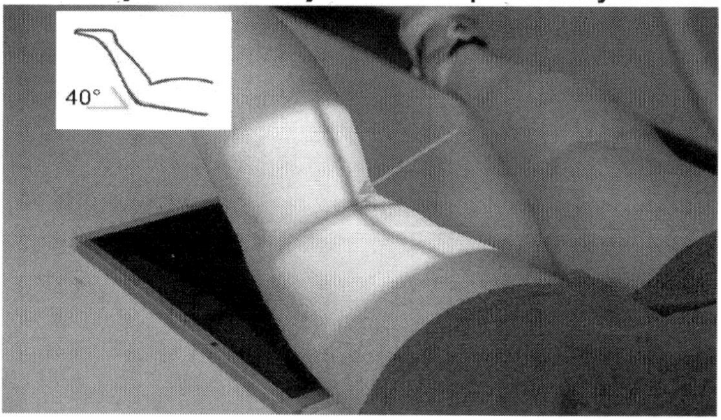

Collimation to include or structures demonstrated

- The knee joint plus 2 inches (5cm) of distal femur and proximal tibia/fibula

Image evaluation

- Intercondyloid fossa of femur, medial and lateral intercondylar tubercles of the intercondylar eminence in profile.
- Apex of patella should not superimpose in fossa
- Condyles symmetrical–fossa open and in center of collimated image.
- In all the intercondylar projections the central ray is directed 90-degree to the tib/fin

Fig. 95b. Radiograph. Knee-Posteroanterior (PA) Axial Intercondylar Fossa Projection. Comp-Coventry method

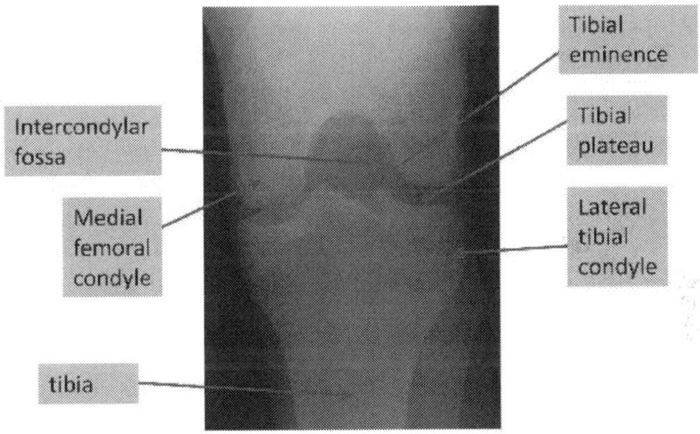

Knee–Posteroanterior (AP) axial, superoinferior intercondylar fossa projection
Béclère method

SID, Technical factors, Shielding

- 40 inches (100 cm). Grid. 70kVp @ 3.2 mAs or AEC. Gonadal shielding

Patient/part position

- Patient seated on the x-ray table

Specific part/body position or rotation

- Flex affected knee and place on sponge supports
- The detector should be in close contact with the knee

Direction and point of entry of CR

- 40 inches (100cm) perpendicular to the long axis of tibia-fibula

Fig. 96a. Position. Knee-Posteroanterior (PA) Axial Intercondylar Fossa Projection. Béclère method

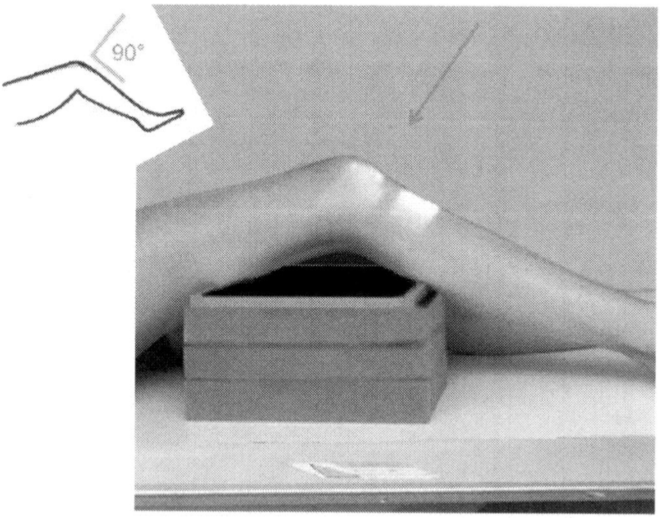

Collimation to include or structures demonstrated

- The knee joint plus 2 inches (5cm) of distal femur and proximal tibia/fibula

Image evaluation

- Intercondyloid fossa of femur, medial and lateral intercondylar tubercles of the intercondylar eminence in profile.
- Apex of patella should not superimpose in fossa
- Condyles symmetrical–fossa open and in center of collimated image.
- In all the intercondylar projections the central ray is directed 90-degree to the tib/fin

Fig. 96b. Radiograph. Knee-Posteroanterior (PA) Axial Intercondylar Fossa Projection. Béclère method

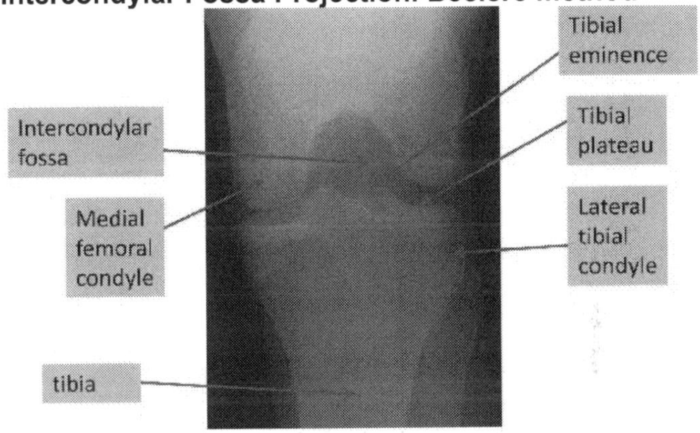

Knee–Anteroposterior (AP) weight-bearing projection, bilateral

SID, Technical factors, Shielding

- 40 inches (100 cm). Grid. 70kVp @ 3.2 mAs or AEC.

Gonadal shielding

Patient/part position

- Standing

Specific part/body position or rotation

- Patient's back to the IR with weigh equally distributed

Direction and point of entry of CR

- Horizontally between the knees ½inch (1.5cm) below level of patella apex

Fig. 97a. Position. Knee-Posteroanterior (PA) Axial Intercondylar Fossa Projection. Weight-Bearing Projection, bilateral

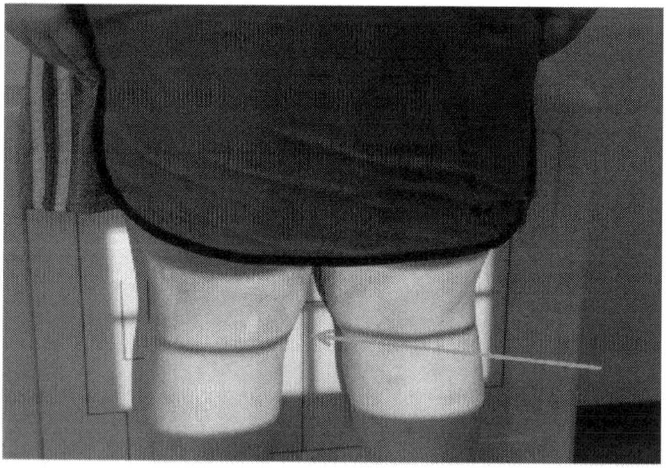

Collimation to include or structures demonstrated

- The knee joint plus 2 inches (5cm) of distal femur and proximal tibia/fibula

Image evaluation

- Include soft tissue and bony trabecular detail of knee
- Condyles should be symmetrical with open joint space
- Patella superimposed on femur

Notes

- This projection can demonstrate arthritis, varus (inward) or valgus (outward) deformity
- Joint narrowing is only demonstrated on erect

Fig. 97b. Radiograph. Knee-Posteroanterior (PA) Axial Intercondylar Fossa Projection. Weight-Bearing Projection, bilateral.

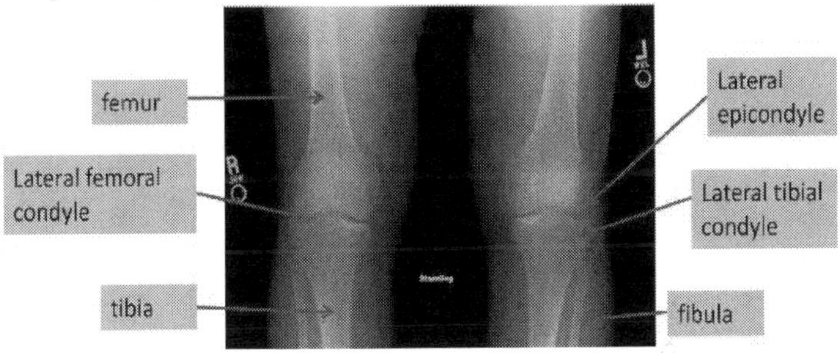

Knee–Posteroanterior (PA) weight-bearing projection, bilateral
Rosenberg method

SID, Technical factors, Shielding

- 40 inches (100 cm). Grid. 70kVp @ 3.2 mAs or AEC.

Gonadal shielding

Patient/part position

- Standing PA

Specific part/body position or rotation

- Patients holds the grid device with knees flexed and femur 45º to IR

Direction and point of entry of CR

- 10 degrees caudally between the knees ½ inch (1.5cm) below level of patella apex

Fig. 98a. Position. Knee-Posteroanterior (PA) Axial. Intercondylar Fossa Projection. Weight-Bearing Projection, Bilateral. Rosenburg Method

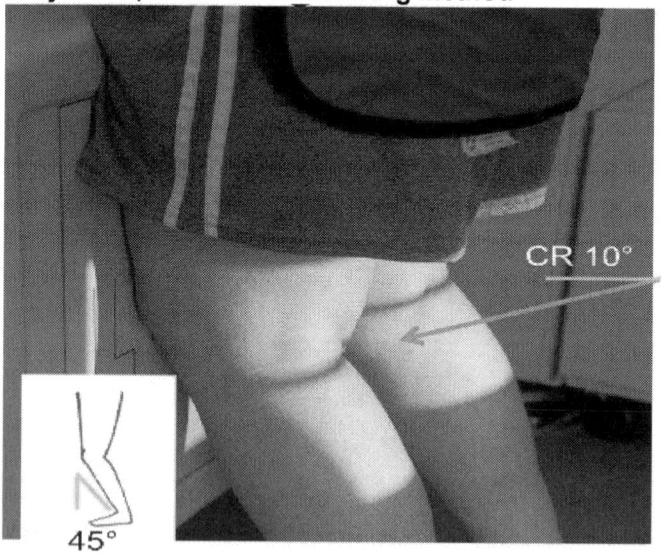

Collimation to include or structures demonstrated

- The knee joint plus 2 inches (5cm) of distal femur and proximal tibia/fibula

Image evaluation

- Intercondyloid fossa of femur, medial and lateral intercondylar tubercles of the intercondylar eminence in profile.
- Apex of patella should not superimpose in fossa

Note: This projection can demonstrate arthritis, joint narrowing, varus (inward) or valgus (outward) deformity

- In all the intercondylar projections the central ray is directed 90-degree to the tib/fin

Fig. 98b. Radiograph. Knee-Posteroanterior (PA) Axial. Intercondylar Fossa Projection. Weight-Bearing Projection, Bilateral. Rosenburg Method

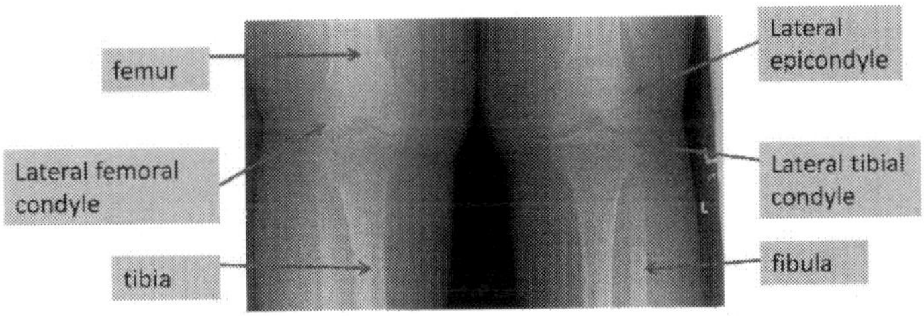

Patella–Posteroanterior (PA) projection

SID, Technical factors, Shielding

- 40 inches (100 cm). Grid. 70kVp @ 3.2 mAs or AEC.

Gonadal shielding

Patient/part position

- Prone to reduce OID with support under femur & lower leg to relieve pressure on patella.

Specific part/body position or rotation

- Heel may be rotated 5º-10º laterally to place patella parallel to IR (or turn patella medially)

Direction and point of entry of CR

- Patella placed in midline of table and parallel to IR. May require 5º–10º lateral rotation

Fig. 99a. Position. Patella- Posteroanterior (PA) projection

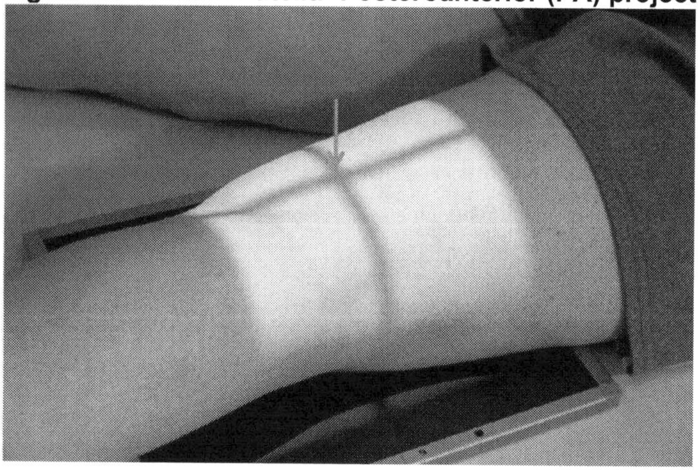

Collimation to include or structures demonstrated

- The knee joint plus 2 inches (5cm) of distal femur and proximal tibia/fibula

Image evaluation

- The PA with smaller OID gives better record detail
- Patella will be superimposed over femur.
- Symmetrical femoral condyles

Fig. 99b. Radiograph. Patella- Posteroanterior (PA) projection

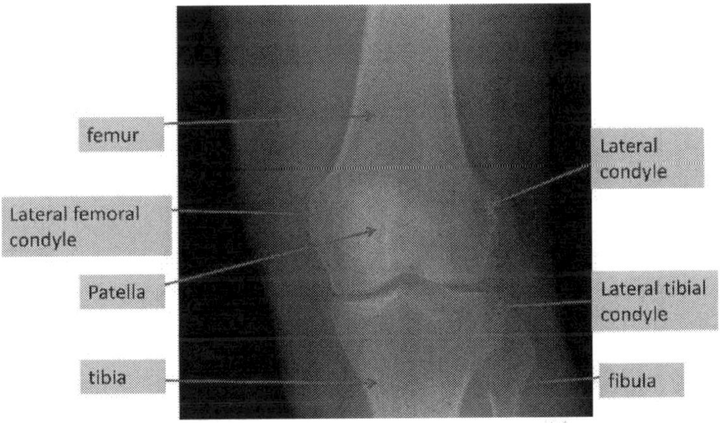

Patella–Lateral (mediolateral) projection

SID, Technical factors, Shielding

- 40 inches (100 cm). Grid. 70kVp @ 3.2 mAs or AEC.

Gonadal shielding

Patient/part position

- Recumbent and lateral on affected side

Specific part/body position or rotation

- Patella true lateral and perpendicular to tabletop. Knee flexed 10°

Direction and point of entry of CR

- Perpendicular CR directed to the patella femoral joint

Fig. 100a. Position. Patella-Lateral (mediolateral) projection

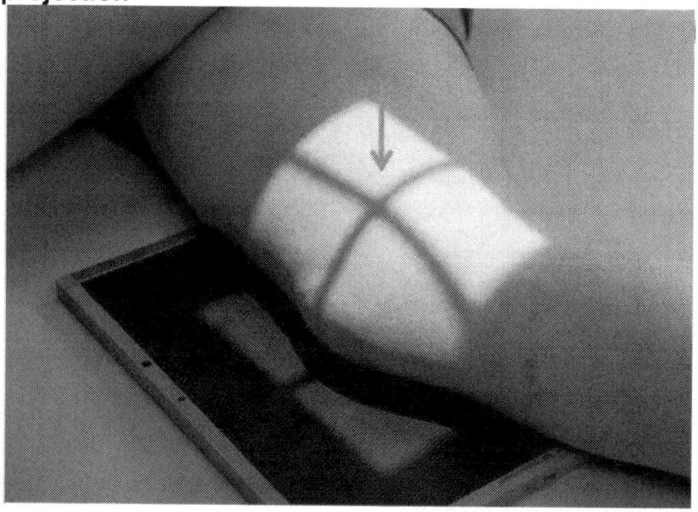

Collimation to include or structures demonstrated

- The knee joint plus 2 inches (5cm) of distal femur and proximal tibia/fibula

Image evaluation

- Open joint space with condyles superimposed/patella in lateral profile.

Note:

- 10º flexion only if know or healing patella fracture to prevent separation of unhealed patellar fragments.

Fig. 100b. Radiograph. Patella-Lateral (mediolateral) projection

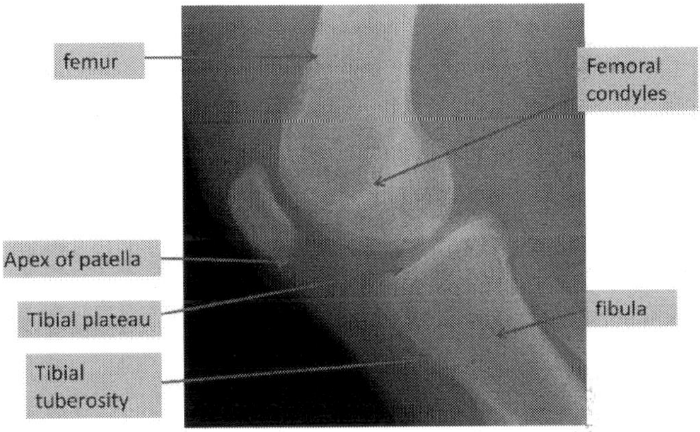

Patella–Tangential (axial or sunrise/skyline) projection
Settegast method

SID, Technical factors, Shielding

- 40 inches (100 cm). No Grid. 65kVp @ 2.3 mAs. No AEC.

Gonadal shielding

Patient/part position

- Prone or supine with knees flexed

Specific part/body position or rotation.

- IR placed to rest against the distal femur
- If patient is supine, flex knee greater than 90
- If patient prone, flex knee less than 90

Direction and point of entry of CR

- Parallel through the patellofemoral joint space, using 15°-20° angulation if needed

Fig. 101a. Position. Patella- Tangential (Axial or Sunrise/Skyline) projection Settegast method. Patient Supine

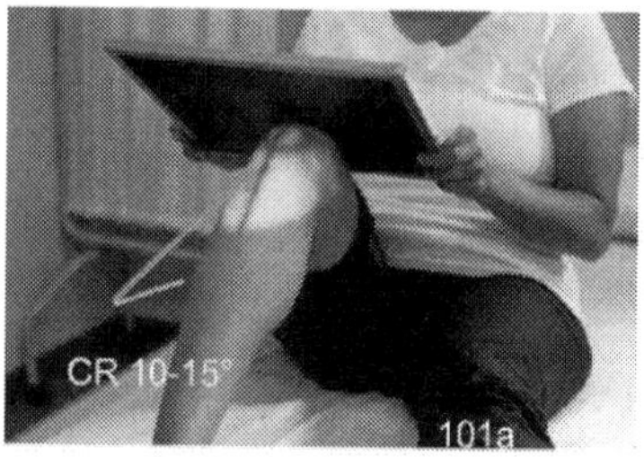

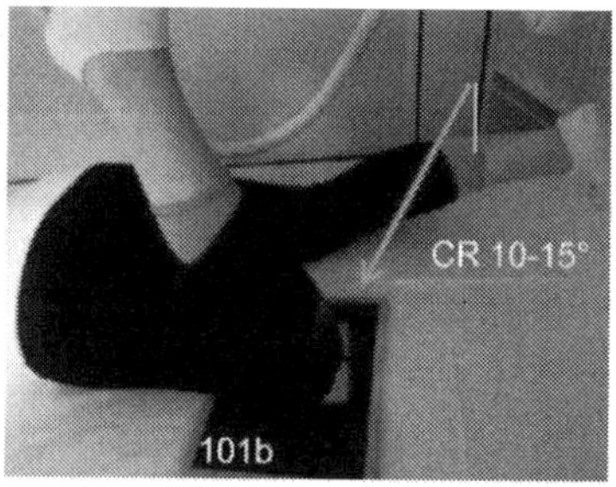

Fig. 101b. Position. Patella- Tangential (Axial or Sunrise/Skyline) projection Settegast method. Patient Prone

Collimation to include

- Patella and distal femur

Image evaluation

- Patella femoral joint space open.

Note:

- This projection will demonstrate longitudinal (vertical) patella fractures.

Fig. 101c. Radiograph. Patella- Tangential (Axial or Sunrise/Skyline) projection. Settegast method.

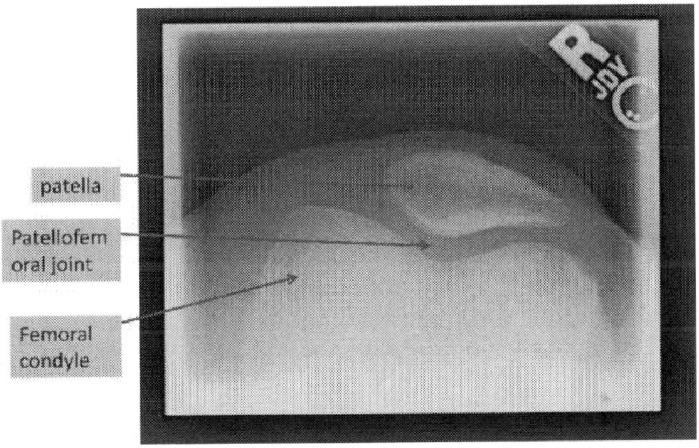

Patella–Tangential Axial Hughston

Hughston method

SID, Technical factors, Shielding

- 40 inches (100 cm). Grid. 70kVp @ 3.2 mAs or AEC.

Gonadal shielding

Patient/part position

- Prone with femur parallel to table

Specific part/body position or rotation

- Tibia/fibula elevated and supported to form an angle of 50° - 60° with the tabletop

Direction and point of entry of CR

- CR 45 degrees to long axis of leg through the patellofemoral joint.

Fig. 101d. Position. Patella- Tangential (Axial or Sunrise/Skyline) projection. Hughston Method

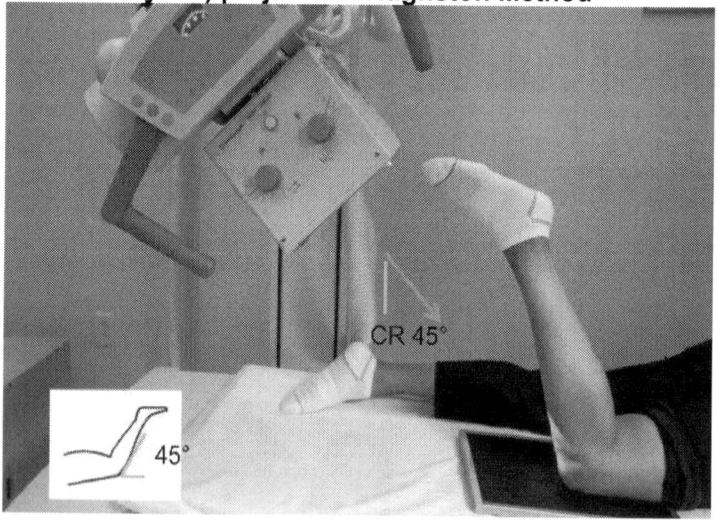

Collimation to include or structures demonstrated

- Patella and distal femur

Image evaluation

- Patella femoral articulation open

Note: This projection is not used for transverse fractures of patella. It will demonstrate longitudinal fracture of patella or subluxation of patella

Fig. 101e. Radiograph. Patella- Tangential (Axial or Sunrise/Skyline) projection. Hughston Method

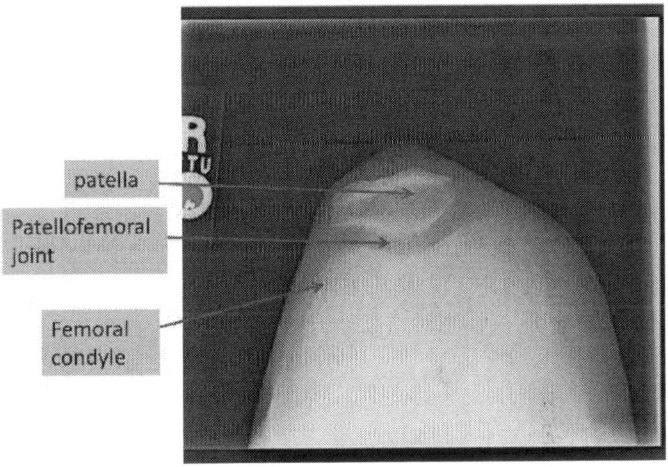

Patella–Tangential (axial or sunrise/skyline) projection

Merchant method

SID, Technical factors, Shielding

- 40 inches (100 cm). No Grid. 65kVp @ 2.3 mAs. No AEC.

Gonadal shielding

Patient/part position

- Supine

Specific part/body position or rotation

- This projection requires an "axial viewer", an adjustable IR holder devise that supports leg and relaxes muscles and allows exact duplication of knee flexion
- 40-degree flexion common. However, knee flexion is determined by physician.

Direction and point of entry of CR

- CR to patella femoral joint space.
- 72 inches (183 cm) to compensate for large OID

Fig. 101f. Position. Patella- Tangential (Axial or Sunrise/Skyline) projection. Merchant Method

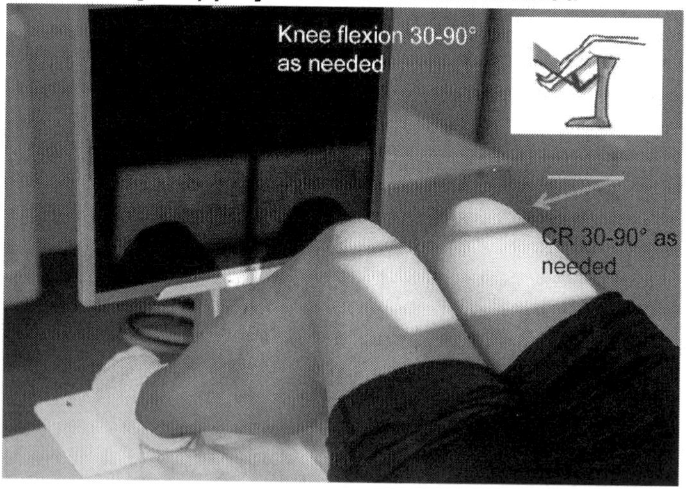

Collimation to include or structures demonstrated

- Patella and distal femur

Image evaluation

- Open patella femoral articulation

Fig. 101g. Radiograph. Patella- Tangential (Axial or Sunrise/Skyline) projection. Merchant Method

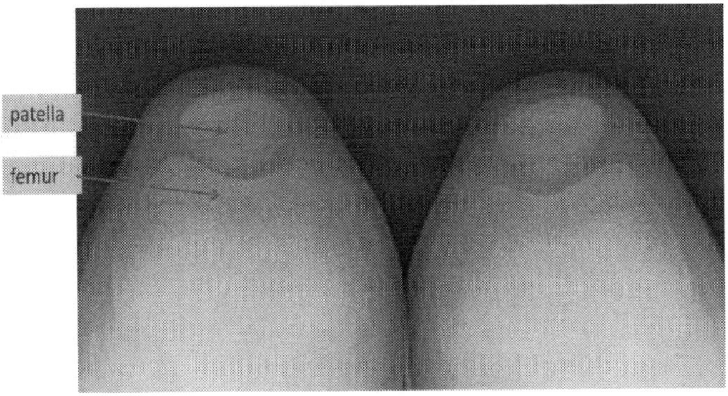

Femur–Anteroposterior (AP) projection

Mid- and distal femur

SID, Technical factors, Shielding

- 40 inches (100 cm). Grid. 75-80kVp @ 7.5 mAs or AEC.

Gonadal shielding

Patient/part position

- Patient supine

Specific part/body position or rotation

- Rotate and immobilize leg/feet 5-degrees internally keeping femoral epicondyle equidistant from the IR
- No manipulation of the leg in fracture suspect cases

Direction and point of entry of CR

- Center to midpoint of IR

Fig. 102a. Position. Femur-Anteroposterior (AP) projection. Mid and Distal Femur

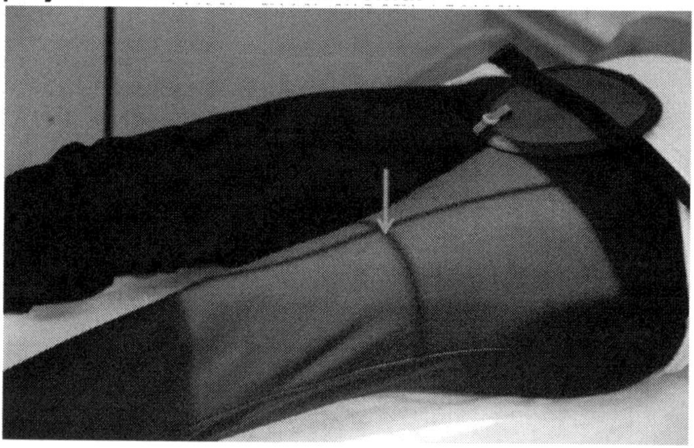

Collimation to include or structures demonstrated

- Mid and distal femur including knee joint

Image evaluation

- Majority of femur and the joint nearest to the pathology or injury
- Epicondyles in profile/medial larger than lateral
- Intercondylar eminence centered within the intercondylar fossa

Note:

- Include orthopedic appliance in their entirety
- Place the thicker part (hip)towards the cathode to reduce heel effect
- When imaging the entire femur, if two IPs are needed, either include knee with distal femur or hip with proximal femur.
- In trauma imaging do not internally rotate of legs/feet to avoid injury to blood vessels and nerves

Fig. 102b. Radiograph. Femur-Anteroposterior (AP) projection. Mid and Distal Femur

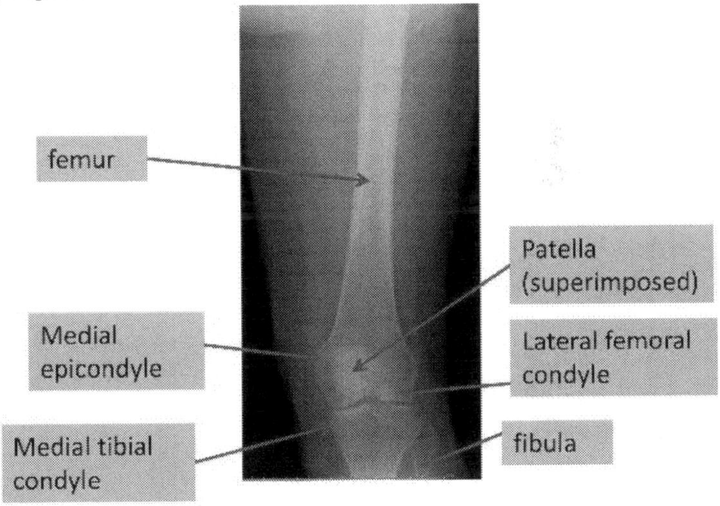

Femur–Lateral projection

Mid- and distal femur

SID, Technical factors, Shielding

- 40 inches (100 cm). Grid. 77-82kVp @ 7.5 mAs or AEC.

Gonadal shielding

Patient/part position

- Patient supine with legs extended and unaffected leg supported

Specific part/body position or rotation

- Roll affected leg 10-15 degrees posteriorly (backward)

Direction and point of entry of CR

- 40 inches (100 cm) CR to mid femur

Fig. 103a. Position. Femur-Lateral projection. Mid and Distal Femur

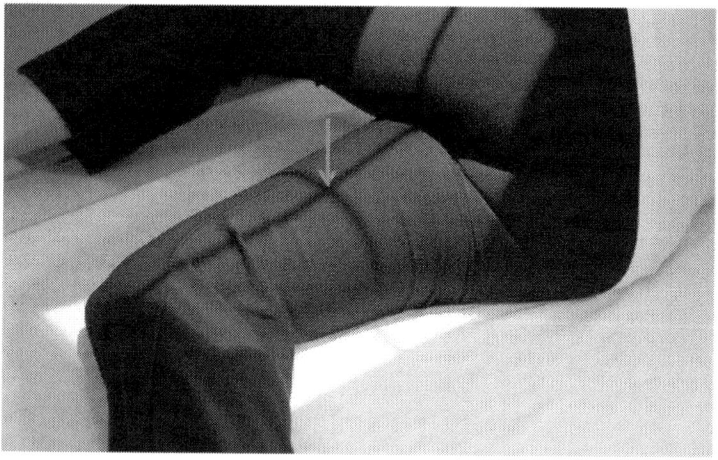

Collimation to include or structures demonstrated

- Mid and distal femur including knee joint

Image evaluation

- Majority of femur and joint nearest to the pathology or injury
- Include orthopedic appliance in their entirety
- Due to divergent rays the inferior surface of the condyles will not be superimposed
- The medial condyle is magnified and projects more distally than the lateral condyle because the medial further from the IR

Fig. 103b. Radiograph. Femur-Lateral projection. Mid and Distal Femur

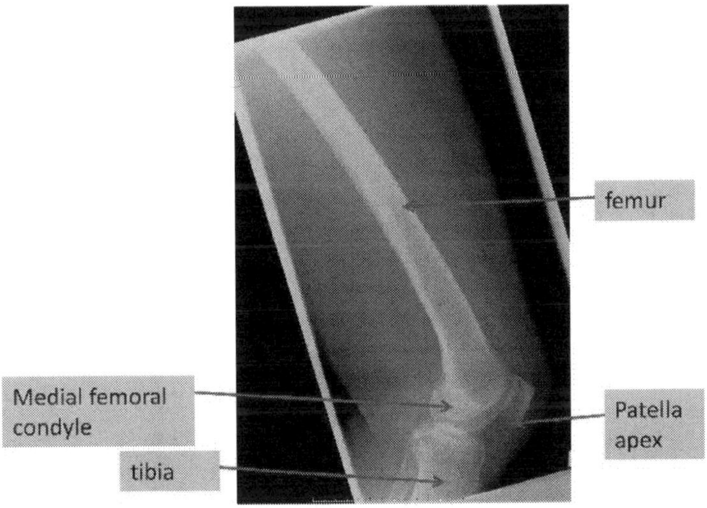

Femur–Lateral projection

Mid- and proximal femur

SID, Technical factors, Shielding

- 40 inches (100 cm). Grid. 77-82kVp @ 7.5 mAs or AEC.

Gonadal shielding

- Patient/part position

Specific part/body position or rotation

- Top of IR at level of ASIS
- Knee flexed, abducted and supported
- Turn patient slightly towards affected side

Direction and point of entry of CR

- 40 inches (100cm) CR to midpoint of shaft

Fig. 104a. Position. Femur-Lateral projection. Mid and Proximal Femur

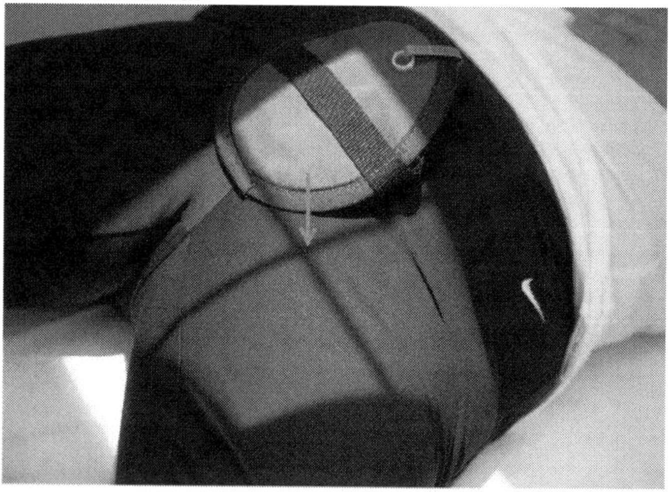

Collimation to include or structures demonstrated

- Entire hip joint and proximal femur

Image evaluation

- Greater trochanter superimposed on femoral neck

Note

- Include orthopedic appliance in their entirety
- This projection is contraindicated in suspected fracture cases

Fig. 104b. Radiograph. Femur-Lateral projection. Mid and Proximal Femur

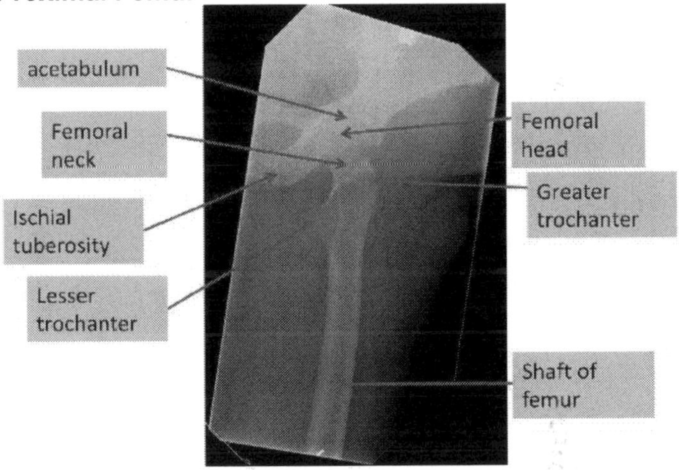

Bone leg length study (bilateral scanograms)

Weight–bearing method

SID, Technical factors, Shielding

- 8 feet(96 inches) or 244 cm. Grid. Hip factors with wedge filter or AEC. Gonadal shielding

Patient/part position

- Patient erect on a 2 inch (5cm) raised support to allow imaging of the ankle.
- Weight equally distributed

Specific part/body position or rotation

- Magnification marker placed on knee to measure magnification or radiographic ruler used
- Toes straight. Legs exactly 20 cm (7.5inches) apart (measured from lateral malleoli)

Direction and point of entry of CR

- CR directed to knee

Fig. 105a. Position. Bone Leg Length Study. (Bilateral Scanograms) Weight-Bearing method

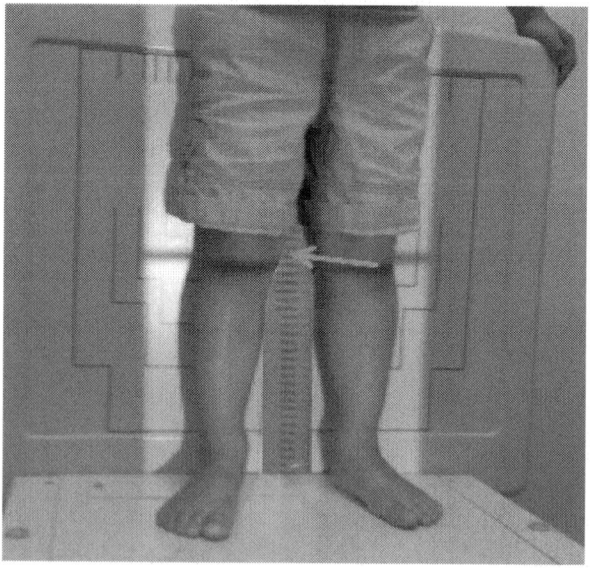

Collimation to include or structures demonstrated

- Hips to ankles on one exposure using 14 X 50"IR (35.4 x 124.5 cm)

Image evaluation

- Entire right and left limbs from the hip to ankle

Note

- In analog imaging a wedge filter will compensate for differences in thickness between the hip joint and ankle join

Fig. 105b. Radiograph. Bone Leg Length Study. (Bilateral Scanograms) Weight-Bearing method

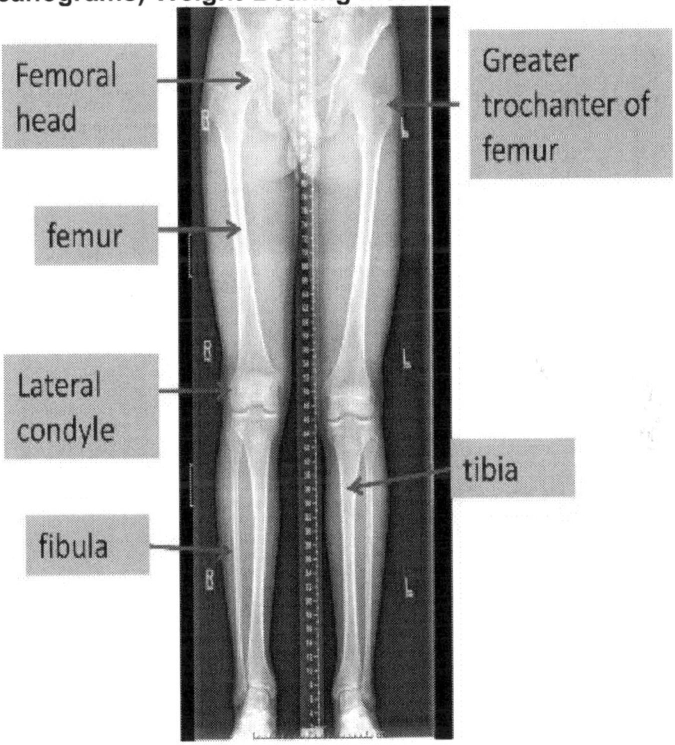

Bone leg length study (bilateral scanograms)

SID, Technical factors, Shielding

- 40 inches (100 cm). Grid. Ankle, knee & hip factors or AEC. Gonadal shielding

Patient/part position

- Patient supine

Specific part/body position or rotation

- Tape radiographic ruler to midline of table or beside patient
- Patients hip's/knees/and ankles image with the ruler

Direction and point of entry of CR

- Center to joint space for each part
- Divide IR into three equal parts & make three exposures to include bilateral of hip, knee & ankle
- Cover, collimate and shield unused portions of IR between exposures

Fig. 106a,b &c. Position. Bone Leg Length Study. (Bilateral Scanograms) Centering to the Hip, Knees and Ankles

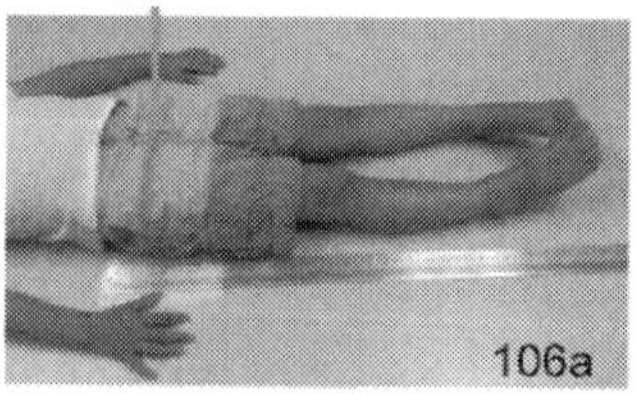

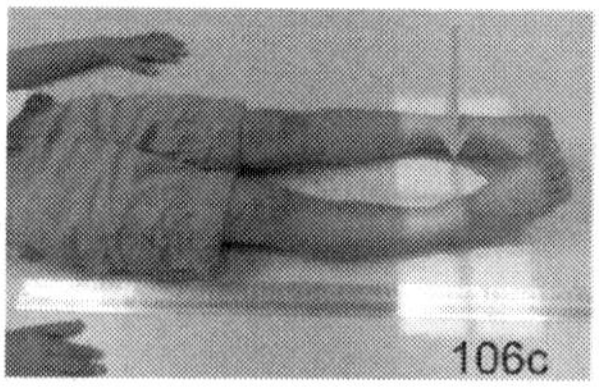

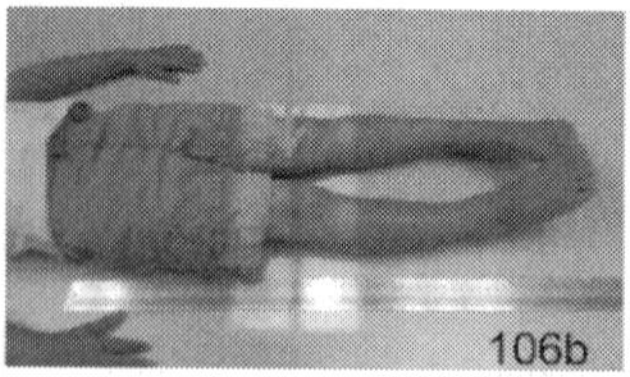

Collimation to include or structures demonstrated

- Bilateral hips, knees and ankles.
- The radiographic ruler included in each exposure

Image evaluation

- The three joints and the ruler seen

Fig. 106d. Radiograph. Bone Leg Length Study (bilateral scanograms)

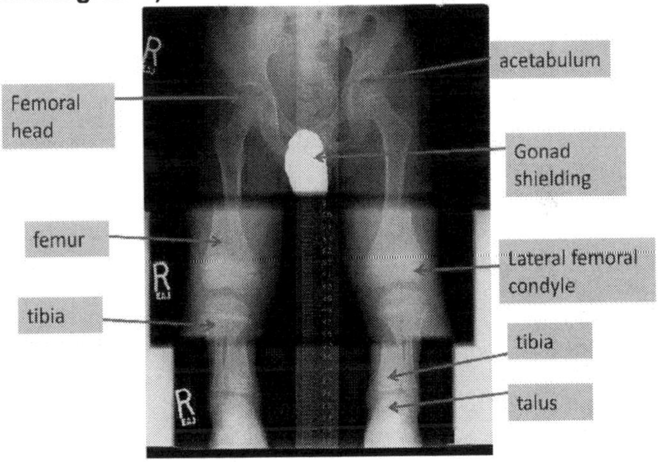

Bones of the Hip & Pelvis

Pelvis has 4 bones—2 hip bones, sacrum and coccyx.

Each hip bones are 3 fused bones—ilium, pubis and ischium that unit to form the acetabulum. The two hip bones unit to form the pubic symphysis anteriorly and posterior with the sacrum to form the sacroiliac joint

Exact location of head and neck of femur

- The perpendicular bisector of the line drawn from the ASIS to the superior margin of the symphysis will pass through the head and neck of the femur, head 1.5 inches (3.8cm) distal on the line and the neck 2.5 inches (6.4 cm) distal on the line)

Fig 106a. Labeled Pelvis

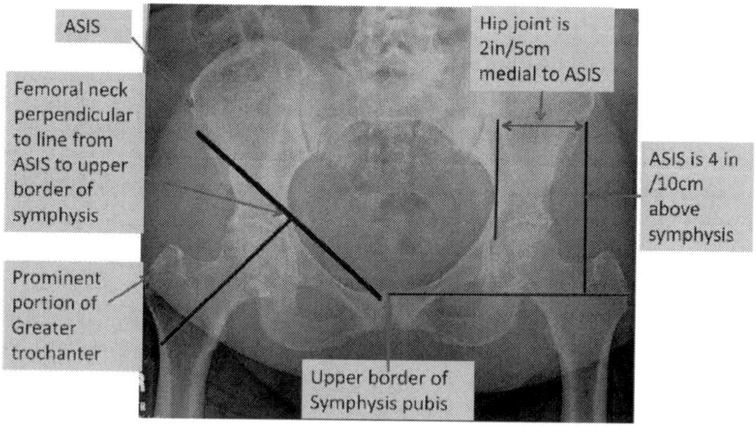

Appearance of proximal femur with the leg rotation:

- In anatomic position foreshortening of neck of femur

Fig. 107b and Fig. 107c

- In internal rotation no foreshortening /anteversion of neck of femur

Fig. 107d and Fig. 107e

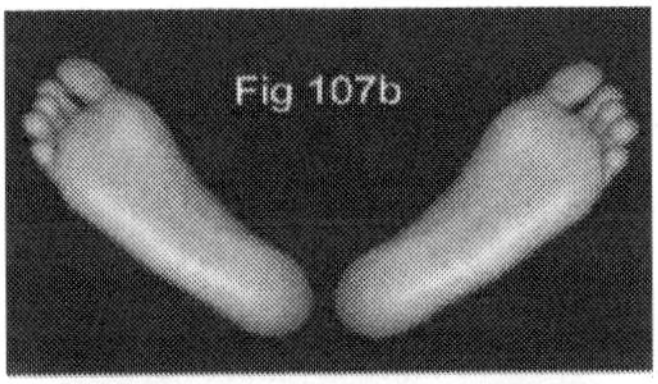

Fig 107b

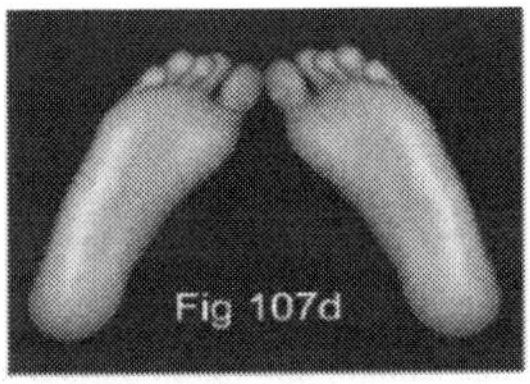

Fig 107d

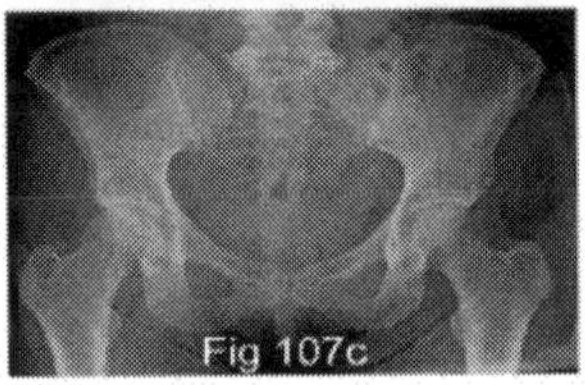

Fig 107c

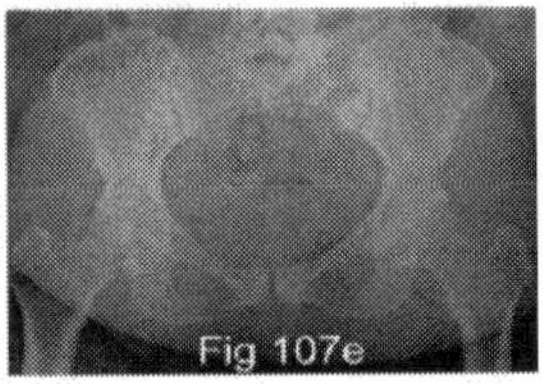

Fig 107e

Position of the foot in cases of hip fracture Foot externally rotated

Positioning Tips for Hip

- Advise patient in advance before palpating for the symphysis to avoid embarrassment or misunderstanding.
- Superior margin of symphysis located on same plane with most prominent point of greater trochanter
- The greater trochanter is best palpated when the feet are internally rotated.
- Hip joint located 2inches (5 cm) medial to ASIS at level of superior aspect of greater trochanter or inguinal crease (just above the level with the symphysis)
- Greater trochanter located 4inches (10 cm) below the ASIS
- Crest located at L4/L5

Hip–Anteroposterior (AP) projection

Hip and proximal femur

SID, Technical factors, Shielding

- 40 inches (100 cm). Grid. 85kVp @ 20-30 mAs or AEC. Gonadal shielding when possible

Patient/part position

- Supine

Specific part/body position or rotation

- Rotate feet 15-20 degree internally

Direction and point of entry of CR

- 2.5inches(6.4 cm) distal to line perpendicular to the midpoint of line from ASIS to symphysis (crease of groin) or 1-2 inches (2.5-5 cm) medial and 3-4 inches (7.6 – 10 cm) distal to ASIS

Fig. 108a. Position. Hip-Anteroposterior (AP) projection. Hip and proximal femur

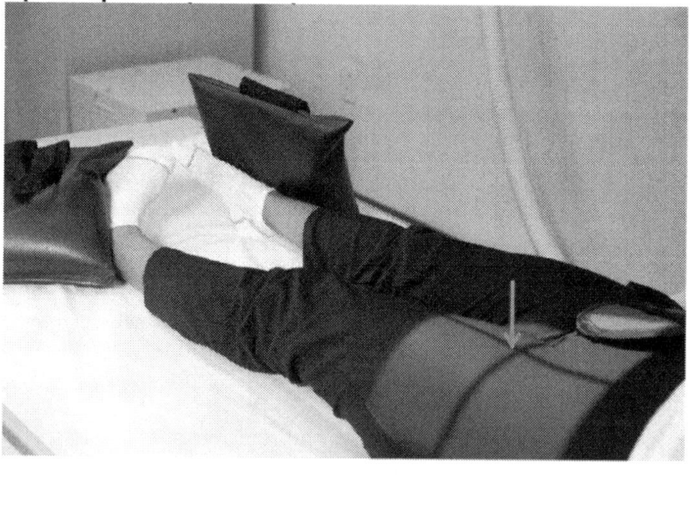

Collimation to include or structures demonstrated

- Hip joint and proximal femur

Image evaluation

- Greater trochanter in profile
- Lesser trochanter superimposed by femoral neck
- Femoral neck without foreshortening

NOTE

- Include any orthopedic appliance in their entirely

Fig. 108b. Radiograph. Hip-Anteroposterior (AP) projection. Hip and proximal femur

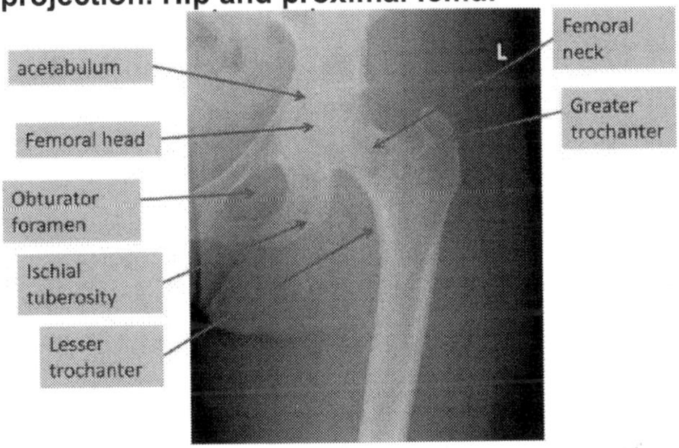

Hip–Lateral (mediolateral) projection

Lauenstein method

SID, Technical factors, Shielding

- 40 inches (100 cm). Grid. 85kVp @ 20-30 mAs or AEC. Gonadal shielding when possible

Patient/part position

- Supine

Specific part/body position or rotation

- Rotate patient to affected side (degree of obliquity depends on patient's ability to abduct leg)
- Flex knees & turn patient slightly towards affected side

Direction and point of entry of CR

- Just below the crest midpoint on line between the ASIS and symphysis pubis

Fig. 109a. Position. Hip-Lateral (mediolateral) projection. Lauenstein method

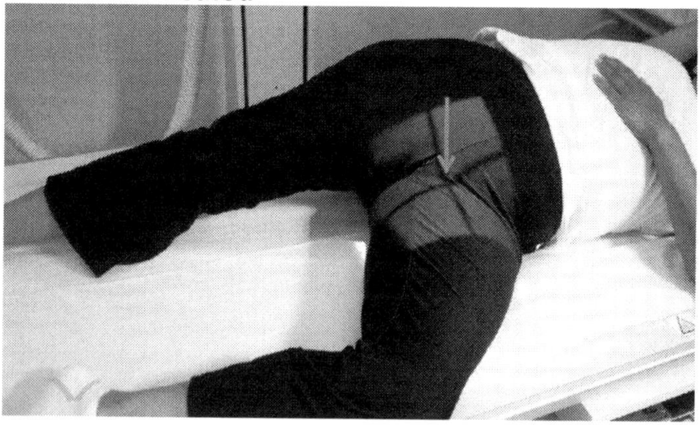

Collimation to include or structures demonstrated

- Hip joint and proximal femur

Image evaluation

- Greater trochanter superimposed on femoral neck

NOTE

- Include any orthopedic appliance in their entirety

Fig. 109b. Radiograph. Hip-Lateral (mediolateral) projection. Lauenstein method

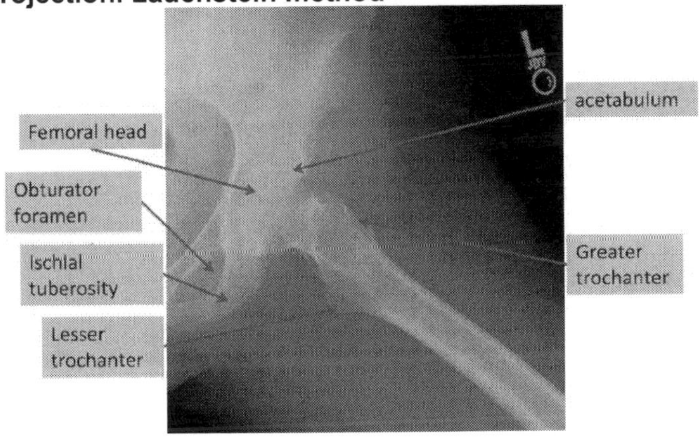

Hip–Axiolateral inferosuperior or Cross-table Lateral projection

Trauma imaging: Danelius-Miller method to include Hip and proximal femur

SID, Technical factors, Shielding

- 40 inches (100 cm). Grid. 90Vp @ 20-30 mAs. No AEC. Gonadal shielding when possible

Patient/part position

- Patient supine, affected leg neutral
- Affected hip raised on a firm support.

Specific part/body position or rotation

- Thighs of unaffected leg vertical with knee flexed
- Affected leg on a firm support that should not extend beyond the side of the patient.
- No internal rotation on suspected fracture cases
- Place and support IR in the crease formed at patient's waist, angled 45 degrees away from the body and parallel to the long axis of the femoral neck

Direction and point of entry of CR

- CR directed horizontally to center of IR and right angle to the femoral neck)

Fig. 110b. Schematic Diagram. Showing CR/Detector Alignment & Position. Trauma Hip-Axiolateral inferiosuperior or cross-table lateral projection, Danelius-Miller method

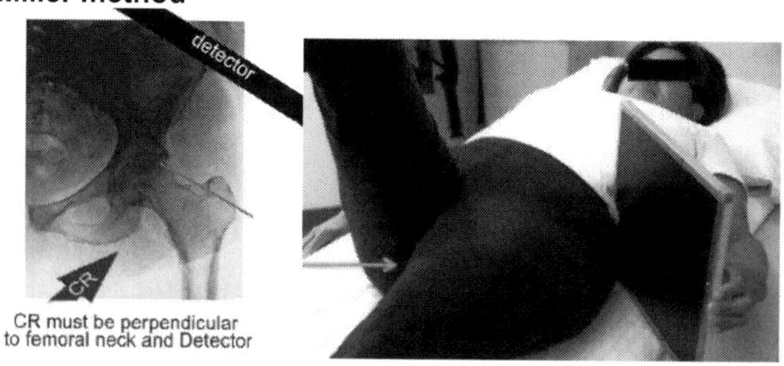

Collimation to include or structures demonstrated

- Hip and proximal femur

Image evaluation

- Visualization of the acetabulum, femoral head and neck

Notes

- Include orthopedic appliance in their entirely
- Thin patients use above placement but on heavier patients place the IR superior to iliac crest–to include the acetabulum and femoral head on IR
- No internal rotation of leg and feet on suspected fracture cases

Fig. 110c. Radiograph. Trauma Hip-Axiolateral inferiosuperior or cross-table lateral projection, Danelius-Miller method

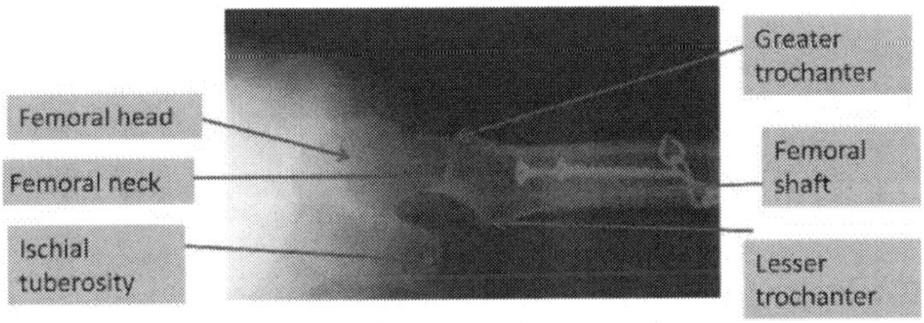

Hip–Modified Axiolateral trauma projection

Trauma Imaging: Clements-Nakayama modification, Transfemoral Lateral Hip to include hip and proximal femur

SID, Technical factors, Shielding

- 40 inches (100 cm). Grid. 90kVp @ 20-30 mAs. No AEC.

Gonadal shielding when possible Patient/part position

- Patient supine leg neutral

Specific part/body position or rotation

- Minimize manipulation of patient in suspected fracture cases

Direction and point of entry of CR

- Support IR at lateral side of affected hip with upper border of IR tilted back 15-degrees
- Direct the CR 15-degrees posteriorly, aligned to femoral neck & IR

Fig. 111a. Position. Trauma Hip-Modified Axiolateral trauma projection, Clements-Nakayama modification, Transfemoral Lateral Hip and proximal femur

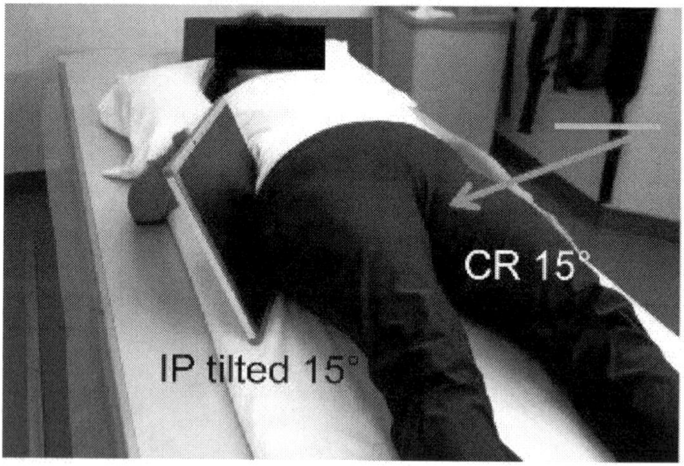

Collimation to include or structures demonstrated

- Hip and proximal femur

Image evaluation

- Visualization of the acetabulum, femoral head and neck

Note

- Include orthopedic appliance in their entirety
- This positioning is used when patient has limited movement of both legs e.g. bilateral hip fracture

Fig. 111b. Radiograph. Trauma Hip-Modified Axiolateral trauma projection, Clements-Nakayama modification, Transfemoral Lateral Hip and proximal femur

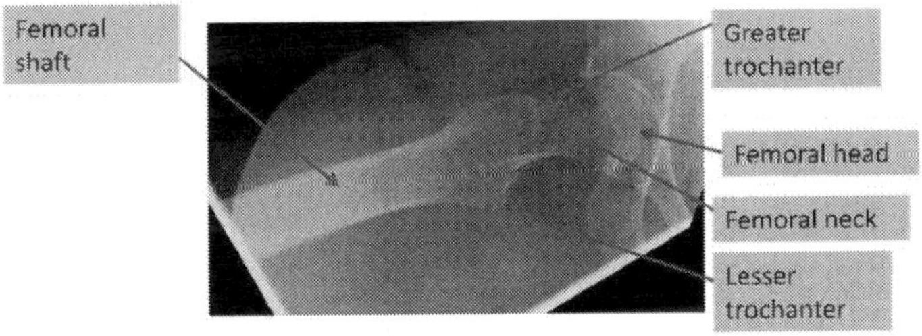

Acetabulum–Internal Oblique, LPO or RPO positions

Judet Method

SID, Technical factors, Shielding

- 40 inches (100 cm). Grid. 80kVp @ 20-30 mAs or AEC.

Gonadal shielding when possible Patient/part position

- Patient semisupine with affected side raised

Specific part/body position or rotation

- Patient rotated 45-degrees

Direction and point of entry of CR

- 40 inches (100 cm). CR directed perpendicular to IR 2 inches (5 cm) inferior to the ASIS of affected side

Fig.112a. Position. Acetabulum-Internal Oblique, LPO position. Judet Method (affected side up)

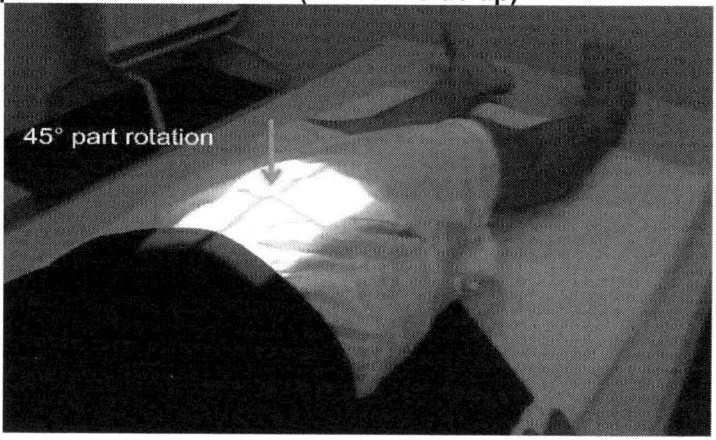

Collimation to include or structures demonstrated

- Acetabulum, femoral head and neck

Image evaluation

- Iliopubic column and posterior rim of affected acetabulum demonstrated

Note

- The projection demonstrates fractures of the posterior rim of the acetabulum also fracture of iliopubic column (anterior)and the posterior rim of the acetabulum

Fig.112b. Radiograph. Acetabulum-Internal Oblique, LPO position. Judet Method (affected side up)

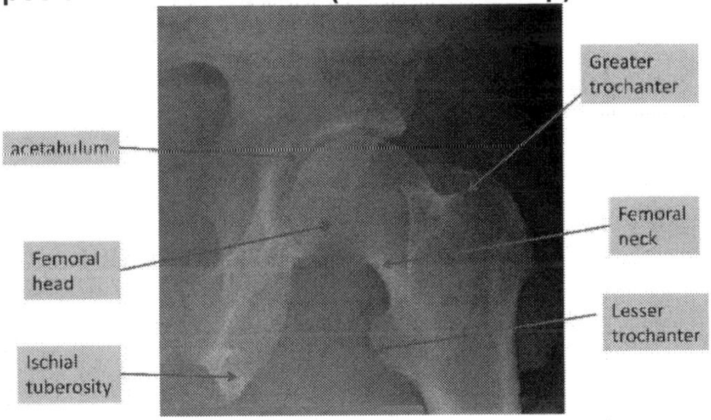

Acetabulum–External Oblique, LPO or RPO positions

Judet Method

SID, Technical factors, Shielding

- 40 inches (100 cm). Grid. 80kVp @ 20-30 mAs or AEC.

Gonadal shielding when possible Patient/part position

- Patient supine

Specific part/body position or rotation

- Patient semisupine with affected hip down

Direction and point of entry of CR

- 2 inches (5 cm) distal and 2 inches medial to the down side ASIS

Fig. 113a. Position. Acetabulum- External Oblique, LPO position (affected side down) Judet Method

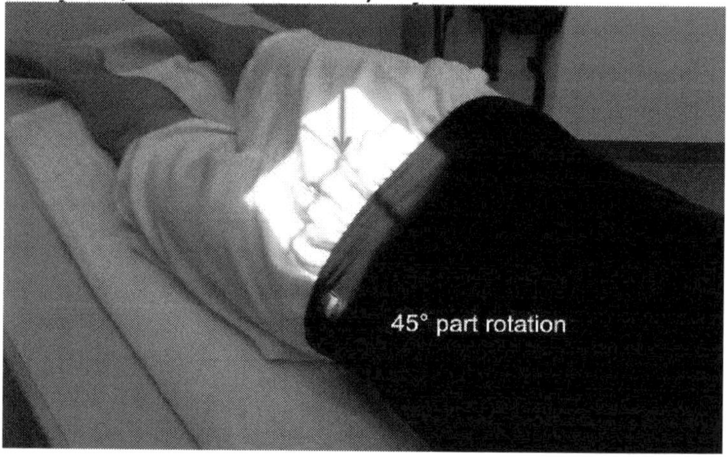

Collimation to include or structures demonstrated

- The acetabulum, femoral head and neck

Image evaluation

- Iliopubic column and posterior rim of the affected acetabulum demonstrated

Note

- This projection will demonstrate the ilioischial column (posterior) and the anterior rim of the acetabulum

Fig. 113b. Radiograph. Acetabulum- External Oblique, LPO position (affected side down) Judet Method

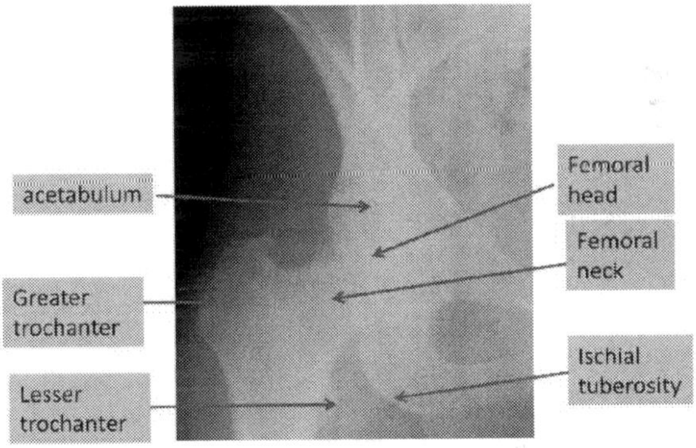

Ilium–Posterior Oblique, RPO & LPO positions

SID, Technical factors, Shielding

- 40 inches (100 cm). Grid. 80kVp @ 20-30 mAs or AEC.

Gonadal shielding when possible Patient/part position

- Patient semisupine with affected side down

Specific part/body position or rotation

- Patient rotated 40 degrees to place the broad wing of ilium of interest parallel to tabletop
- Hips abducted with knee slightly flexed

Direction and point of entry of CR

- CR directed at the level of ASIS in the midline of IR

Fig. 114a. Position. Ilium – Posterior Oblique, LPO position (affected side down)

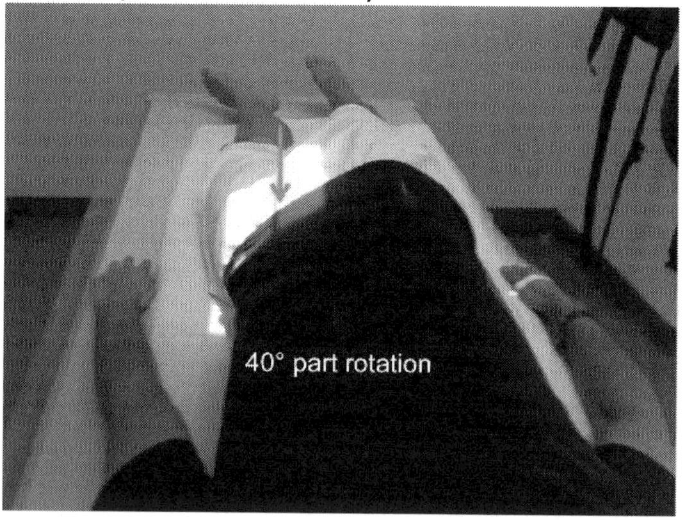

Collimation to include or structures demonstrated

- Upper border of IR placed 1 inch (2.5 cm) above the crest

Image evaluation

- RPO& LPO (posterior oblique) demonstrates an unobstructed projection of iliac wing and profile of acetabulum

Fig. 114b. Radiograph. Ilium – Posterior Oblique, LPO position (affected side down)

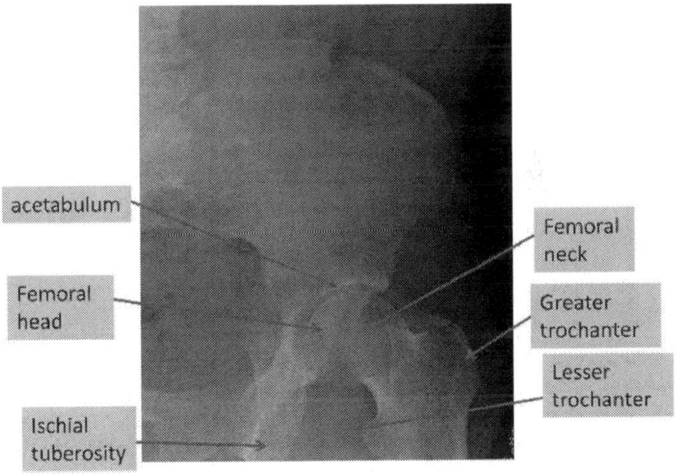

Ilium–Anterior Oblique, RAO & LAO positions

SID, Technical factors, Shielding

- 40 inches (100 cm). Grid. 80kVp @ 20-30 mAs or AEC.

Gonadal shielding when possible

Patient/part position

- Patient semiprone with affected side down
- Hips abducted and knees flexed

Specific part/body position or rotation

- Patient rotated 40 degrees
- Top of IR 1 inch (2.5 cm) above the crest

Direction and point of entry of CR

- CR to ASIS in midline of IR

Fig. 115a Position. Ilium – Anterior Oblique, RAO position

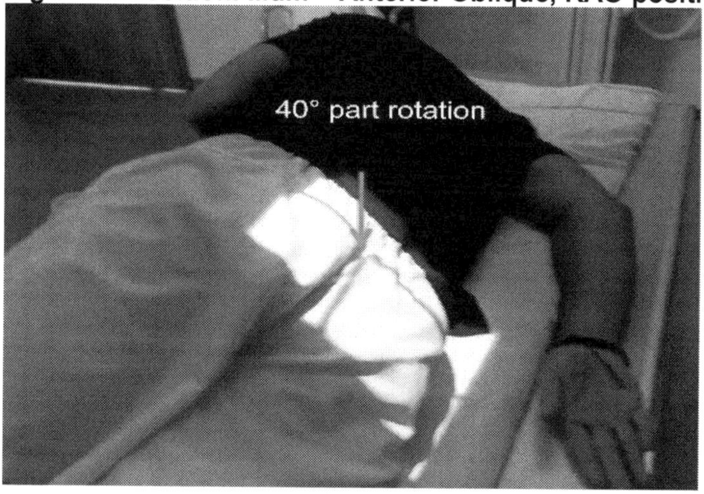

Collimation to include or structures demonstrated

- The acetabulum, femoral head and neck

Image evaluation

- RAO& LAO (anterior oblique) demonstrates ilium profile and proximal end of femur

Fig. 115b. Radiograph. Ilium – Anterior Oblique, RAO position

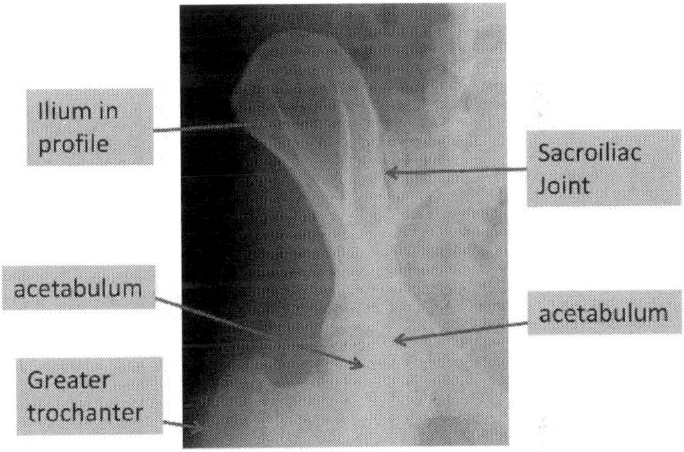

Pelvis–Anteroposterior (AP) projection (bilateral hips)

SID, Technical factors, Shielding

- 40 inches (100 cm). Grid. 80kVp @ 20-30 mAs or AEC.

Gonadal shielding when possible Patient/part position

- Supine

Specific part/body position or rotation

- Legs extended with feet internally rotated to avoid foreshortening of the femoral neck
- Upper border of IR placed cross-wise 1.5-2 inches (3.8–5cm) above the crest

Direction and point of entry of CR

- 2 inches (5cm) above the symphysis pubis or 2inches (5 cm) below the ASIS in the midline.
- If centering for a hip the centering point can be lower to include more of the proximal femur

Fig. 116a. Position. Pelvis- Anteroposterior (AP) projection (bilateral hips)

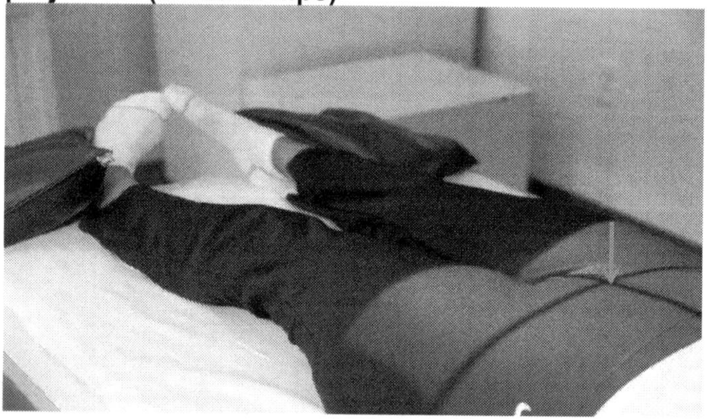

Collimation to include or structures demonstrated

- Entire pelvis from the crest to the symphysis plus the proximal femur

Image evaluation

- Greater trochanter in profile
- Lesser trochanter superimposed by femoral neck
- Femoral neck without foreshortening
- Ischial spine symmetrical
- Sacrum & coccyx midline

Fig. 116b. Radiograph. Pelvis- Anteroposterior (AP) projection (bilateral hips)

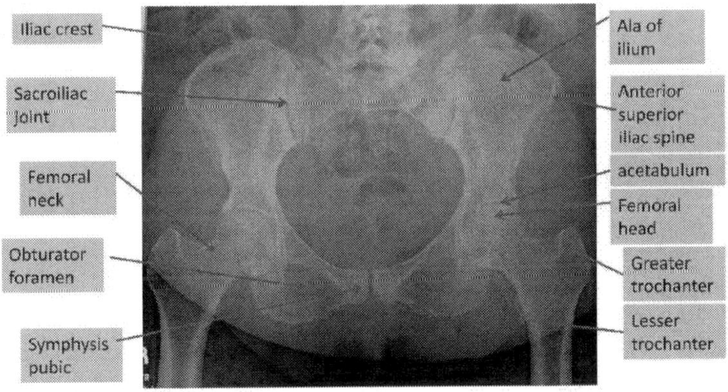

Pelvis–Anteroposterior projection, unilateral or bilateral

Modified Cleaves or frog-leg method

SID, Technical factors, Shielding

- 40 inches (100 cm). Grid. 80kVp @ 20-30 mAs or AEC.

Gonadal shielding when possible Patient/part position

- Patient supine with ASIS equal distance from tabletop on both sides

Specific part/body position or rotation

- Knees flexed; soles of feet together & legs abducted 20-45-degrees from vertical (symmetrical)

Direction and point of entry of CR

- Midline about 1inch (2.5 cm) above the symphysis or 3inches (7.6 cm) below ASIS

Fig. 117a. Position. Pelvis- Anteroposterior projection, bilateral. Modified Cleaves or Frog-leg method

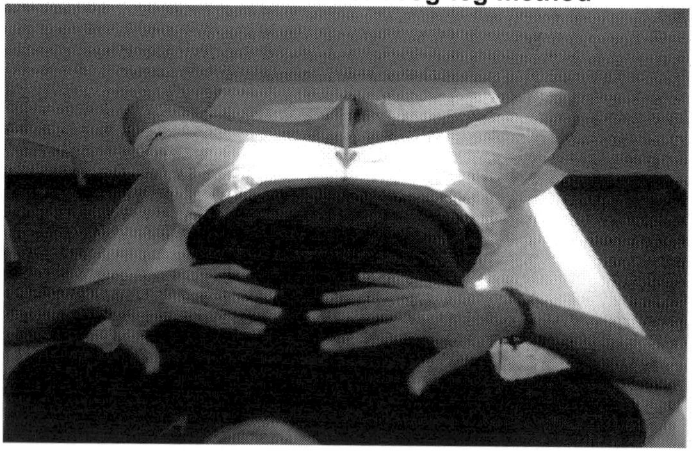

Collimation to include or structures demonstrated

- Entire pelvis from the crest to the symphysis plus the proximal femur

Image evaluation

- Inferior sacrum, ilia, symphysis, acetabulum, femoral neck and head plus greater and lesser trochanters symmetrical in appearance and position
- Size of obturator foramen symmetrical
- Sacrum & coccyx aligned with symphysis

Notes:

- This projection is contraindicated in cases of fracture
- Abduction will affect how the femoral neck is seen.
- With 45 degrees abduction from the vertical, the neck is only partially foreshortened.
- 20 degrees abduction from the vertical gives no foreshortening.
- 70-degree abduction from the vertical give maximum foreshortening of neck but shaft is seen without foreshortening.

Fig. 117b. Radiograph. Pelvis- Anteroposterior projection, bilateral. Modified Cleaves or Frog-leg method

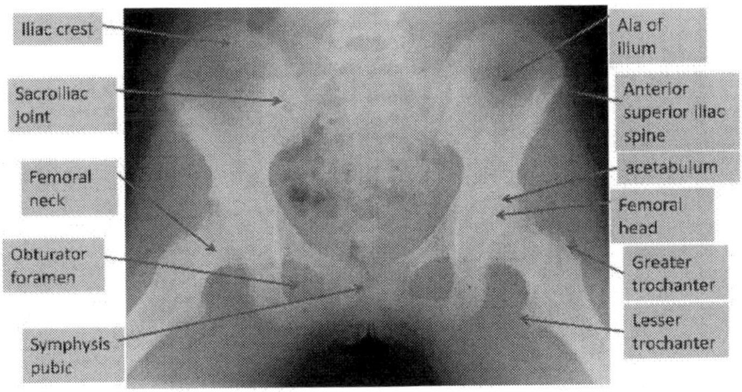

Pelvis–Anteroposterior (AP) axial projection, Outlet
Taylor Method

SID, Technical factors, Shielding

- 40 inches (100 cm). Grid. 80kVp @ 20-30 mAs or AEC. Gonadal shielding when possible

Patient/part position

- Patient supine

Specific part/body position or rotation

- ASIS to tabletop distance and pelvis symmetrical

Direction and point of entry of CR

- CR directed perpendicular to pubic rami
- Males: 20-35° cephalic; 2inches (5 cm) **distal** to superior border of symphysis.
- Females: 30-45° cephalic. 2inches (5 cm) **distal** to upper border of symphysis

Fig. 118a. Position. Pelvis – Anteroposterior (AP) Axial projection, Outlet Taylor method

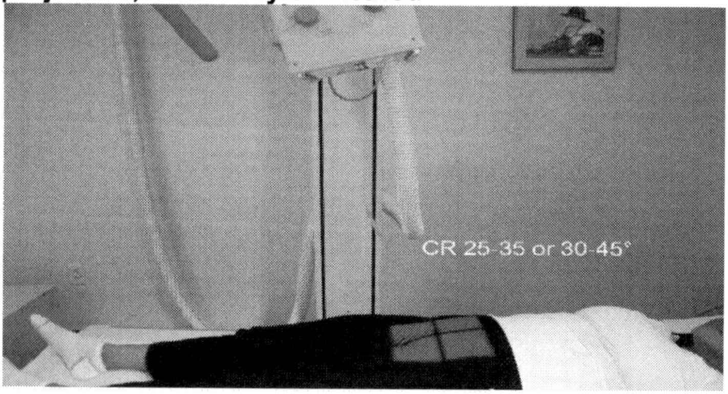

Collimation to include or structures demonstrated

- Lower pelvis

Image evaluation

- Superior and inferior rami of symphysis without foreshortening
- Pubic and ischial bones magnified and pubic bones superimposed on sacrum and coccyx

Fig. 118b. Radiograph. Pelvis – Anteroposterior (AP) Axial projection, Outlet Taylor method

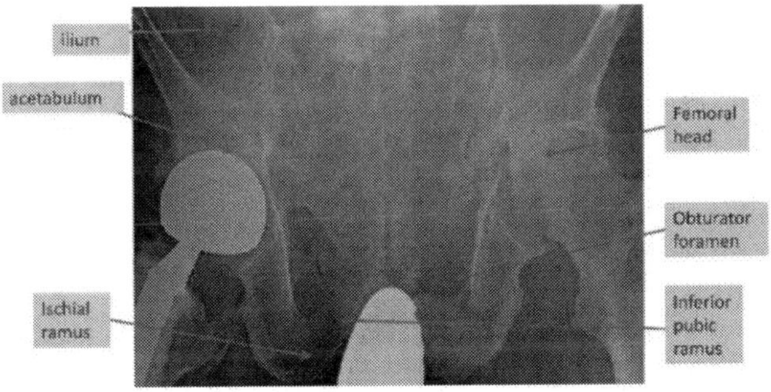

Pelvis–Anteroposterior (AP) axial projection, Inlet
Bridgeman method

SID, Technical factors, Shielding

- 40 inches (100 cm). Grid. 80kVp @ 20-30 mAs or AEC.

Gonadal shielding when possible Patient/part position

- Patient supine

Specific part/body position or rotation

- ASIS to tabletop distance and pelvis symmetrical
- Knees flexed slightly to relieve back strain

Direction and point of entry of CR

- CR to the midpoint at level of the ASIS
- 40° caudal tube angulation

Fig. 119a. Position. Pelvis – Anteroposterior (AP) Axial projection, Inlet

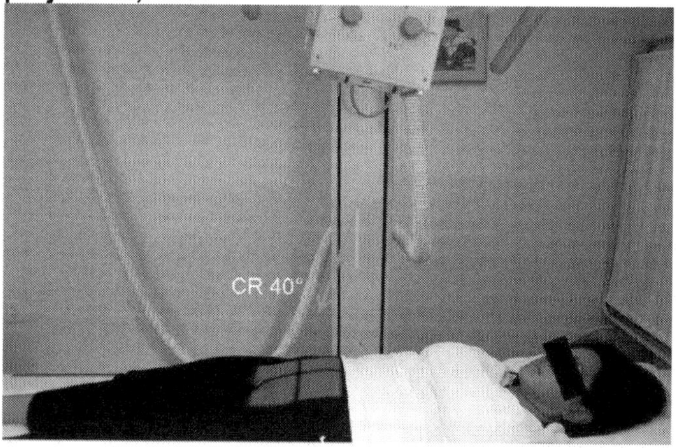

Collimation to include or structures demonstrated

- Lower pelvis

Image evaluation

- Axial projection of pelvic ring or inlet
- Medially superimposed superior and inferior rami of pubic bones
- Nearly superimposed lateral 2/3 of pubic and ischial bones
- Symmetric pubis and ischial spines

Fig. 119b. Radiograph. Pelvis – Anteroposterior (AP) Axial projection, Inlet

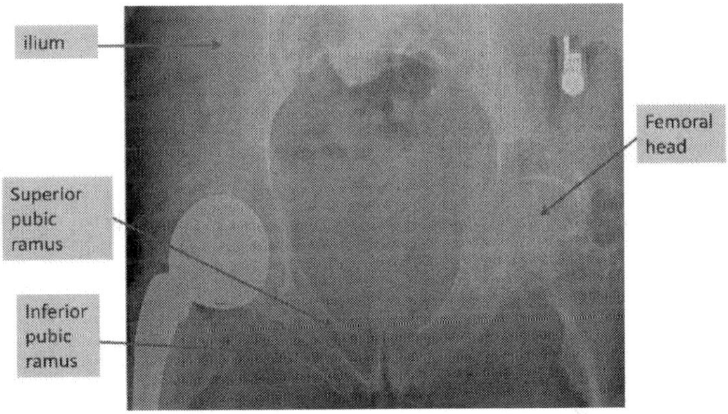

Imaging the Bony Thorax

The thorax includes the sternum, twelve thoracic vertebrae and twelve pairs of ribs.
Sternum has three parts: manubrium, body and xiphoid.
The sternal angle location: at the junction of the manubrium and body.
Suprasternal or jugular notch location: on the superior surface of manubrium
The manubrium of the sternum: articulates with the clavicles on either side

Fig. 120a – Bones of the Thorax

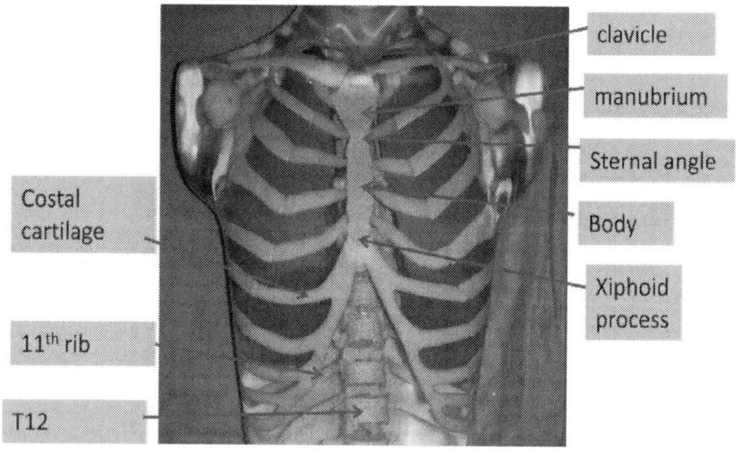

Considerations When Imaging the Sternum

- Imaging is best oblique because of sternum superimposed on the spine in the AP or PA projection
- Patient is rotated to project the sternum on the homogenous heart shadow
- Breathing technique can be used to blur out the rib shadows

Considerations when imaging the sternoclavicular (S/C) joints

- A 10-15-degree patient rotation will demonstrate the downside S/C joint on the anterior oblique position

Considerations when imaging the ribs

- Each rib is attached to a thoracic vertebra.
- There are seven true ribs attaching directly to the sternum and five false ribs, 8-12.
- Ribs 8-10 connect to the costocartilage of the 7th rib. Ribs 11 & 12 are floating ribs with no costocartilage attachment.

Fig. 120b – Sternum

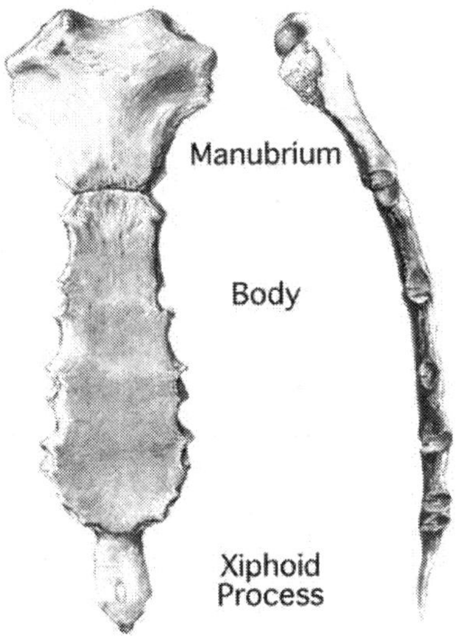

Sternum–Right Anterior Oblique, RAO positions

SID, Technical factors, Shielding

- 40 inches (100 cm). Grid. 75-80kVp @ 10 mAs or AEC. Gonadal shielding

Patient/part position

- Recumbent or erect

Specific part/body position or rotation

- From the PA position, rotate patient 15 –20° just enough to separate the sternum and vertebral column. Thin patient need more rotation than heavier patients
- Arms in swimmers' position or away from body

Direction and point of entry of CR

- Perpendicular to midpoint of sternum at level of T7, 1inch (2.5 cm) to left (lateral to MSP) on elevated side

Fig. 121a. Position. Sternum- Anterior Oblique (RAO) position

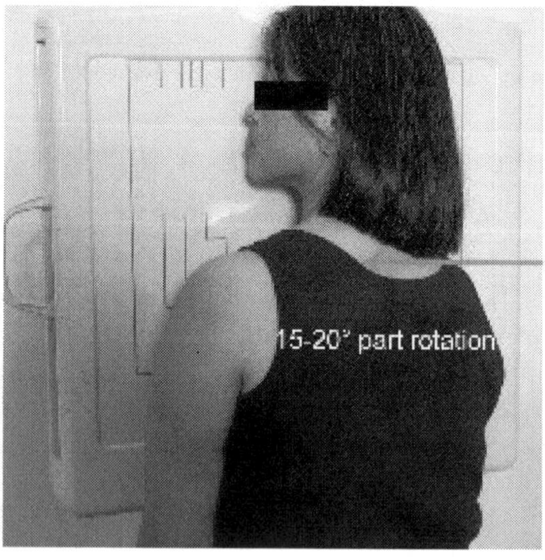

Collimation to include or structures demonstrated

- Entire sternum from jugular notch to xiphoid

Breathing Instructions

- Breath slowly(breathing technique) to blur out the ribs or exposure on arrested expiration

Image evaluation

- Sternum adequately penetrated/bony details clearly seen
- RAO will project the sternum over the heart shadow-provides uniform density
- Sternal ends of clavicles and entire sternum included
- Sternum separated from the vertebral column
- Sternum superimposed over the cardiac shadow
- Right sternoclavicular joint open and left closed

Fig. 121b. Radiograph. Sternum- Anterior Oblique (RAO) position

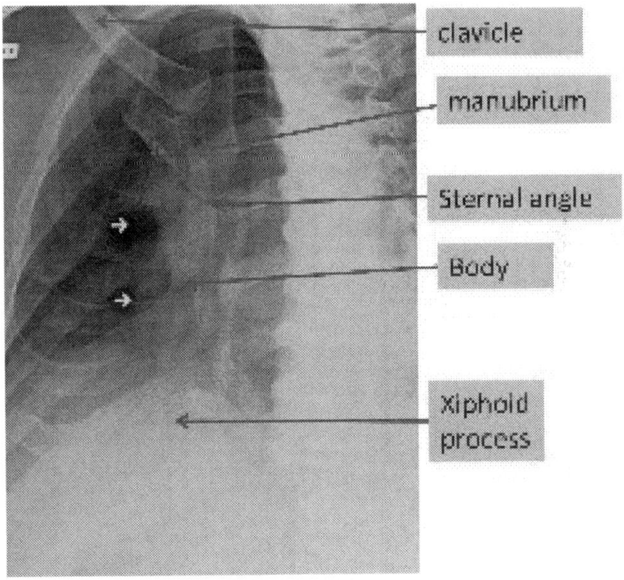

Sternum–Lateral projection, right or left

SID, Technical factors, Shielding

- 72inches (183 cm). Grid. 75-80kVp @ 25mAs or AEC.

Gonadal shielding

Patient/part position

- Erect or lateral recumbent position (or supine with a horizontal beam)

Specific part/body position or rotation

- Arms raised above the head for recumbent position

Direction and point of entry of CR

- Perpendicular CR to midpoint of sternum

Fig. 122a. Position. Sternum – Lateral projection, right

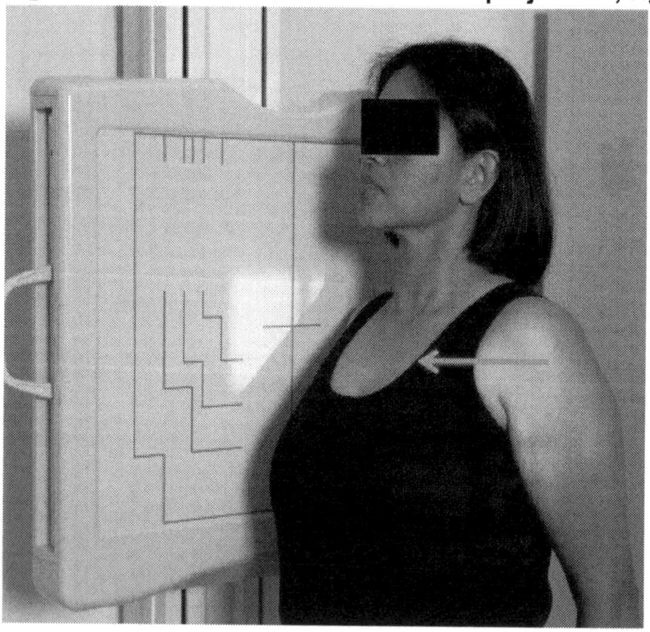

Collimation to include or structures demonstrated

- Place upper border of image plate 11/2 inches above the jugular notch to include the entire sternum

Breathing Instructions

- Exposure on arrested deep inspiration

Image evaluation

- Sternum adequately penetrated
- Entire sternum included
- Sternal ends of clavicles superimposed
- Sternum seen separated from the ribs and soft tissue of shoulder

Fig. 122b. Radiograph. Sternum – Lateral projection, right

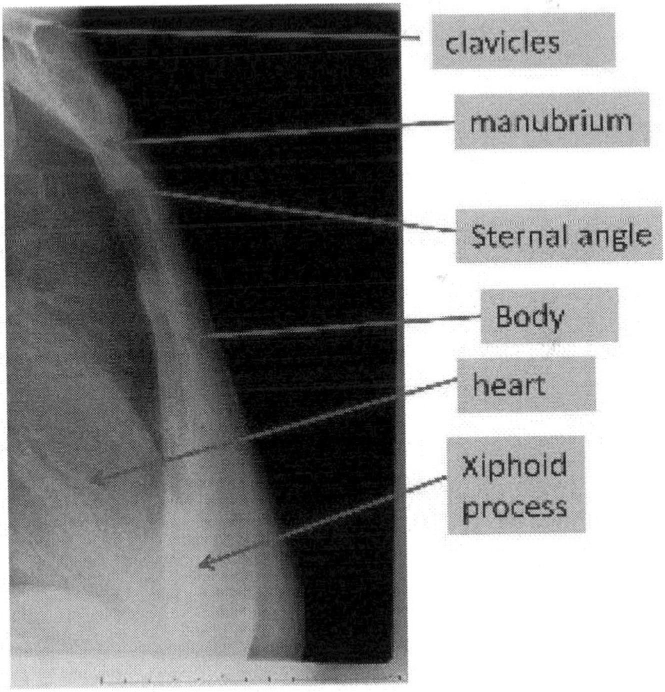

Sternoclavicular (S/C) joint–Posteroanterior (PA) projection

SID, Technical factors, Shielding

- 40 inches (100 cm). Grid. 75-80kVp @ 10mAs or AEC. Gonadal shielding

Patient/part position

- Prone or erect PA

Specific part/body position or rotation

- True PA with MSP perpendicular to IR and shoulder on same transverse plane

Direction and point of entry of CR

- Perpendicular to midpoint of T2 or T3, 3 inches (7.6cm) below vertebral prominence

Fig. 123a. Position. Sternoclavicular (S/C) joint – Posteroanterior (PA) projection

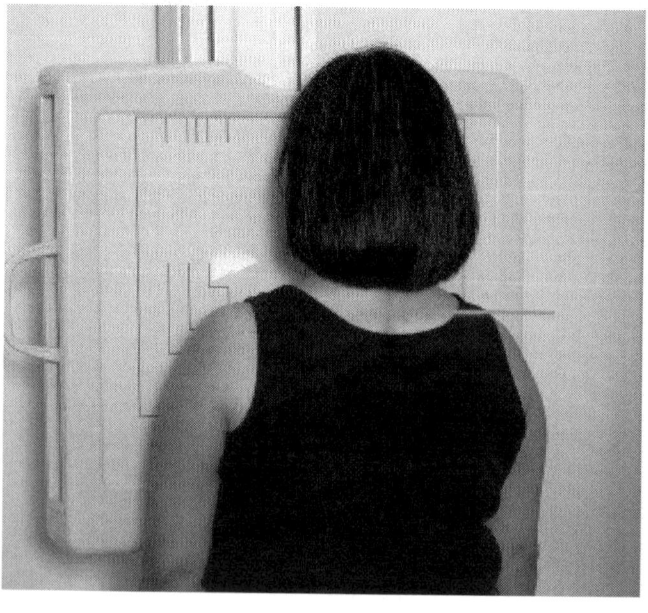

Collimation to include or structures demonstrated

- To include the sternoclavicular joints and medial clavicle

Breathing Instructions

- Arrested expiration–for uniform density

Image evaluation

- Manubrium adequately penetrated with bony details clearly seen
- Sternal ends of clavicles equidistant from vertebral column

Fig. 123b. Radiograph. Sternoclavicular (S/C) joint – Posteroanterior (PA) projection

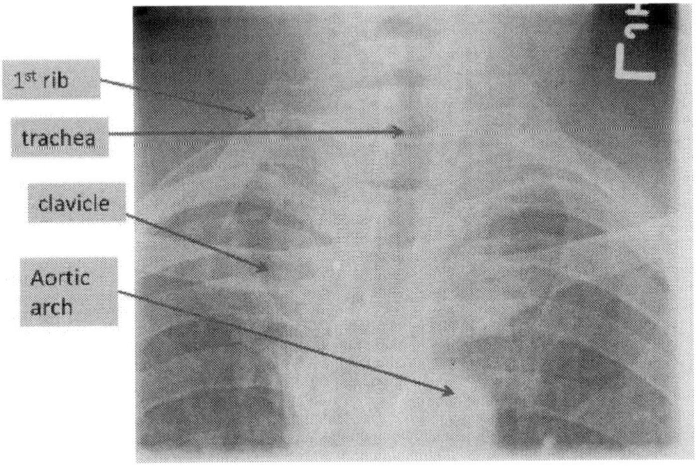

Sternoclavicular (S/C) joint–Anterior Oblique, RAO & LAO positions

SID, Technical factors, Shielding

- 40 inches (100 cm). Grid. 75-80kVp @ 10mAs or AEC. Gonadal shielding

Patient/part position

- Erect or prone with head on pillow

Specific part/body position or rotation

- Rotate patient 10–15 degrees, keeping side of interest nearest table
- Patient rotated only enough to position the interested sternoclavicular joint anterior to the vertebral column (thin patient need more rotation than large)

Direction and point of entry of CR

- Affected joint placed at midline of table
- CR perpendicular to level of T2-3 (jugular notch) or 3inches (7.6 cm) distal to the vertebral prominence (C7) & 1-2inches (2.5-5 cm) lateral to MSP on the UP SIDE

Fig. 124a. Position. Sternoclavicular (S/C) joint- Anterior Oblique (LAO) position

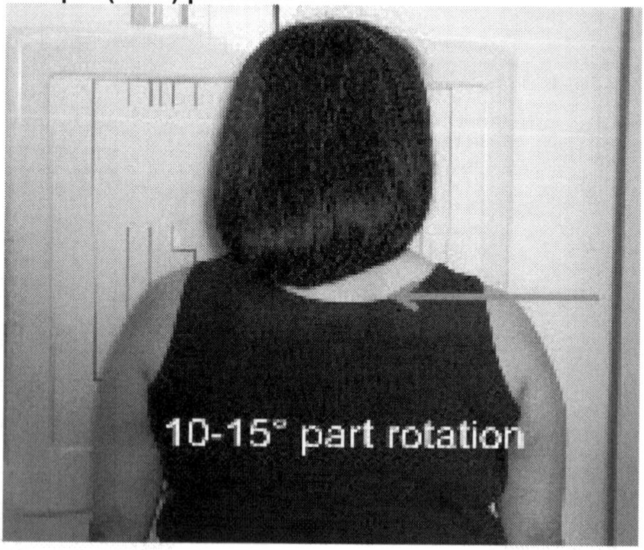

Collimation to include or structures demonstrated

- Sternoclavicular joint nearest the IR open and seen clearly with sternoclavicular joint adequately penetrated

Breathing Instructions

- Exposure on arrested expiration (breath in/breath out/ hold)

Image evaluation

- Sternal ends of clavicles, manubrium and bony detail seen
- Sternoclavicular joint nearest the IR open and seen clearly with sternoclavicular joint adequately penetrated

Note

- Both sides done for comparison

Fig.124b &c. Radiograph. Sternoclavicular (S/C) joint – Anterior Oblique, RAO and LAO positions.

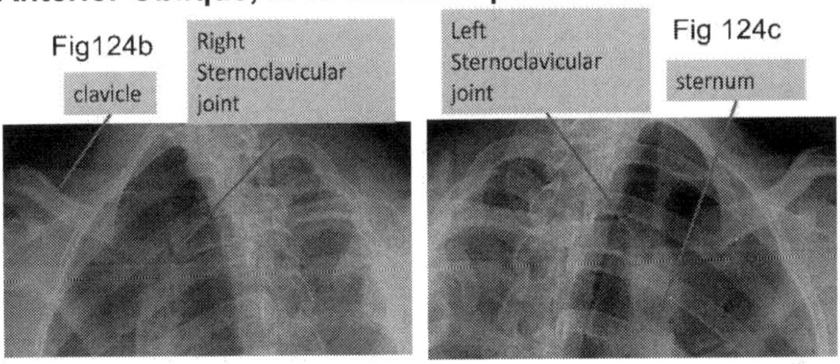

Ribs–Anteroposterior (AP) or Posteroanterior (PA) projection

Upper ribs

SID, Technical factors, Shielding

- 40 inches (100 cm). Grid. 70-75kVp @ 10mAs or AEC. Gonadal shielding

Patient/part position

- Supine or erect (if supine move pillow away from thorax

Specific part/body position or rotation- AP

- Lift chin to prevent superimposition on thorax
- Arm away from body with palms turned outwards to move scapulae away from the ribs
- Shoulder equal distance from the tabletop

Direction and point of entry of CR

- Perpendicular at midpoint level of T7

Fig.125a. Position. Ribs -Anteroposterior (AP) projection-Upper Ribs

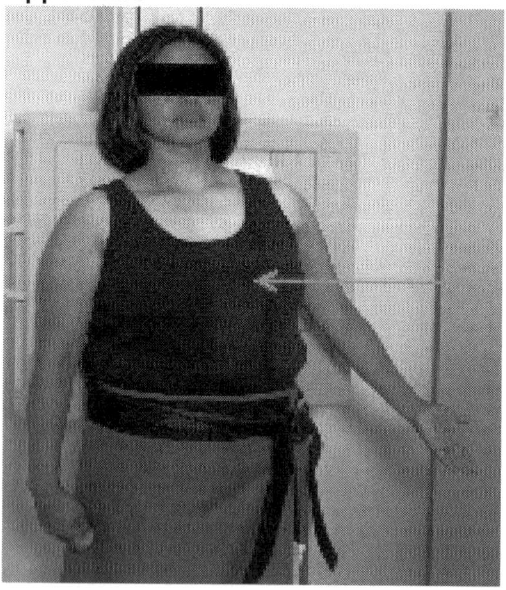

Collimation to include or structures demonstrated

- 2inches (5 cm) above upper top of shoulder
- PA used to demonstrate anterior ribs
- AP used to demonstrate posterior ribs

Breathing Instructions

- Arrested inspiration

Image evaluation

- Upper 1-10th ribs/ sternoclavicular joint (upper ribs)
- Sternoclavicular joints symmetrical
- Ribs are clearly seen without over exposure and through the lungs and heart
- Anterior or posterior ribs

Notes:

- Chest x-ray often performed with rib series to evaluate for collapse lungs or evaluation of lungs prior to surgery
- BB markers can indicate area of interest

Fig.125b. Radiograph. Ribs -Anteroposterior (AP) projection- Upper Ribs

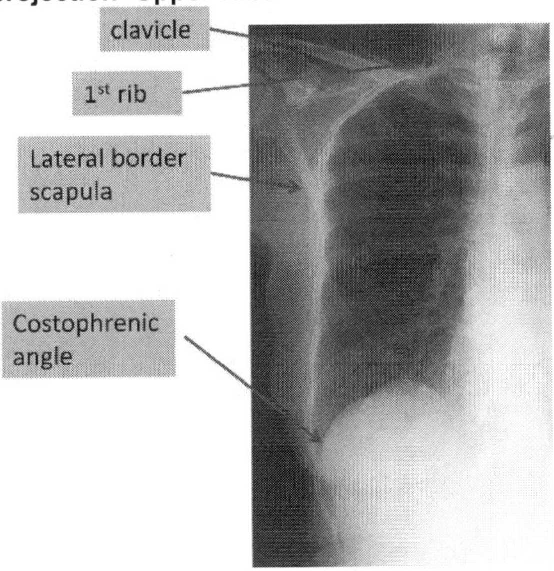

Ribs–Anteroposterior (AP) projection

Ribs lower

SID, Technical factors, Shielding

- 40 inches (100 cm). Grid. 70-80kVp @ 20mAs or AEC. Gonadal shielding

Patient/part position

- Supine or erect (if supine move pillow away from thorax)

Specific part/body position or rotation

- Shoulder equal distance from the tabletop./chin slightly elevated

Direction and point of entry of CR

- Midpoint between xiphoid and crest

Fig.126a. Position. Ribs -Anteroposterior (AP) projection-Lower Ribs

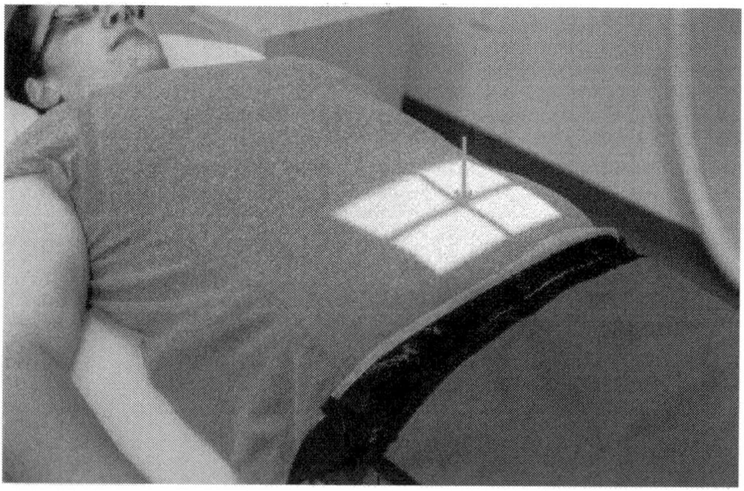

Collimation to include or structures demonstrated

- Top 0.5 of crest and ribs 8 though 12
- Position so lower border of IR at level of iliac crest

Breathing Instructions

- Arrested expiration

Image evaluation

- This position best demonstrates posterior ribs
- Lower 8-12th ribs and top of iliac crest seen through the abdomen
- Spine should not be rotated

Notes:

- Chest x-ray often performed with rib series to evaluate for collapse lungs or to evaluate lungs prior to surgery
- BB markers can indicate area of interest

Fig.126b. Radiograph. Ribs -Anteroposterior (AP) projection- Lower Ribs

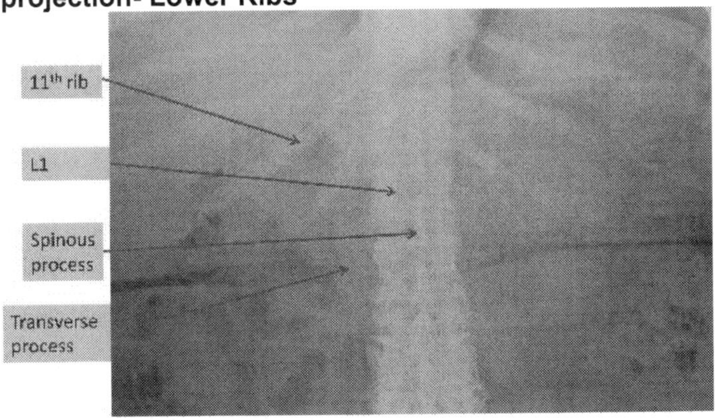

Ribs–Anterior Oblique, LAO or RAO positions

Upper and Lower ribs

SID, Technical factors, Shielding

- 40 inches (100 cm). Grid. 70-75kVp @ 10mAs or AEC.

Gonadal shielding

Patient/part position

- Supine or erect rotate 45°

Specific part/body position or rotation

- Affected side raised and rotated away from the IR
- Arm on affected side raised above head– to move scapula away from rib cage
- Unaffected arm lowered and supported behind thorax

Direction and point of entry of CR

- Upper–perpendicular to midpoint of IR–level of T7
- Lower–T10

Fig. 127a. Position. Ribs- LAO position, Upper or Lower Ribs

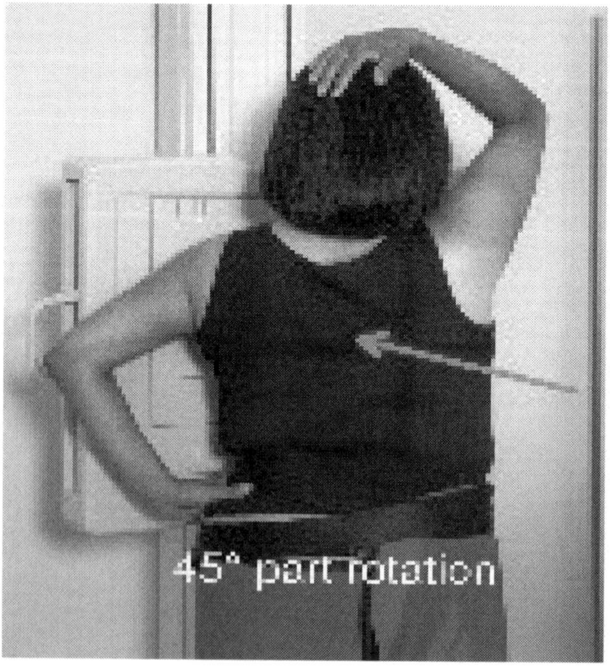

Collimation to include or structures demonstrated

- Upper–upper border of image plate 1 ½ inches (3.8cm) above top of shoulder
- Lower–lower border of image plate at iliac crest to include top of crest

Breathing Instructions

- Upper ribs–exposure during arrested inspiration
- Lower ribs–deep breath/blow it out, exposure during expiration

Image evaluation

- LAO–right side up with the patient PA–show the right axillary ribs and the left vertebral ribs
- RAO–left side up with the patient PA–shows the **left** axillary ribs and the **right** vertebral ribs.
- Ribs 1-10 should be clearly seen through the lungs without overexposure
- Ribs 8-12 seen without overexposure through the abdomen

Fig. 127b. Radiograph. Ribs- LAO position, Upper or Lower Ribs

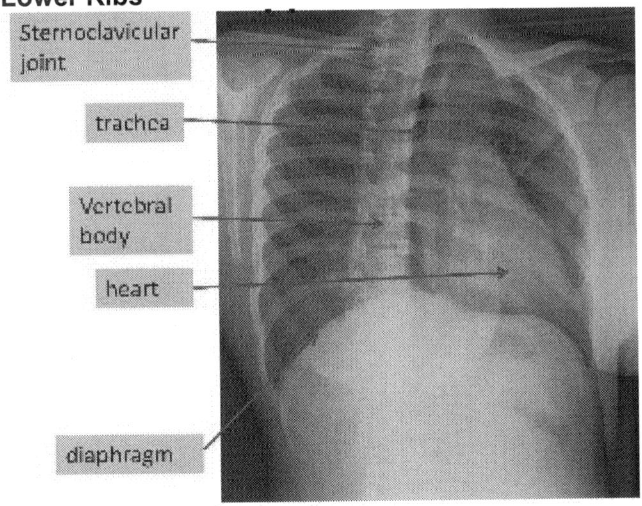

Ribs–Posterior Oblique, LPO or RPO positions

Upper and Lower ribs

SID, Technical factors, Shielding

- 40 inches (100 cm). Grid. 70-75kVp @ 10mAs or AEC.

Gonadal shielding

Patient/part position

- Supine or erect rotate 45°

Specific part/body position or rotation

- For LPO or RPO the affected side is the lowered side
- Hand on the lowered side raised above the head–to move scapula away from rib cage
- Unaffected arm lowered and supported behind thorax

Direction and point of entry of CR

- Upper–perpendicular to midpoint of IR–level of T7
- Lower–at T10

Fig 128a. Position. Ribs- LPO position, upper or lower ribs

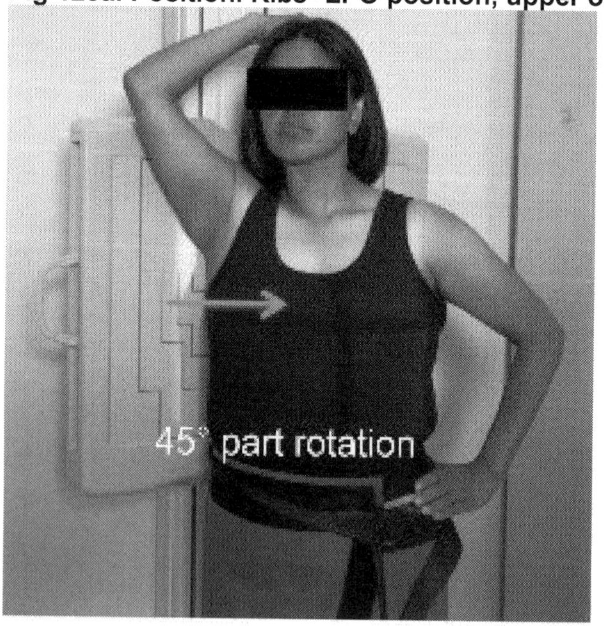

Collimation to include or structures demonstrated

- Upper–upper border of image plate 1 ½ inches (3.8cm) above top of shoulder
- Lower–lower border of image plate at iliac crest (lower ribs)

Breathing Instructions

- Upper ribs–exposure during arrested inspiration
- Lower ribs–deep breath/blow it out, exposure during expiration

Image evaluation

- RPO–right side down with the patient AP–shows the right axillary ribs and the left vertebral ribs
- LPO–Left side down with the patient AP - Shows the **left** axillary ribs and **right** vertebral ribs.
- Ribs 1-10 should be clearly seen through the lungs without overexposure
- Ribs 8-12 seen without overexposure through the abdomen

Fig. 128b. Radiograph. Ribs- LAO position, Upper or Lower Ribs

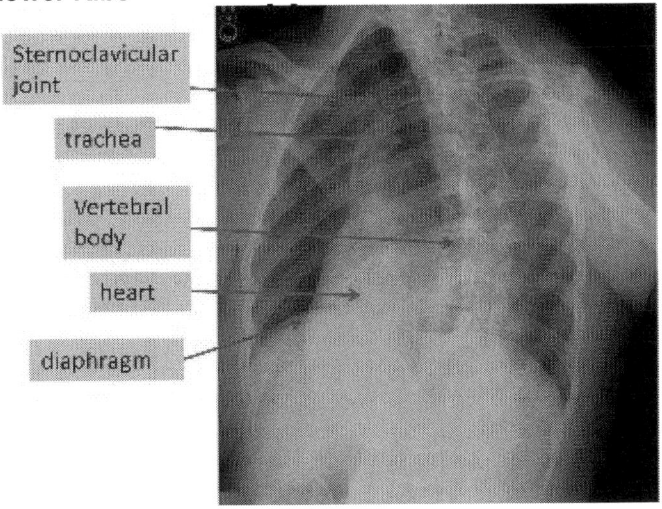

Imaging the Vertebral Spine

Structural differences between cervical, thoracic and lumbar vertebrae

Cervical–seven: C1 C2 & C7 are atypical

- C1–atlas, ring like with no body or spinous process.
- C2–axis, has dens (odontoid) process
- Bifid tips on spinous processes/Transverse foramina/ Concave posterior (lordotic) curve

Thoracic–twelve

- Costal facet on transverse process of T1, T10–T12 for ribs articulation
- Demifacets only on T1, T2–T 9–for the head of a rib
- Convex posterior (kyphotic) curve

Lumbar–five largest vertebral body

- Concave posterior (lordotic) curve

Sacrum–five fused sacral segments, completely fuses between ages 20-30. Before fusion, the segments are separated by cartilage.

- First sacral segment similar to L5
- Base, apex and alae/ Sacral foramina/ Forms posterior pelvis/ Articulates with ilia

Coccyx–three to five fused coccygeal segments
Base of apex/ Cornua (horns)/ Curves anteriorly and inferiorly

Similarities between cervical, thoracic and lumbar vertebrae

- Body or centrum, Vertebral arch,Vertebral foramen,Vertebral canal
- Pedicles, Superior & inferior vertebral notches, Intervertebral foramina
- Laminae, Transverse process, Spinous process, Articular process or zygopophyses, Superior and inferior articular processes

Parts of the Scotty Dog

Fig. 129a.Parts of the "Scotty Dog" – seen on the oblique lumbar spine

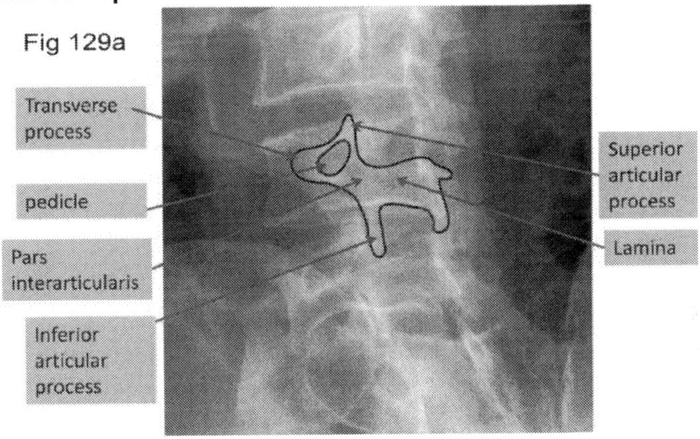

Parts of the "Scotty Dog"
Ear – Superior articular process
Nose- Transverse process
Eye= Pedicle
Neck- Par Interarticularis
Body- Lamina
Foot- Inferior Articular process

Spine Anatomy

Fig. 129b. Labeled Lumbar spine

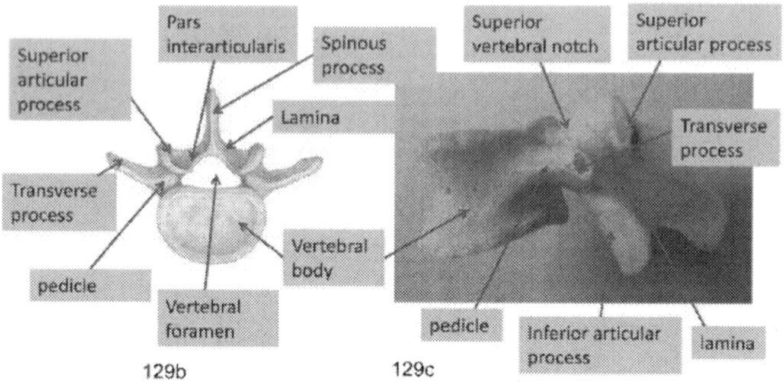

129b 129c

Fig. 129c. Spine Anatomy

Procedural adaptations necessary for radiography of the spine in trauma situations

- Immobilization is critical
- Do not remove any immobilization devices until a negative diagnosis has been confirmed or a physician supervises the removal.
- In cases of suspected neck injuries movement of the head will contribute to spinal cord damage.
- Cross table projections may be necessary

Curves of The Vertebral Column

Primary curves

- Located in thoracic and sacral regions
- Appear in the later stages of fetal development

Secondary curves (compensatory curves)

- Cervical and lumbar curves develop after birth
- Kyphosis–exaggerated thoracic curvature
- Lordosis–exaggerated lumbar curvature
- Scoliosis–abnormal lateral curvature

Spinal Terminology

- Spondylolysis/vertebral ankylosis: Breaking down of a vertebral structure; bony defect occurring in the pars interarticularis area of the lamina. Results in spondylolisthesis
- Spondylolisthesis: body of the lumbar vertebra slip forward over the vertebra beneath it.
- Sacralization: first sacral segment fused to L5. It looks like lumbar spines and larger sacrum.
- Lumbarization: first sacral segment not fused. It looks like a sixth lumber and smaller sacrum
- Herniated nucleus pulposus: "slipped disk" tearing or rupturing of the posterior portion of the **annulus fibrosis** (outer ring of the intervertebral disk) which causes the **nucleus pulposus** (inner semifluid, gelatinous substance which makes up the intervertebral disk) to protrude through the tear and press on the spinal cord or nerve roots

Cervical Spine, C1-2–Anteroposterior (AP) projection
Open mouth method

SID, Technical factors, Shielding

- 1 (100 cm). Grid. 75kVp @ 20mAs or AEC. Gonadal shielding

Patient/part position

- Erect or supine with long axis of patient parallel to long axis of table

Specific part/body position or rotation

- Instruct patient to open mouth as wide as possible
- The line between the lower margin of the upper incisors and the base of the patient's skull (level of mastoid tips) is perpendicular to IR plane

Direction and point of entry of CR

- Perpendicular to C1 through the open mouth

Fig 130a. Position. Cervical Spine, C1-2- Anteroposterior (AP) Projection. Open Mouth method

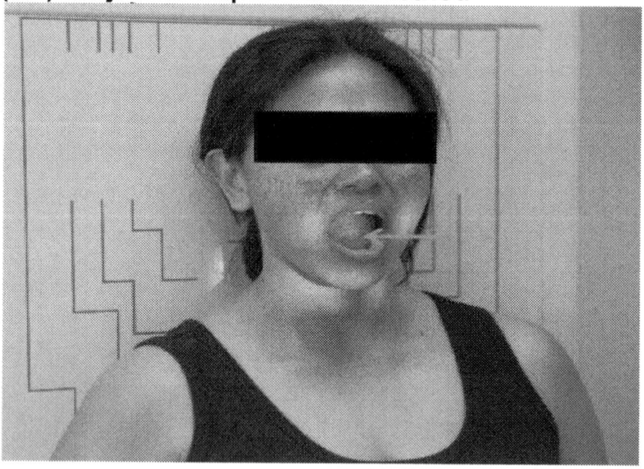

Collimation to include or structures demonstrated

- Atlas (C1) and axis (C2)

Breathing Instructions

- Patient should keep mouth open and say "ah" during the exposure

Image evaluation

- Odontoid process of axis
- C1/C2 articulation seen without superimposition
- Mandibular rami equidistant from odontoid process (dens)

Fig 130b. Radiograph. Cervical Spine, C1-2- Anteroposterior (AP) Projection

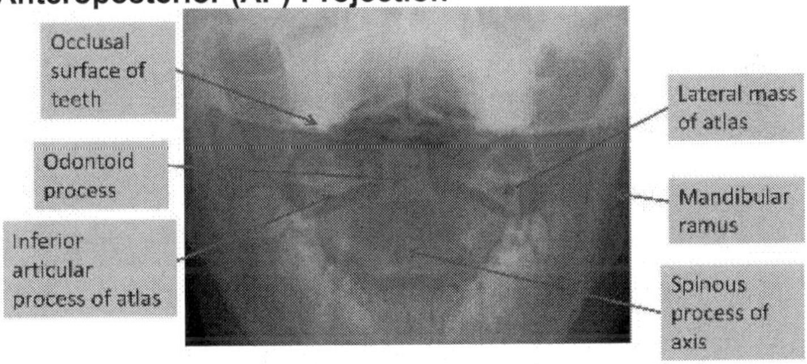

Cervical Spine, C1-2–Anteroposterior (AP) or Posteroanterior (PA) projection

Fuchs (AP) and Judd (PA) Methods

SID, Technical factors, Shielding

- 40 inches (100 cm). Grid. 75kVp @ 10mAs or AEC.

Gonadal shielding

Patient/part position

- Erect, supine or prone
- MSP perpendicular to IR and centered

Specific part/body position or rotation

- Patient AP for the Fuchs and PA for the Judd

AP positioning: Patient's chin elevated (tip of mastoid process and tip of chin vertical). Shoulders on same plane with support under knees for comfort

PA positioning: Neck extended. Chin resting on table. Chin & mastoid tips are vertical, with OML 37-degree to plane of IR. Elbows flexed to support head & shoulder.

Direction and point of entry of CR

- CR perpendicular to midpoint of IR, just distal to chin & passing just distal to the tip of the mastoid process

Fig. 131a. Position. Cervical Spine -C1-2. Anteroposterior (AP), Fuch method

Fig. 131b. Position. Cervical Spine -C1-2. Posteroanterior (PA)Judd method

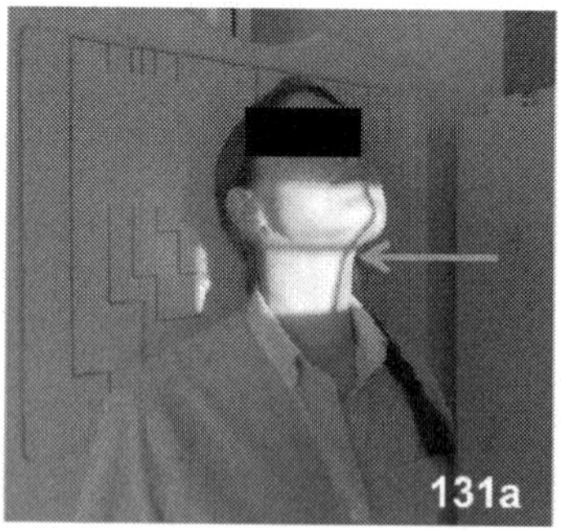

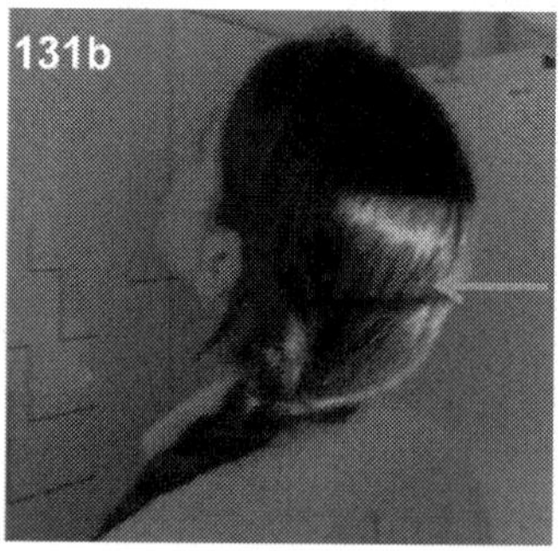

Collimation to include or structures demonstrated

- C1 and C2
- Place the lower border of IR at level of the upper margin of the thyroid cartilage.

Breathing Instructions

- Arrested expiration

Image evaluation

- Odontoid process (dens) within the foramen magnum.
- Symmetry of mandible, cranium & vertebrae.

Note:

- These projections demonstrate the odontoid process when its upper half is not clearly see using the open-mouth position.
- NOT recommended for patient with trauma or degenerative disease

Fig. 131b. Radiograph. Cervical Spine -C1-2. Anteroposterior (AP), Fuch method

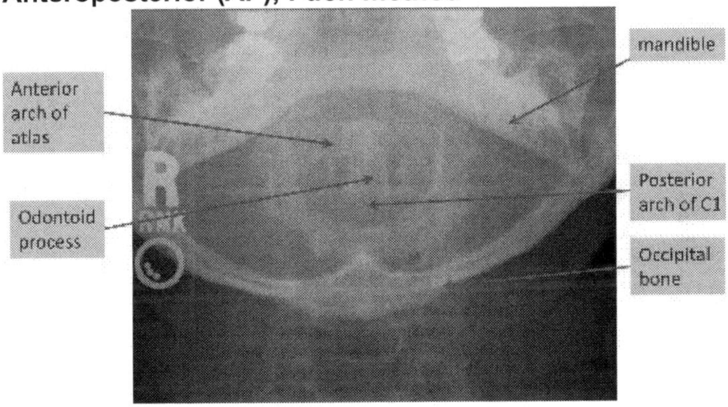

Cervical Spine–Anteroposterior (AP) Axial projection

SID, Technical factors, Shielding

- 40 inches (100 cm). Grid. 70kVp @ 10mAs or AEC. Gonadal shielding

Patient/part position

- Erect vs. supine, depends on patient condition
- Long axis of patient parallel to long axis of table

Specific part/body position or rotation

- Midsagittal plane of patient centered to midline of table with no rotation of head and shoulder

Direction and point of entry of CR

- 15-20 degrees cephalic to thyroid cartilage (C4).Angulation depends on cervical curvature. Generally supine 15-degrees & erect 20-degrees

Fig. 132a. Position. Cervical Spine-Anteroposterior (AP) Axial projection

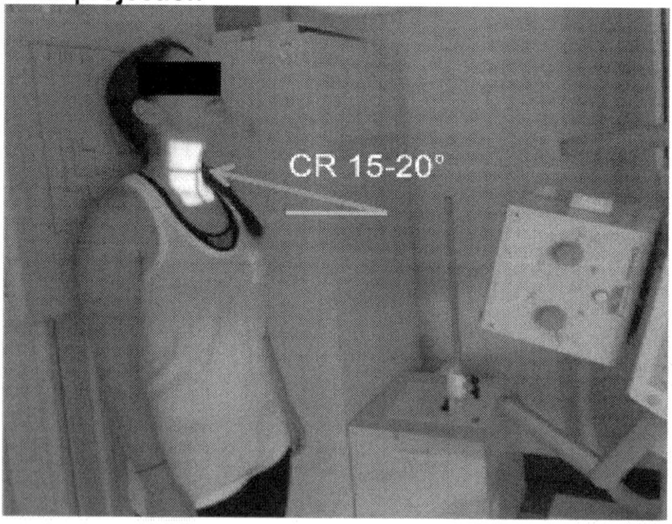

Collimation to include or structures demonstrated

- C3 to T2
- Open intervertebral disk

Breathing Instructions

- Arrested respiration

Image evaluation

- Symmetrical mastoid tips & gonia
- This position best demonstrates C3-T2
- The mandible and occiput superimposed on C1 and most of C2

Fig. 132b. Radiograph. Cervical Spine-Anteroposterior (AP) Axial projection

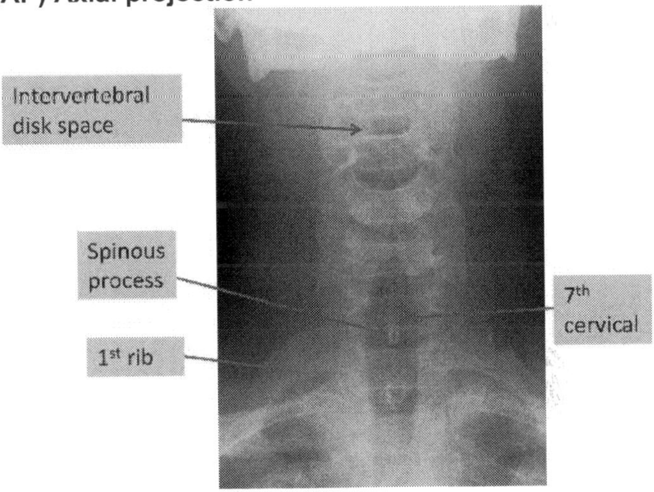

Cervical Spine–Lateral

SID, Technical factors, Shielding

- 60-72inches, 150 to 183 cm. No Grid. 80kVp @ 12mAs. Gonadal shielding

Patient/part position

- Erect
- Supine using a horizontal ray for trauma cases

Specific part/body position or rotation

- Chin up–to prevent superimposition of mandible over anterior arch of C1
- Shoulders rolled back with hands behind body or shoulders depressed by patient holding 5-10 lb. (2.3-4.5 kg) weights

Direction and point of entry of CR

- Perpendicular to C4 at level of thyroid cartilage

Fig. 133a. Position. Cervical Spine – Lateral

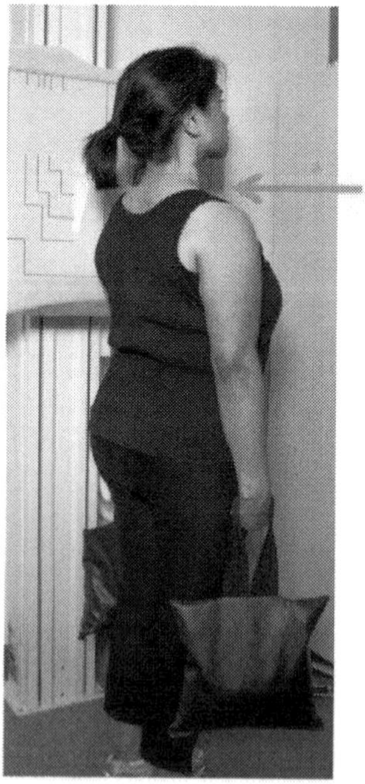

Collimation to include or structures demonstrated

- C1 to T1
- Cervical bodies, articular pillars, zygapophyseal joints of C3- C7 and spinous process

Breathing Instructions

- Arrested expiration to relax shoulders and move them inferiorly

Image evaluation

- C1 through C7 including the C7/T1 junction.
- Superimposed EAMs
- Open zygapophyseal joints and intervertebral disk spaces
- No overlapping of atlas or axis on mandibular rami

Notes

- This position best demonstrates the zygapophyseal joints, spinous process and intervertebral disk spaces
- If C7/T1 junctions not seen a lateral cervicothoracic projection is needed
- **No grid used.** The Air gap will reduce scatter.

Fig. 133b. Radiograph. Cervical Spine – Lateral

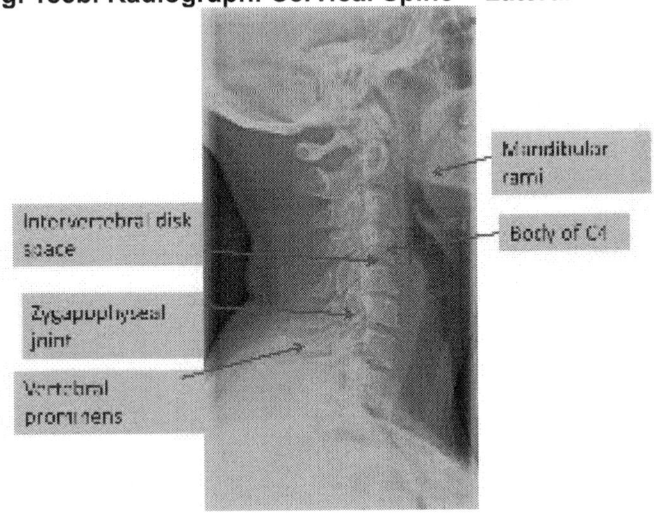

Cervical Spine–Posterior Oblique, LPO and RPO positions

SID, Technical factors, Shielding

- 60-72inches, 150 to 183 cm. No Grid. 80kVp @ 10mAs. Gonadal shielding

Patient/part position

- Patient erect or supine
- Patients positioned AP with back to the IR for the posterior oblique

Specific part/body position or rotation

- From the AP position rotate patient 45-degrees with the left side raised for the RPO
- From the AP position rotate patient 45-degrees with the right side raised for the LPO
- Elevate chin to prevent superimposition of mandible over the spine

Direction and point of entry of CR

- 15-20° cephalic at C4 for the RPO or LPO

Fig. 134a. Position. Cervical Spine – Posterior Oblique, LPO position

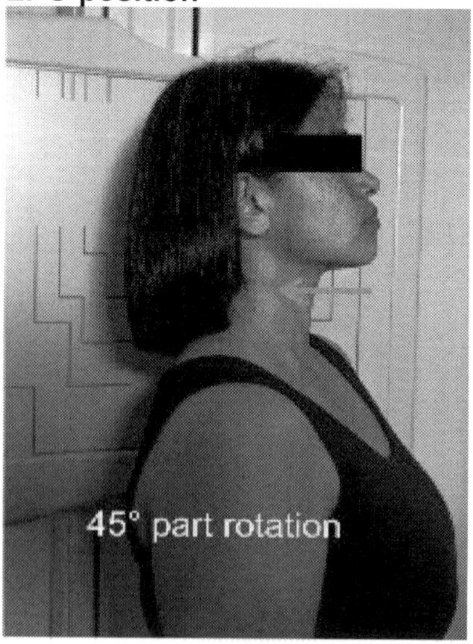

Collimation to include or structures demonstrated

- C1 – T1
- Open intervertebral foramina farthest from the IR

Breathing Instructions

- Arrested respiration

Image evaluation

- No superimposition of the chin or occipital bone on C1 & C2
- Open intervertebral disk spaces & intervertebral foramina
- Posterior oblique, **LPO or RPO** demonstrated the intervertebral foramina furthest from the IR

Fig. 134b. Radiograph. Cervical Spine – Posterior Oblique, LPO position

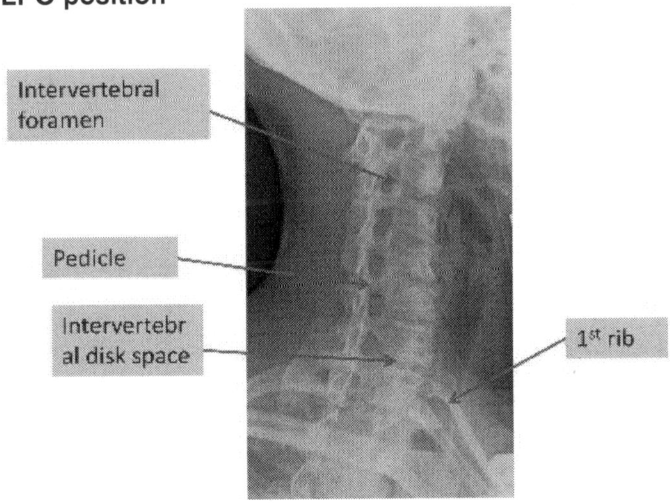

Cervical Spine–Anterior oblique, LAO and RAO positions

SID, Technical factors, Shielding

- 60-72inches, 150 to 183 cm. No Grid. 80kVp @ 10mAs. Gonadal shielding

Patient/part position

- Patient erect or supine
- Patients positioned PA with front to the IR for the anterior oblique

Specific part/body position or rotation

- From the PA position rotate patient 45-degrees with the left side raised for the RAO
- From the PA position rotate patient 45-degrees with the right side raised for the LAO
- Elevate chin to prevent superimposition of mandible over the spine

Direction and point of entry of CR

- 15-20° cephalic at C4 for the RPO or LPO

Fig. 135a. Position. Cervical Spine – Anterior Oblique, RAO position

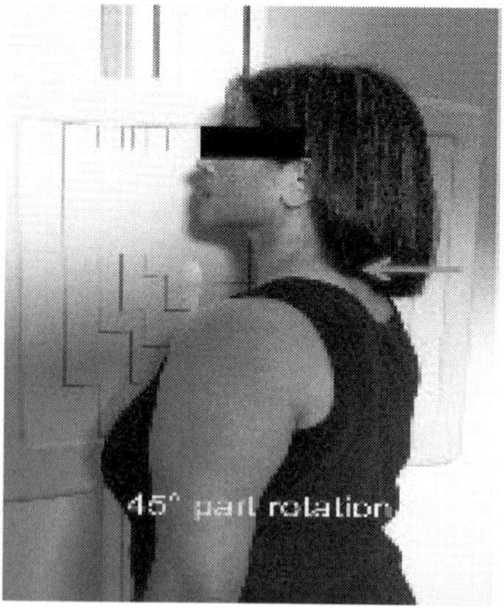

Collimation to include or structures demonstrated

- C1 – T1
- Open intervertebral foramina closest to the IR

Breathing Instructions

- Arrested respiration

Image evaluation

- No superimposition of the chin or occipital bone on C1 & C2
- Open intervertebral disk spaces & intervertebral foramina
- Anterior oblique, **LAO or RAO** demonstrates intervertebral foramina and pedicles closest to IR

Fig. 135. Radiograph. Cervical Spine – Anterior Oblique, RAO position

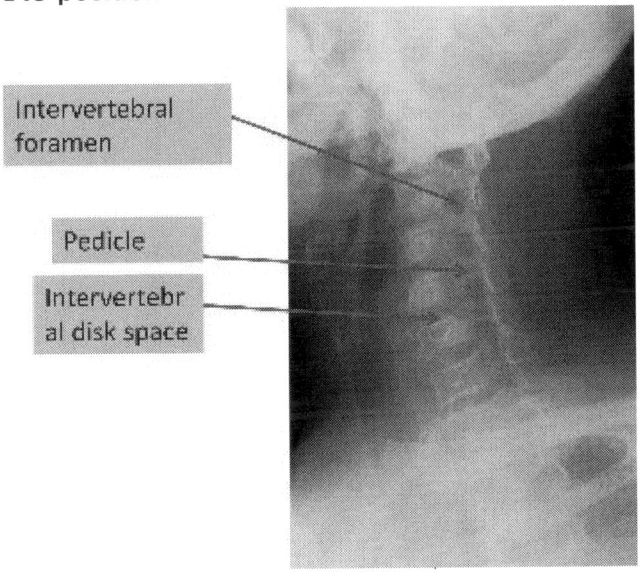

Cervical Spine–Hyperflexion Lateral

SID, Technical factors, Shielding

- 60-72inches, 150 to 183 cm. No Grid. 80kVp @ 10mAs.

Gonadal shielding

Patient/part position

- Erect only

Specific part/body position or rotation

- Bent forward, chin as close to chest as possible

Direction and point of entry of CR

- C4 at level of uppermost part of thyroid cartilage

Fig. 136a.Position. Cervical Spine-Hyperflexion Lateral

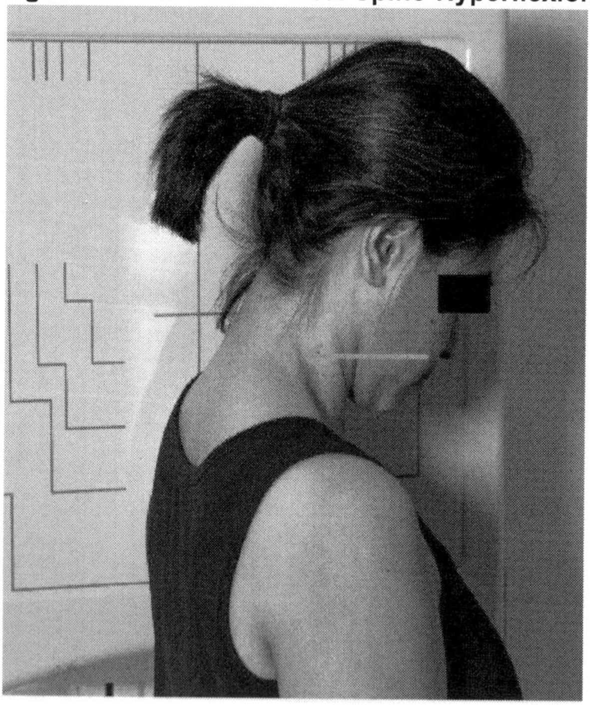

Collimation to include or structures demonstrated

- True lateral of C1 to C7

Breathing Instructions

- Arrested respiration

Image evaluation

- Normal anteroposterior movement will be demonstrated
- Spinous process separated
- Body of mandible vertical and angled to lower corner of IR
- Zygapophyseal joint demonstrated
- EAMs should be superimposed

Fig. 136b. Radiograph. Cervical Spine-Hyperflexion Lateral

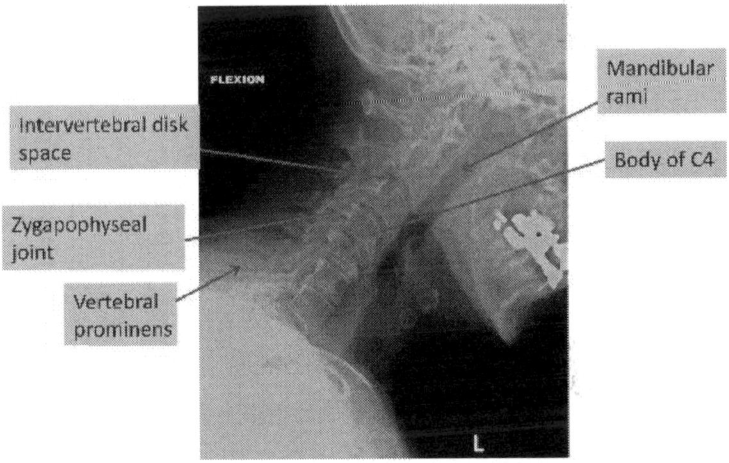

Cervical Spine–Hyperextension Lateral

SID, Technical factors, Shielding

- 60-72inches, 150 to 183 cm. No Grid. 80kVp @ 10mAs.

Gonadal shielding

Patient/part position

- Erect only

Specific part/body position or rotation

- Head bent backward with chin elevated as much as possible

Direction and point of entry of CR

- C4 at level of uppermost part of thyroid cartilage

Fig.137a. Position. Cervical Spine- Hyperextension Lateral

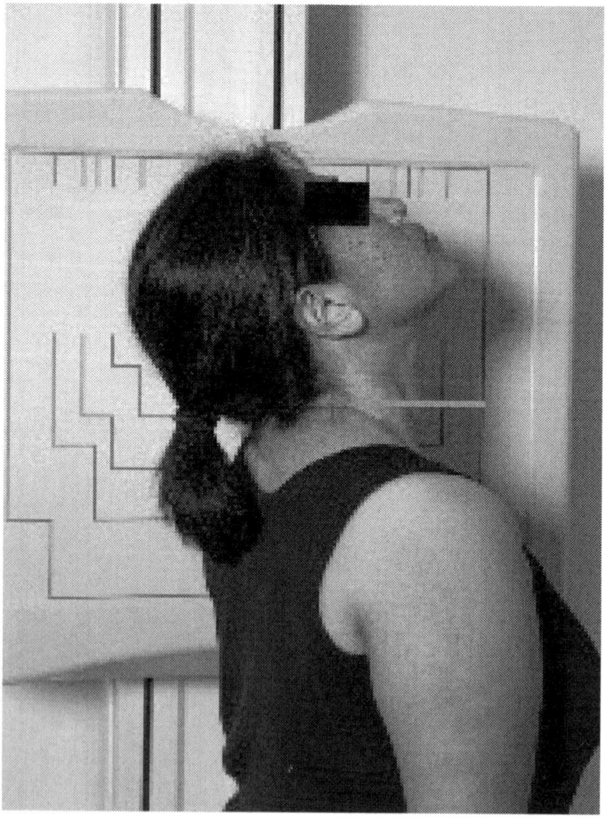

Collimation to include or structures demonstrated

- True lateral of C1 to C7

Breathing Instructions

- Arrested respiration

Image evaluation

- EAMs should be superimposed
- Spinous process together
- Body of mandible at almost 45° angle with horizontal and pointing to upper corner of IR
- Intervertebral disk

Fig.137b. Radiograph. Cervical Spine- Hyperextension Lateral

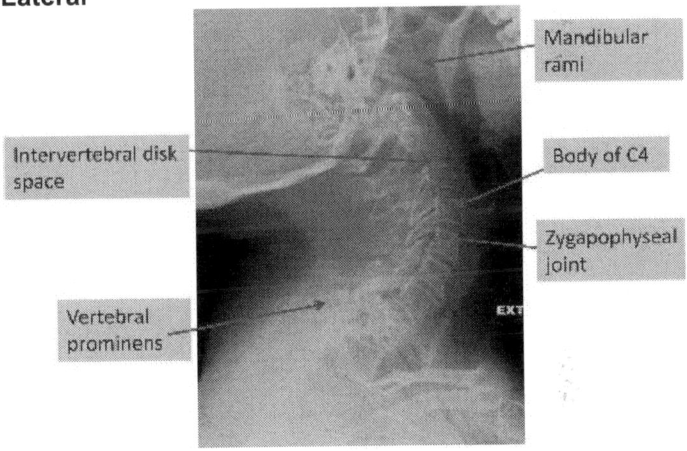

Cervical Spine–Lateral Cervicothoracic (C7-T1) region

Swimmers method

SID, Technical factors, Shielding

- 40 inches (100 cm). Grid. 75-80 kVp @ 10mAs or AEC. Gonadal shielding

Patient/part position

- Recumbent, supine or erect
- Supine using a horizontal bean for trauma cases.
- Erect and recumbent with patient in the lateral position

Specific part/body position or rotation

- Depress the shoulder furthest from the IR & raise the arm nearest the IR above the head

Direction and point of entry of CR

- CR horizontal through T1, 2 inches (5 cm) below the jugular notch
- Use 3-5° caudal angulation through T1 if patient is unable to depress the shoulder away from the IR

Fig. 138a. Position. Cervical Spine – Lateral Cervicothoracic (C7-T1) region. Swimmers method

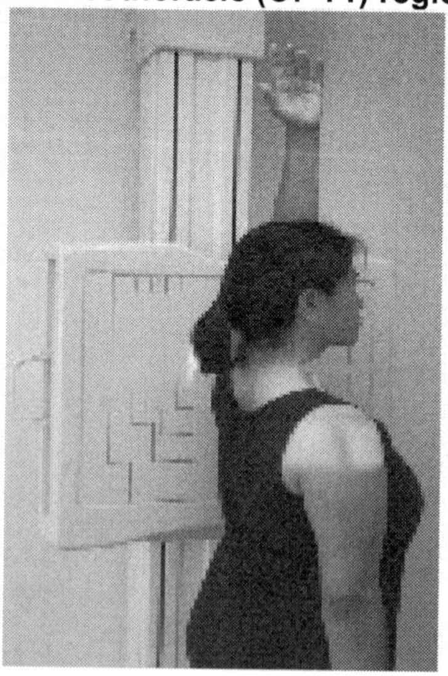

Collimation to include or structures demonstrated
Breathing Instructions

- Arrested expiration

Image evaluation

- Humeral heads separated
- C7/T1
- Vertebral bodies should appear box-like
- This position best demonstrates C7T1 junction and entire C7

Fig. 138b. Radiograph. Cervical Spine – Lateral Cervicothoracic (C7-T1) region. Swimmers method

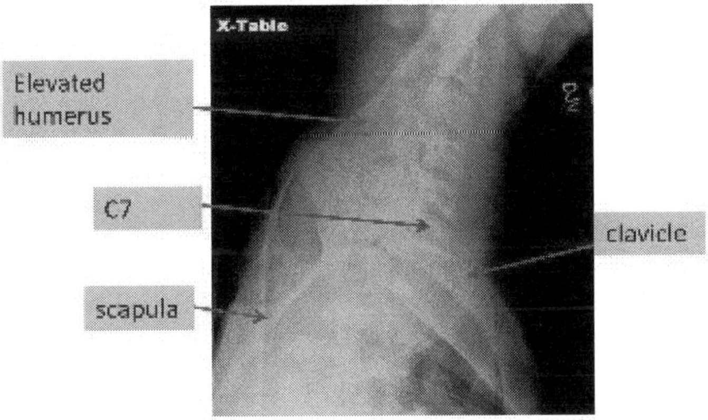

Thoracic spine–Anteroposterior (AP) projection

SID, Technical factors, Shielding

- 40 inches (100 cm). Grid. 80kVp @ 10mAs or AEC. Gonadal & Breast shielding

Patient/part position

- Erect or supine. Erect for patients with severe kyphosis and unable to lie supine

Specific part/body position or rotation

- Upper thoracic positioned to the anode end tube to minimize anode heel effect
- Weight equally distributed to avoid spine rotation
- If supine, flex knees with plantar surface of feet flat on table to reduce dorsal kyphosis

Direction and point of entry of CR

- Perpendicular to T7

Fig. 139a. Position. Thoracic spine- Anteroposterior (AP) projection

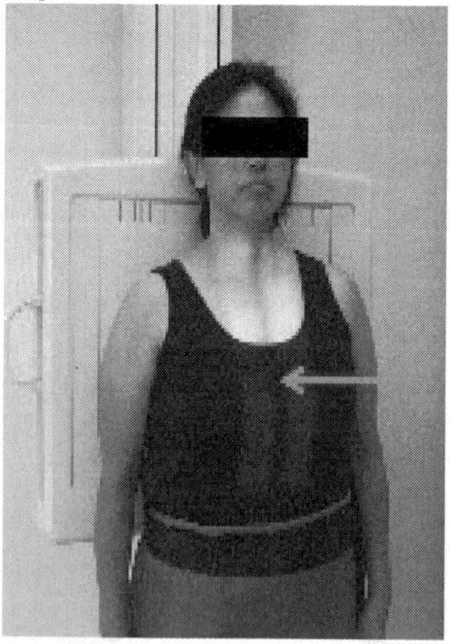

Collimation to include or structures demonstrated

- Top edge of IR at least 1.5-2 inches (3.8-5cm) above the top of shoulders
- C7 – L1, intervertebral disk space, transverse process, costovertebral articulations

Breathing Instructions

- Breathing technique or arrested expiration

Image evaluation

- C7-L1 demonstrated
- Spinous processes in midline of vertebrae
- Sternoclavicular joints symmetrical

Fig. 139a. Position. Thoracic spine- Anteroposterior (AP) projection

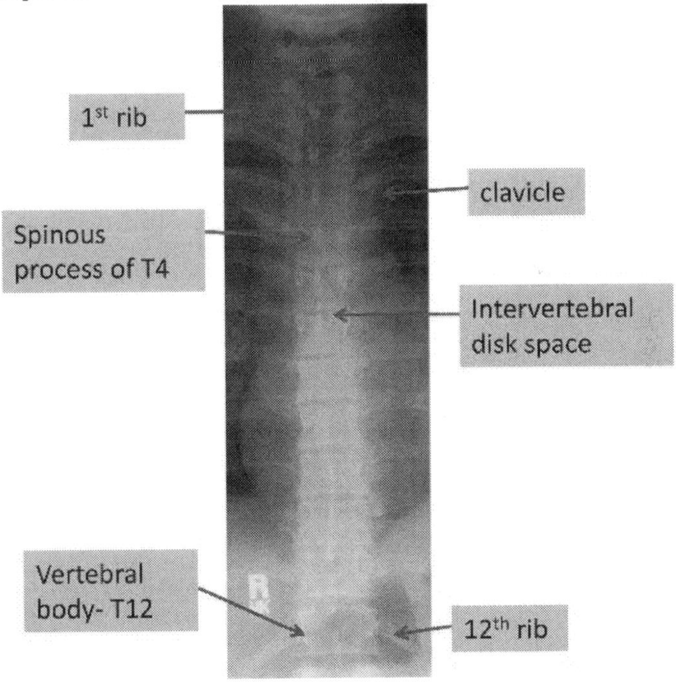

Thoracic Spine–Lateral projection

SID, Technical factors, Shielding

- 40 inches (100 cm). Grid. 90kVp @ 10mAs or AEC.

Gonadal & Breast shielding

Patient/part position

- Either erect or supine. Left lateral is preferred to minimize magnified of the heart. The magnified heart will overlap the spine.

Specific part/body position or rotation

- Hands raised to elevate ribs, allowing ribs to clear the intervertebral foramina
- Pillow under patient's head & radiolucent support under waist and lower thoracic if needed to keep long axis of spine parallel to long axis of table.

Direction and point of entry of CR

- Perpendicular to IR at T7, the inferior angle of scapula
- Cephalic angulation if needed to direct CR perpendicular to the long axis of spine. Generally 10° for females and 15° for males because of greater shoulder width

Fig. 140a. Position. Thoracic Spine – Lateral projection

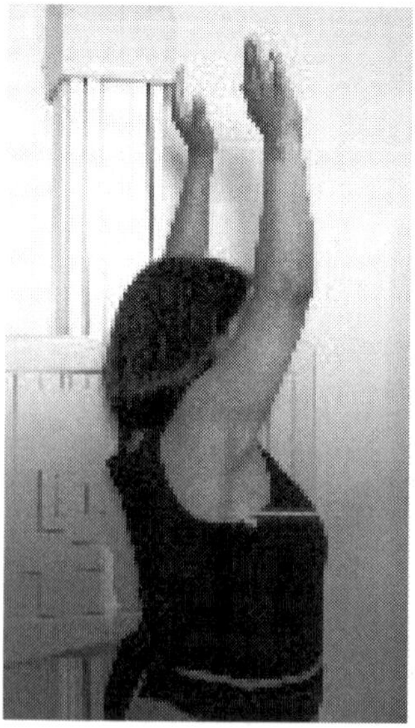

Collimation to include or structures demonstrated

- Top of IR placed 1.5 to 2 inches (3.8-5cm) above shoulder
- This position best demonstratesT3/4 to L1, because the upper thoracic are obscured by the shoulders
- Intervertebral foramina and spinous process demonstrated

Breathing Instructions

- Breathing technique to blur ribs or arrested expiration to provide even density

Image evaluation

- Box like vertebral bodies
- Open intervertebral disk spaces
- Superimposed posterior ribs

Note:

- Lead rubber placed on the table behind the patient will improved image contrast by reducing scatter to the IR

Fig 140 b. Radiograph. Thoracic Spine-Lateral. Breathing Technique

Fig. 140c. Radiograph. Thoracic Spine-Lateral. Non-Breathing Technique

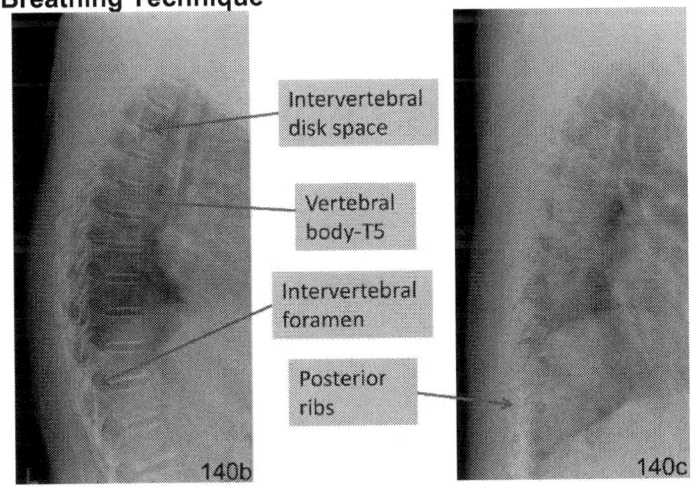

Thoracic Spine– Posterior Oblique, LPO and RPO positions

Or **Anterior Oblique, LAO and RAO position**

SID, Technical factors, Shielding

- 40 inches (100 cm). Grid. 80kVp @ 10mAs or AEC.

Gonadal & Breast shielding

Patient/part position

- Erect or supine, weight equally distributed if standing

Specific part/body position or rotation

- 70° angle between the coronal plane and IR
- Posterior oblique (LPO or RPO) raise the arm away from the IR and support. Flex elbow of arm closest to IR with back of hand resting on hip.

Direction and point of entry of CR

- Perpendicular to IR at T7, 3-4 inches (7.6-10 cm) inferior to jugular notch)

Fig 141a. Position. Thoracic Spine – Posterior Oblique, LPO position

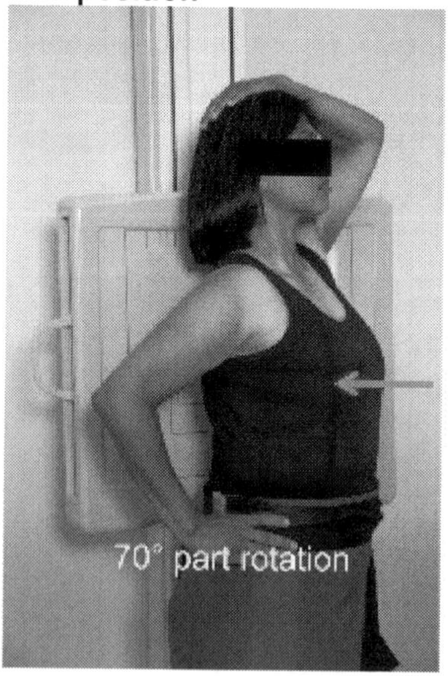

Collimation to include or structures demonstrated

- Upper border of IR 1.5-2 inches (3.8-5 cm) above the shoulders

Breathing Instructions

- Suspend expiration

Image evaluation

- Posterior oblique, LPO or RPO shows thoracic zygapophyseal joints farthest from IR.
- Anterior oblique, LAO or RAO shows joints closest to IR.

Fig 141b. Radiograph. Thoracic Spine – Posterior Oblique, LPO position

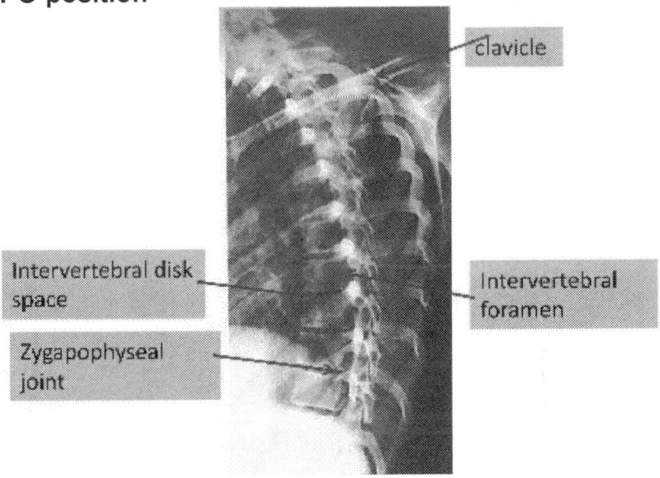

Lumbar Spine–Anteroposterior (AP) or Posteroanterior (PA) projection

SID, Technical factors, Shielding

- 40 inches (100 cm). Grid. 85kVp @ 20mAs or AEC.

Gonadal shielding

Patient/part position

- Supine or erect. Patient with acute back pain may prefer to stand or image PA

Specific part/body position or rotation

- AP with knees flexed to reduce lordotic curve and place divergent rays parallel to intervertebral disk spaces–reducing distortion of bodies.
- PA gives increase OID but places intervertebral disk parallel to divergent beams
- PA will help reduce radiation dose on obese patients

Direction and point of entry of CR

- CR directed to L3, 1-1.5 inches (2.5-3.8 cm) above the crest when imaging lumbar spine or directed to L4-5 at the level of the crest when imaging the lumbosacral spine

Fig. 142a. Position. Lumbar Spine- Anteroposterior (AP) projection

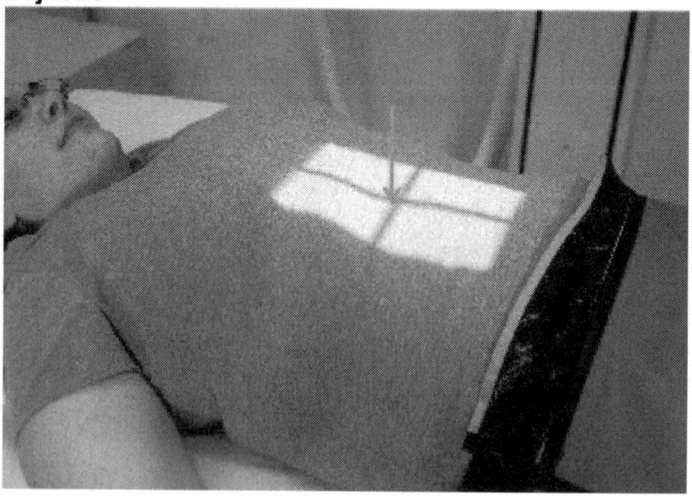

Collimation to include or structures demonstrated

- T12-S2 including the intervertebral disk spaces, laminae, spinous and transverse process

Breathing Instructions

- Arrested expiration

Image evaluation

- Iliac crest symmetrical & S/I joint equidistant from vertebral column
- Spinous process seen in midline of the vertebrae and middle of IR
- This position best demonstrates bodies, intervertebral disk spaces, laminae, spinous and transverse processes

Note:

- 48inches (122 cm) SID can be used to reduce distortion and open intervertebral disk spaces
- Both sacrum and coccyx demonstrated when imaging the lumbosacral spine

Fig. 142b. Radiograph. Lumbar Spine- Anteroposterior (AP) projection

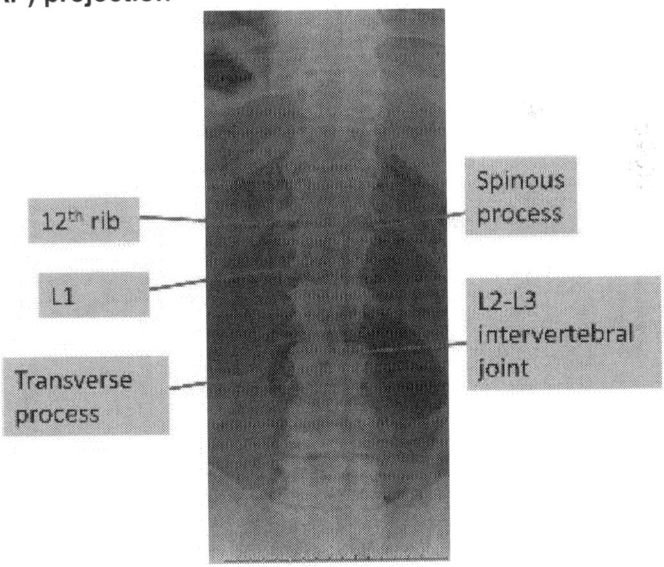

Lumbar Spine–Posterior oblique, RPO and LAO positions

SID, Technical factors, Shielding

- 40 inches (100 cm). Grid. 85kVp @ 20mAs or AEC. Gonadal shielding

Patient/part position

- Supine or erect
- One arm raised and one lowered, patient oblique
- If recumbent, one leg flexed one and one straight

Specific part/body position or rotation

- Support the shoulder, thorax, upper thigh and knee on the raised side
- From the AP position rotate patient 45-degrees with the left side raised for the RPO
- From the PA position rotate patient 45-degrees with the right side raised for the LPO

Direction and point of entry of CR

- 2 inches (5cm) medial to ASIS of raised sided

Fig. 143a Position. Lumbar Spine – Posterior Oblique, LPO position

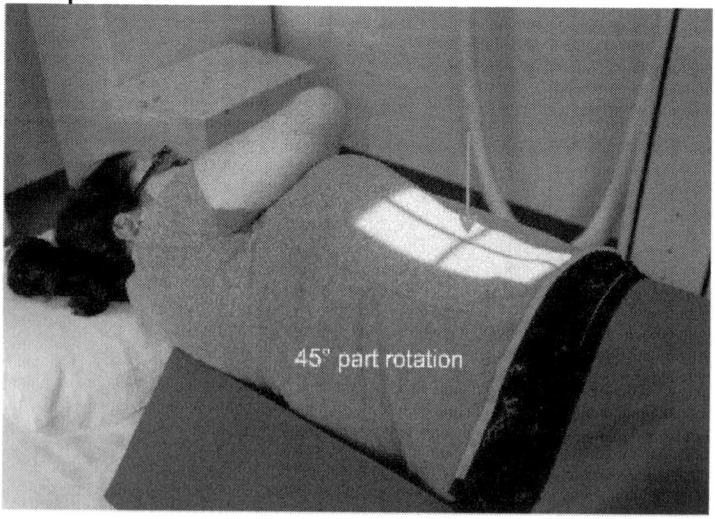

Collimation to include or structures demonstrated

- Zygapophyseal joints, appearance of the 'Scottie dog'

Breathing Instructions

- Arrested expiration

Image evaluation

- Ilia symmetrical on both obliques
- Pedicles demonstrated in the middle of the vertebral body
- Parts of the "Scotty dog" clearly demonstrated.
- The posterior oblique shows the joints closest to the IR

Notes:

- If not enough patient rotation, angle between MCP & IR less than 45– pedicles seen on anterior part of vertebral body
- If too much patient rotation, angle between MCP & IR greater than45– pedicle seen on posterior part of vertebral body

Fig. 143b Radiograph. Lumbar Spine – Posterior Oblique, LPO position

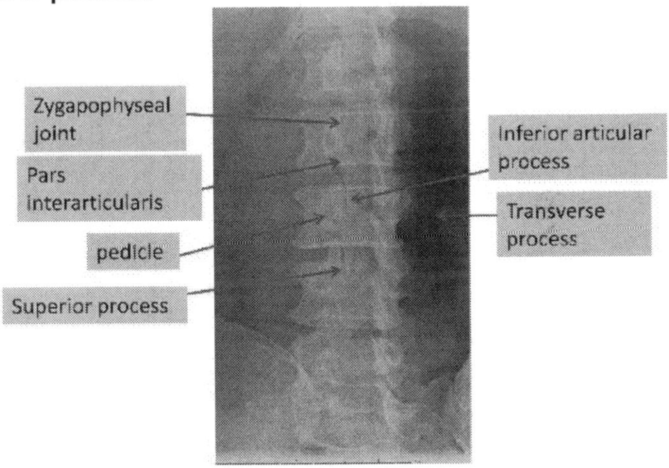

Lumbar Spine–Anterior oblique, RAO and LPO position

SID, Technical factors, Shielding

- 40 inches (100 cm). Grid. 85kVp @ 20mAs or AEC.

Gonadal shielding

Patient/part position

- Prone or erect
- One arm raised and one lowered, patient oblique
- If recumbent, one leg flexed one and one straight

Specific part/body position or rotation

- Support the shoulder, thorax, upper thigh and knee on the raised side
- From the PA position rotate patient 45-degrees with the left side raised for the RAO
- From the AP position rotate patient 45-degrees with the right side raised for the LPO

Direction and point of entry of CR

- Through L3, 1-1.5 inches (2.5-3.8 cm) above the iliac crest

Fig. 144a Position. Lumbar Spine – Anterior Oblique, LAO position

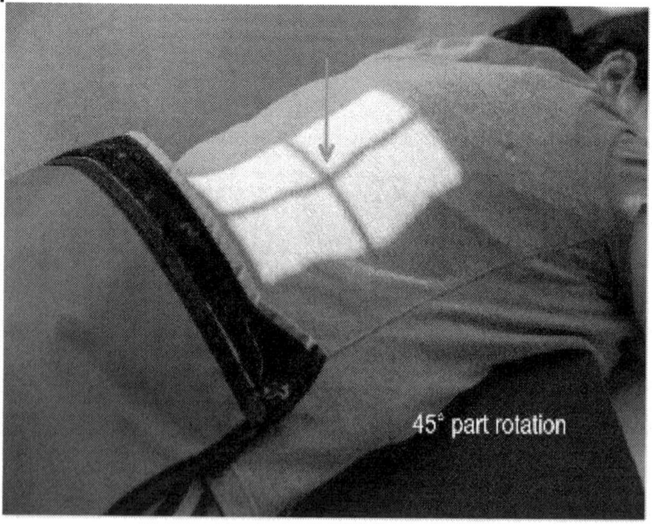

Collimation to include or structures demonstrated
Breathing Instructions

- Arrested expiration

Image evaluation

- Ilia symmetrical on both obliques
- Pedicles demonstrated in the middle of the vertebral body
- Parts of the "Scotty dog" clearly demonstrated.
- The anterior obliques best demonstrates the zygapophyseal joints farthest from the IR

Notes:

- If not enough patient rotation, angle between MCP & IR less than 45– pedicles seen on anterior part of vertebral body
- If too much patient rotation, angle between MCP & IR greater than45– pedicle seen on posterior part of vertebral body

Fig. 144b. Radiograph. Lumbar Spine – Anterior Oblique, LAO position

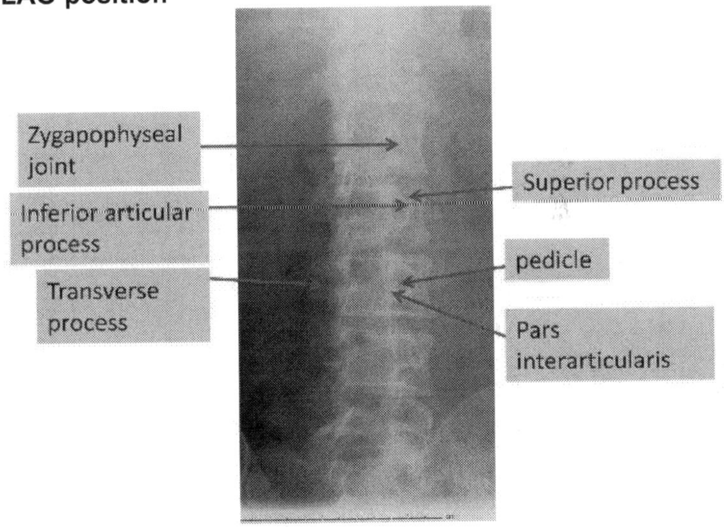

Lumbar Spine–Lateral

SID, Technical factors, Shielding

- 40 inches (100 cm). Grid. 95kVp @ 20mAs or AEC. Gonadal shielding

Patient/part position

- Lateral, recumbent or erect with arms raised

Specific part/body position or rotation

- Men with broad shoulders and narrow hip may need support under the hips.
- Women with wide hips and narrow shoulders will need support under the shoulders.

Direction and point of entry of CR

- Perpendicular through the L3 joint space
- Keep CR perpendicular to the long axis of spine using tube angulation if needed (average 8° for women with wide pelvis and 5° for men)
- Knees flexed with a sponge between knees to prevent rotation

Fig. 145a. Position. Lumbar Spine – Lateral

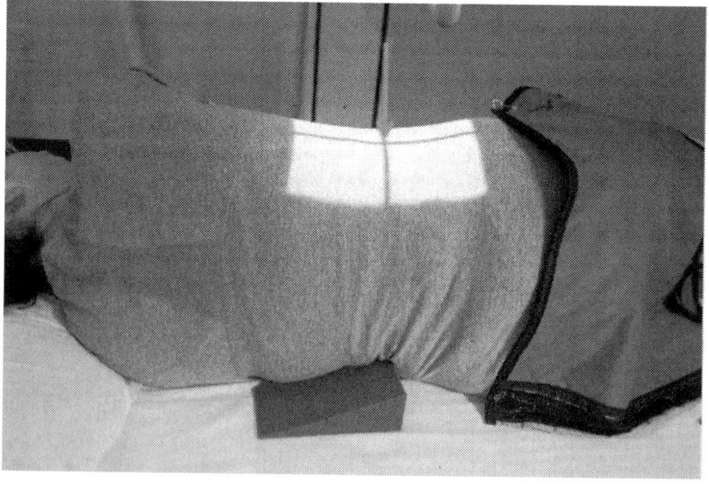

Collimation to include or structures demonstrated

- L1 to upper sacrum
- This position best demonstrates the bodies, interspaces, spinous processes, L/S junction & intervertebral foramina (L1-4)

Breathing Instructions

- Arrested expiration

Image evaluation

- Intervertebral disk spaces and pedicles clearly seen
- Vertebral bodies boxlike
- Superimposed posterior margins of bodies
- Superimposed crest–if no angulation used

Notes:

- The oblique and not the lateral will visualize the intervertebral foramina of L5.
- Lead rubber placed on the table behind the patient will improved image contrast by reducing scatter to the IR

Fig. 145b. Radiograph. Lumbar Spine – Lateral

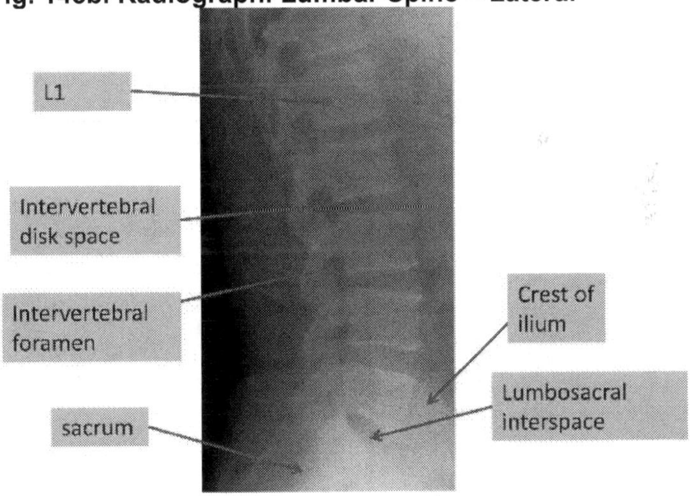

Lumbosacral junction (L5/S1)–Lateral projection

"Spot" projection

SID, Technical factors, Shielding

- 40 inches (100 cm). Grid. 100-110kVp @ 20mAs or AEC.

Gonadal shielding when possible

Patient/part position

- Recumbent or erect with arms raised

Specific part/body position or rotation

- Patient lateral, head supported with spine parallel to the IR

Direction and point of entry of CR

- CR should pass through the dimples, PSIS, through the coronal plane 2 inches (5 cm) posterior to the ASIS and 1½ inches (3.8 cm) inferior to the iliac crest
- Direct CR caudal, if spine not parallel to the long axis of IR use average 8° for women with wide pelvis and 5° for men

Fig. 146a. Position. Lumbosacral Junction (L5/S1) – Lateral projection, "Spot" projection

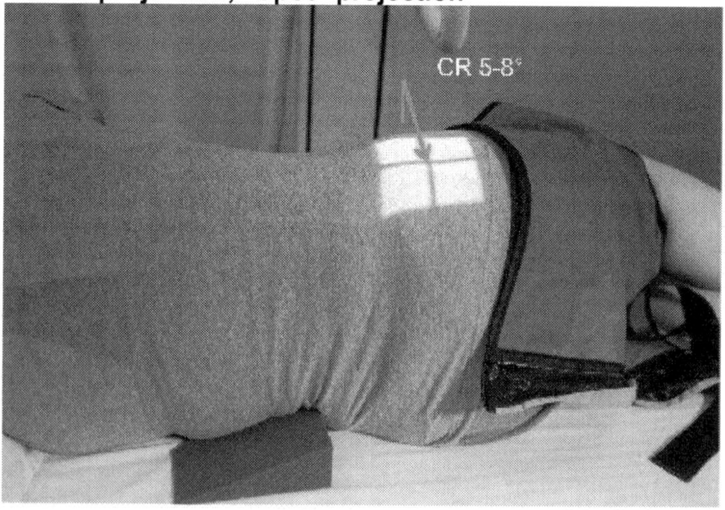

Collimation to include or structures demonstrated

- Include L5 and upper sacrum
- Open lumbosacral intervertebral joint

Breathing Instructions

- Arrested respiration

Image evaluation

- Crest of ilia closely superimposing each other

Note:

- Lead rubber placed on the table behind the patient will improved image contrast by reducing scatter to the IR

Fig. 146b. Radiograph. Lumbosacral Junction (L5/S1) – Lateral projection, "Spot" projection

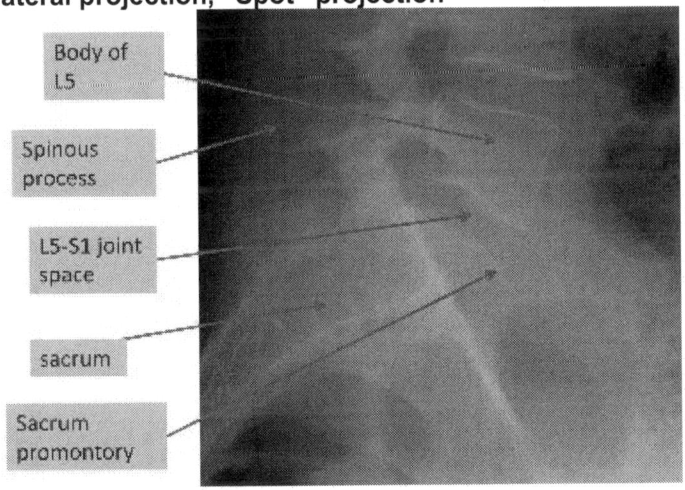

Lumbosacral junction (L5/S1) & Sacroiliac joint–Anteroposterior (AP) axial

SID, Technical factors, Shielding

- 40 inches (100 cm). Grid. 85kVp @ 20mAs or AEC.

Gonadal shielding when possible

Patient/part position

- Supine

Specific part/body position or rotation

- Arms raised, folded on chest or by side with shoulders on same plane.

Direction and point of entry of CR

- Cephalic tube angulation 30-degree males and 35° females
- CR directed 2 inches (5 cm) above symphysis

Fig. 147a. Position. Lumbosacral Junction (L5/S1) and Sacroiliac Joint – Anteroposterior (AP) Axial

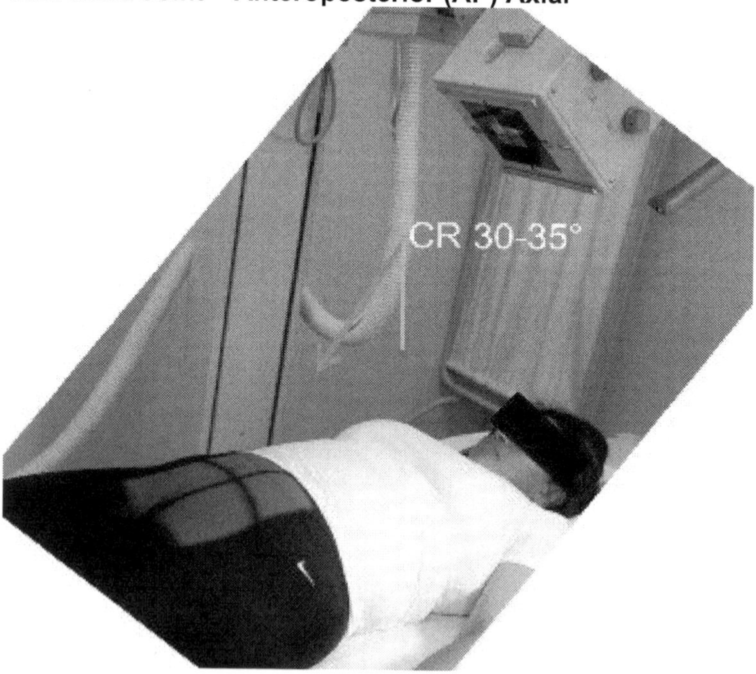

Collimation to include or structures demonstrated

- Lumbosacral junction and upper sacrum
- Open sacroiliac joints and L5/S1 interspace

Breathing Instructions

- Arrested respiration

Image evaluation

- Spinous processes seen in the midline of the vertebrae and middle of IR
- Sacroiliac joint symmetrical with minimal overlap of the ilium and sacrum
- Ilium should not superimpose the sacrum

Fig. 147b. Radiograph. Lumbosacral Junction (L5/S1) and Sacroiliac Joint – Anteroposterior (AP) Axial

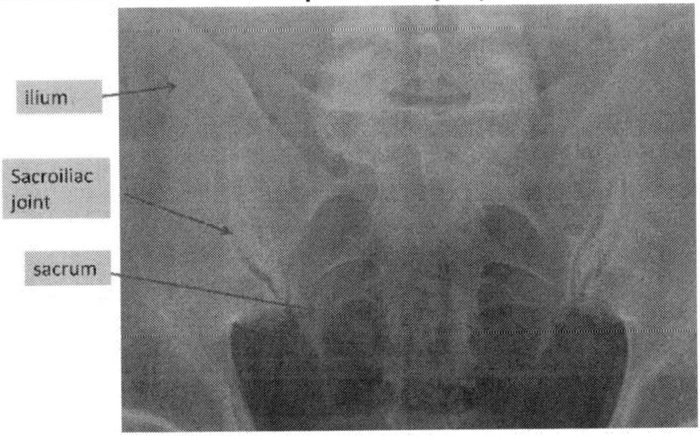

Lumbosacral junction (L5/S1) & Sacroiliac joint– Posteroanterior (PA) axial projection

SID, Technical factors, Shielding

- 40 inches (100 cm). Grid. 75-85kVp @ 10mAs or AEC. Gonadal shielding when possible

Patient/part position

- Prone with shoulders on same plane.

Specific part/body position or rotation

- The prone position, utilizes the divergent rays to clearly show the joint but will increase OID

Direction and point of entry of CR

- Caudal tube angulation, 30-degree males and 35° females
- Center to L/S junction at L4 spinous process

Fig. 148a. Position. Lumbosacral Junction (L5/S1) and Sacroiliac Joint – Posteroanterior (PA) Axial projection

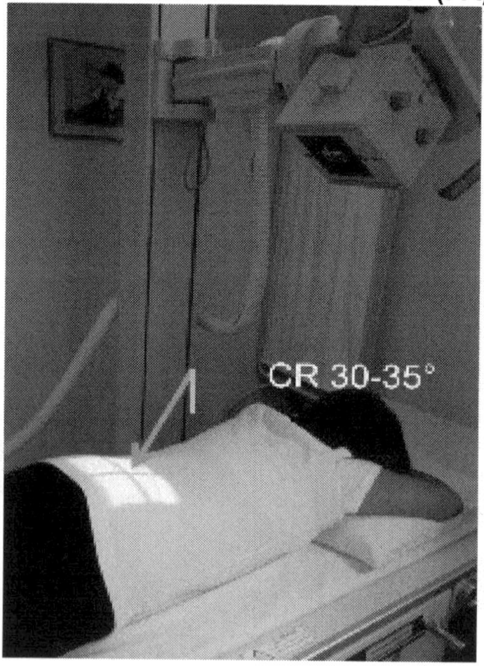

Collimation to include or structures demonstrated

- Upper border of IR 1inches (2.5 cm) above crest with joints in center of IR

Breathing Instructions

- Arrested respiration

Image evaluation

- Spinous processes seen in the midline of the vertebrae and middle of IR
- Sacroiliac joint symmetrical with minimal overlap of the ilium and sacrum
- Ilium should not superimpose the sacrum

Notes:

- Gonadal shielding on male patients only

Fig. 148b. Radiograph. Lumbosacral Junction (L5/S1) and Sacroiliac Joint – Posteroanterior (PA) Axial projection

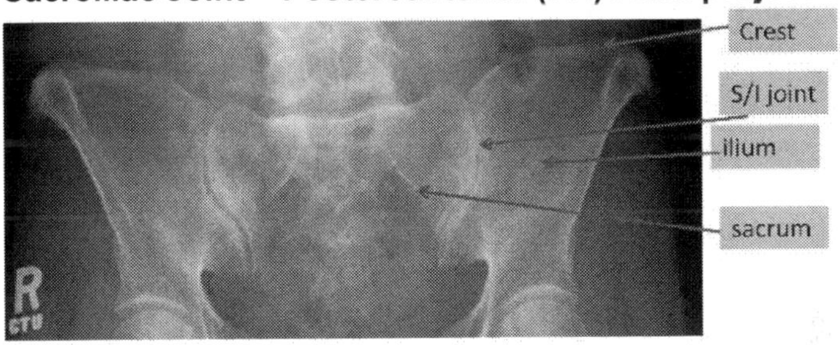

Sacro-Iliac (S/I) Joint–Posterior oblique, LPO or RPO positions

Or Anterior oblique, LAO or RAO positions

SID, Technical factors, Shielding

- 40 inches (100 cm). Grid. 75-85kVp @ 10mAs or AEC.

Gonadal shielding when possible

Patient/part position

- Supine or prone then rotated to the oblique position

Specific part/body position or rotation

- MCP 25–30 degrees with the tabletop.
- Support the shoulder, thorax, upper thigh and knee on the raised side

Direction and point of entry of CR

- LPO or RPO, CR 1inch (2.5 cm) medial to ASIS of raised side

Fig. 149a. Position. Sacro-Iliac (S/I) Joint- Anterior Oblique, RPO

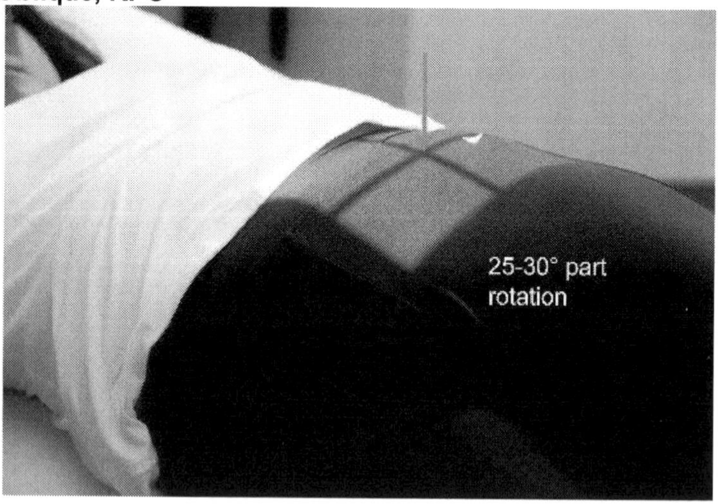

Collimation to include or structures demonstrated

- Upper border of IR 1inch (2.5cm) above crest with joint of interest in center of IR(RPO or LPO)

Breathing Instructions

- Arrested respiration

Image evaluation

- Posterior oblique (RPO or LPO) demonstrates raised side

Notes

- Precise positioning and centering is best if the patient is placed in the AP position, even though the joint is closer to in the PA and would result in less magnification
- Anterior oblique (RAO or LAO)demonstrates lowered side
- For the LAO or RAO, CR to the level 1½ inches (3.8 cm) distal to 5th lumbar spinous process to exit at level of ASIS

Fig. 149b. Radiograph. Sacro-Iliac (S/I) Joint- Anterior Oblique, RPO

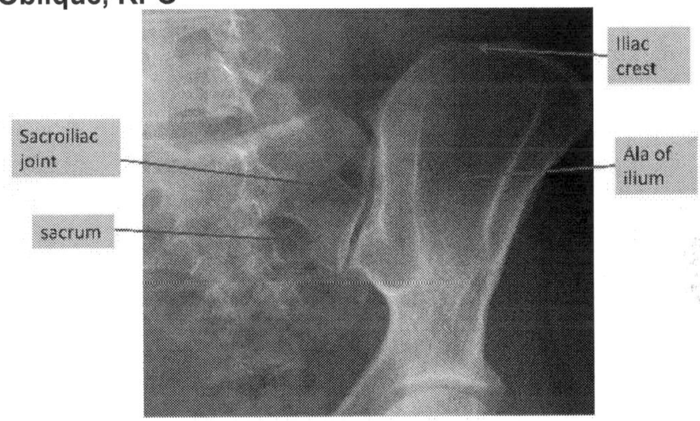

Sacrum–Anteroposterior (AP) axial projection

SID, Technical factors, Shielding

- 40 inches (100 cm). Grid. 85kVp @ 20mAs or AEC.

Gonadal shielding when possible

Patient/part position

- Supine

Specific part/body position or rotation

- Patient should have bowel prep and empty bladder before imaging
- Arms raised, folded on chest or by side
- Extend legs– **flexing legs will tip the pelvis-up,** superimposing symphysis on coccyx.

Direction and point of entry of CR

- Supine: 15° cephalic at point 2inches (5 cm) superior to symphysis pubis

Fig. 150a. Position. Sacrum- Anteroposterior (AP) Axial projection

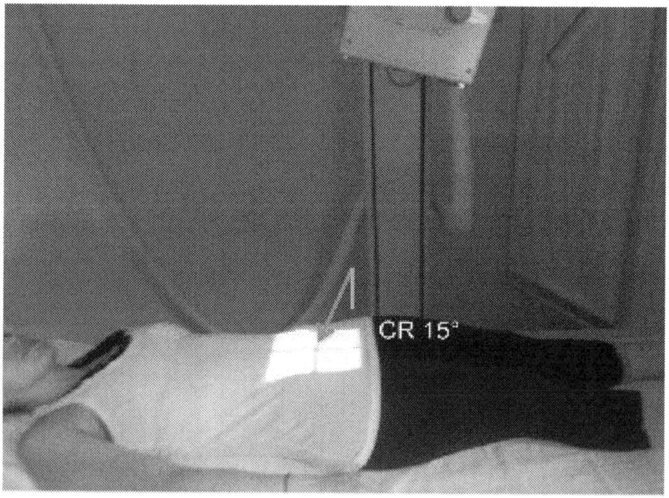

Collimation to include or structures demonstrated
Breathing Instructions

- Arrested respiration

Image evaluation

- Alae of sacrum symmetrical with sacrum directly above symphysis
- Sacrum free of foreshortening

Note

- Patient with painful injury or destructive lesions can be imaged prone
- Prone imaging uses 15° caudal. Center to sacral curve

Fig. 150b. Radiograph. Sacrum- Anteroposterior (AP) Axial projection

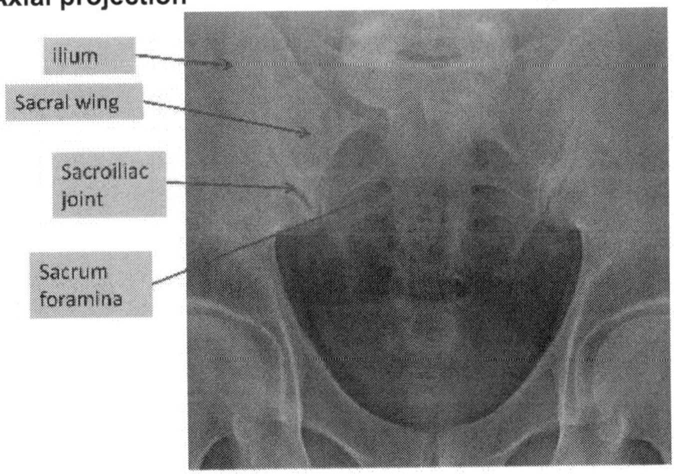

Coccyx–Anteroposterior projection (AP)

SID, Technical factors, Shielding

- 40 inches (100 cm). Grid. 85kVp @ 20mAs or AEC.

Gonadal shielding when possible

Patient/part position

- Supine
- Patient should have bowel prep and should empty bladder before imaging

Specific part/body position or rotation

- Arms raised, folded on chest or by side

Direction and point of entry of CR

- AP–10˚ caudal 2inches (5 cm) superior to symphysis

Fig. 151a. Position. Coccyx – Anteroposterior (AP) projection

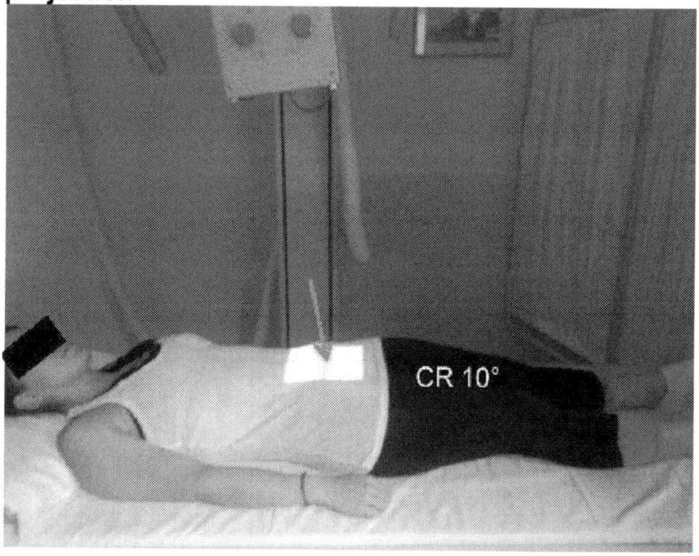

Collimation to include or structures demonstrated
Breathing Instructions

- Arrested respiration

Image evaluation

- Coccyx directly above symphysis

Notes

- Patient can be image prone
- If PA use10°cephalad, CR to coccyx

Fig. 151b. Radiograph. Coccyx – Anteroposterior (AP) projection

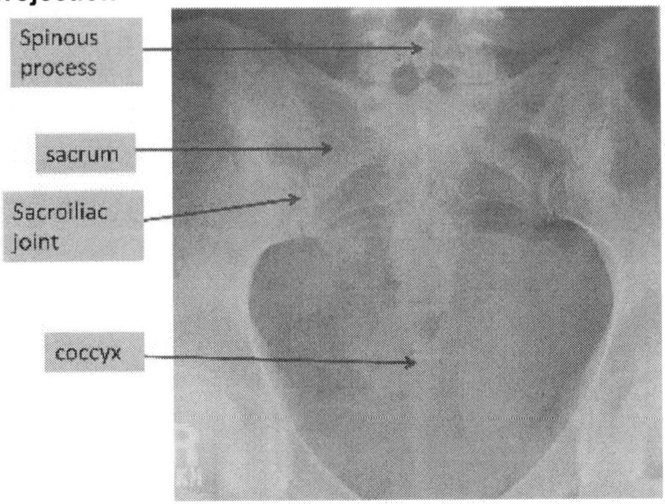

Sacrum & Coccyx–Lateral projection

SID, Technical factors, Shielding

- 40 inches (100 cm). Grid. 70kVp @ 10mAs or AEC.

Gonadal shielding when possible

Patient/part position

Specific part/body position or rotation

- Raised, right angle to body
- A pillow under head or support at lower thoracic and waist will keep spine parallel to tabletop

Direction and point of entry of CR–**Lateral sacrum & coccyx**

- Perpendicular at level of ASIS, 3½ inches (9 cm) posterior to ASIS

Direction and point of entry of CR–**Lateral coccyx**

- Perpendicular, center to coccyx, 3 ½inches (9 cm) posterior & 2 inches (5 cm) below the ASIS

Fig. 152a. Position. Sacrum and Coccyx- Lateral projection

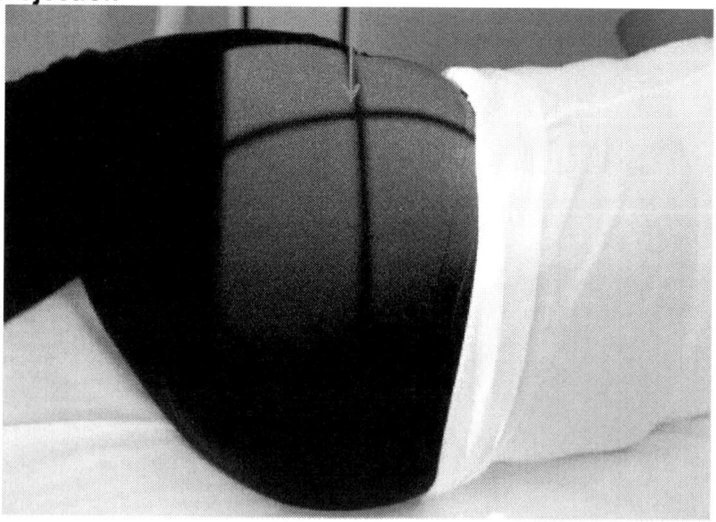

Collimation to include or structures demonstrated

- A true lateral of the entire sacrum and coccyx

Breathing Instructions

- Arrested respiration

Image evaluation

- Femoral head nearly superimposed
- Superimposed margins of ilia and ischia
- Superimposed greater sciatic notches

Note:

- Lead rubber placed on the table behind the patient will reduce scatter to the IR

Fig. 152b. Radiograph. Sacrum and Coccyx- Lateral projection

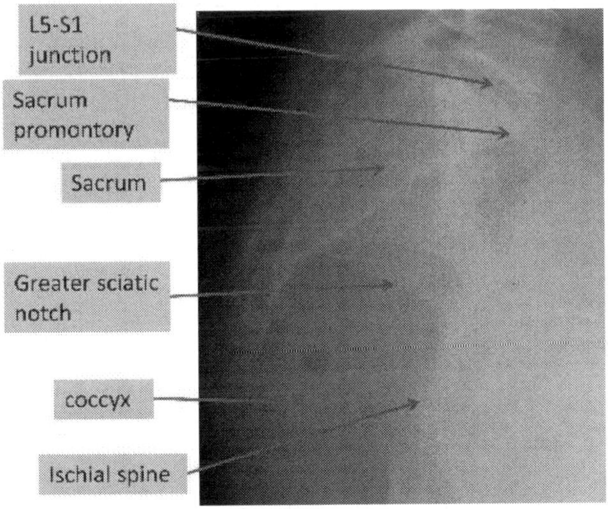

Scoliosis–Posteroanterior (PA) projection

SID, Technical factors, Shielding

- 72inches (183 cm). Grid. 75-85kVp @ 7.5-12.5 mAs or AEC. Gonadal & Breast shielding

Patient/part position

- **PA,** erect with weight distributed equally on both feet

Specific part/body position or rotation

- Extra-long IR needed

Direction and point of entry of CR

- To midpoint of the IR (approx. T10)

Fig. 153a. Position. Scoliosis – Posteroanterior (PA) projection

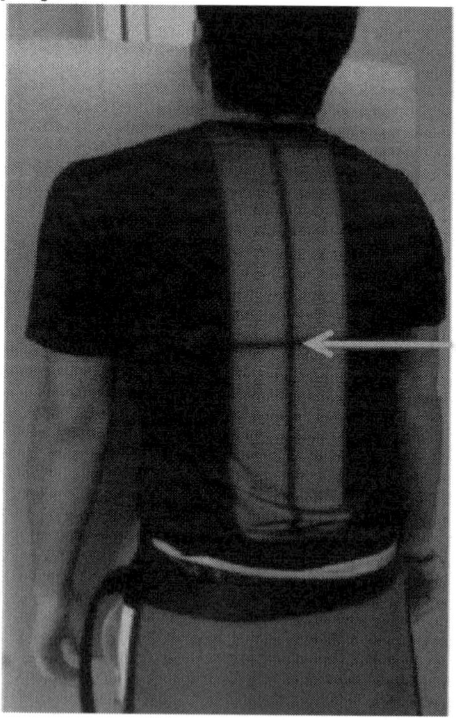

Collimation to include or structures demonstrated

- Bottom edge of IR at level of ASIS, to include 1inch (2.5 cm) of crest

Breathing Instructions

- Arrested respiration

Image evaluation

- Thoracic and lumbar spine plus 1inch (2.5 cm) of crest

Notes

- 14 x 34 inch or 35.4 x 83 cm IR used

Fig. 153b. Radiograph. Scoliosis – Posteroanterior (PA) projection

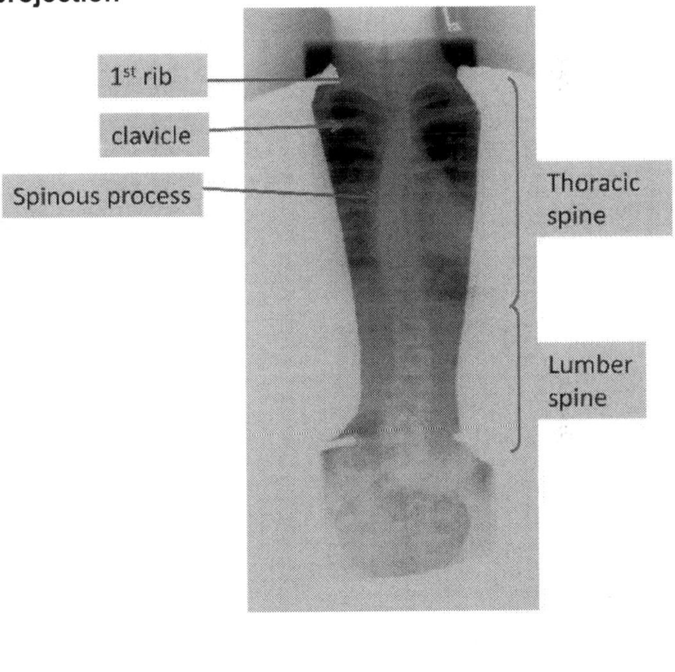

Scoliosis–Lateral projection

SID, Technical factors, Shielding

- 72inches (183 cm). Grid. 85-95kVp @ 7.5-12.5 mAs or AEC. Gonadal & Breast shielding

Patient/part position

- Erect, lateral with weight equally distributed body straight

Specific part/body position or rotation

- Extra-long IR
- Arms extended, holding support

Direction and point of entry of CR

- To midpoint of the IR (approx. T10)

Fig. 154a. Position. Scoliosis – Lateral projection

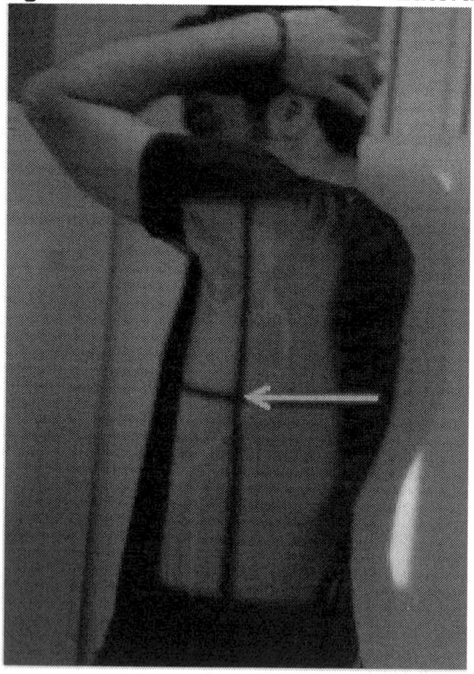

Collimation to include or structures demonstrated

- Bottom edge of IR at level of ASIS, to include 1inch (2.5 cm) of crest

Breathing Instructions

- Arrested respiration

Image evaluation

- Thoracic and lumbar spine plus 1inch (2.5 cm) of crest

Note

- The position best demonstrates abnormal kyphosis or the presence of spondylolisthesis
- 14 x 34 inches or 35.4 x 83 cm IR used

Fig. 154b. Radiograph. Scoliosis – Lateral projection

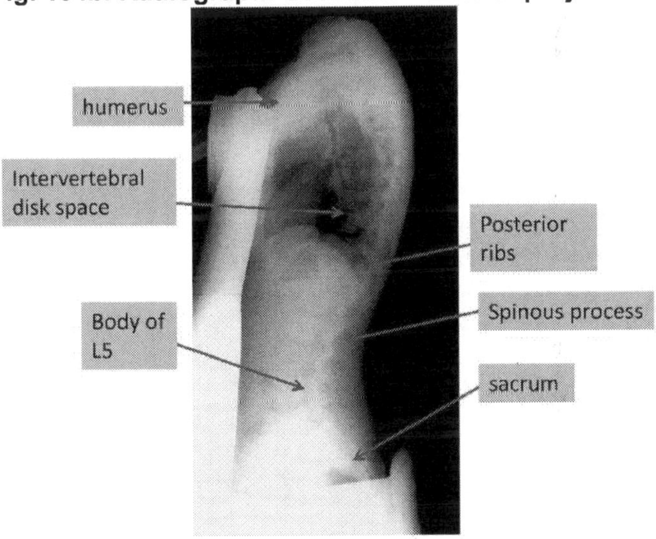

Scoliosis–Posteroanterior (PA) projection, Right and left Bending

SID, Technical factors, Shielding

- 40 inches (100 cm). Grid. 75-85kVp @ 7.5-12.5 mAs or AEC. Gonadal & Breast shielding

Patient/part position

- Erect or supine

Specific part/body position or rotation

Right bending

- Maximum bending to the right without rotation the pelvis

Left bending

- Maximum bending to the left without rotating the pelvis

Direction and point of entry of CR

- To L3, 1½inch (3.8 cm) above crest

Fig. 155a. Position. Scoliosis – Posteroanterior (PA) projection, Left Bending

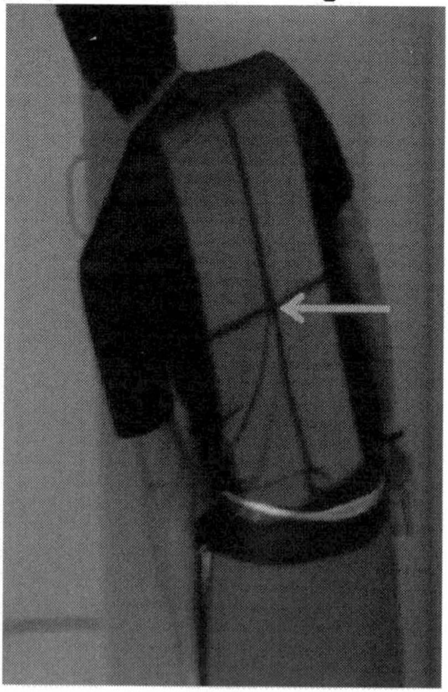

Collimation to include or structures demonstrated

- Bottom edge of IR at level of ASIS to include 1inch (2.5 cm) of crest

Breathing Instructions

- Arrested respiration

Image evaluation

- This position demonstrates herniated disk, spinal fusion and structural changes in early scoliosis

Note

- Bending images can help to differentiate structural from nonstructural curves

Fig. 155b. Radiograph. Scoliosis – Posteroanterior (PA) projection, Left Bending

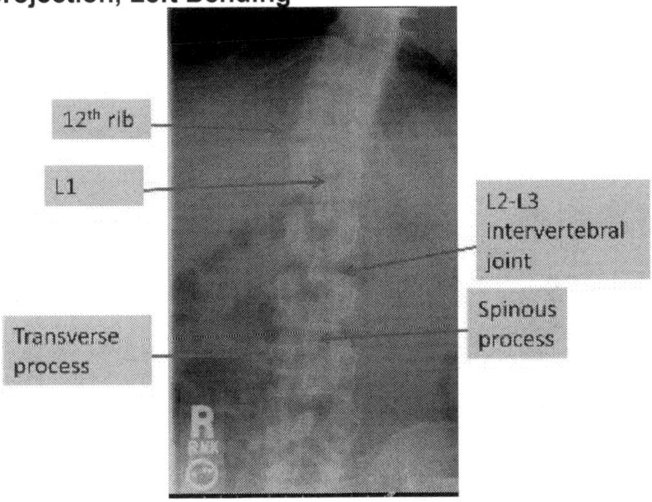

Scoliosis–Lateral hyperflexion projection

Spinal fusion series

SID, Technical factors, Shielding

- 40 inches (100 cm). Grid. 85-95kVp @ 7.5-12.5 mAs or AEC. Gonadal & Breast shielding

Patient/part position

- Erect or supine

Specific part/body position or rotation

- Have patient bend at the waist–knees up and shoulders down if recumbent

Direction and point of entry of CR

- L3

Fig. 156a. Position. Scoliosis – Lateral Hyperflexion projection

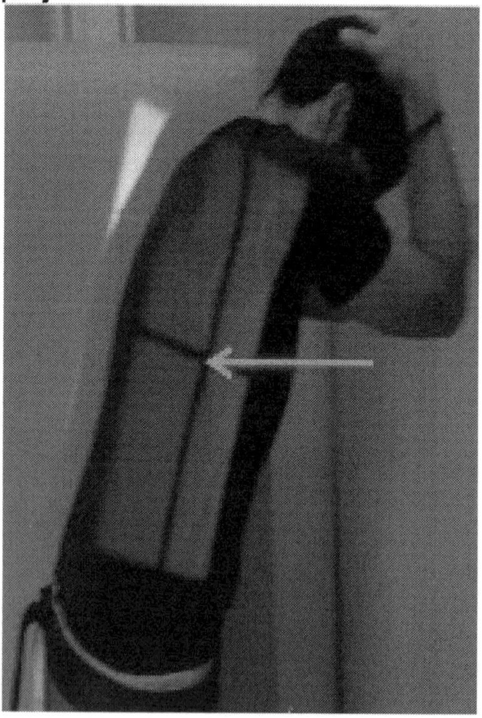

Collimation to include or structures demonstrated

- Bottom edge of IR at level of ASIS, to include 1inch (2.5 cm) of crest

Breathing Instructions

- Arrested expiration

Image evaluation

- Vertebral bodies appear boxlike
- Intervertebral disk spaces and pedicles clearly seen

Notes

- This position best demonstrates mobility of intervertebral joints
- Can be used in cases of disk protrusion to localize the involved joint

Fig. 156b. Radiograph. Scoliosis – Lateral Hyperflexion projection

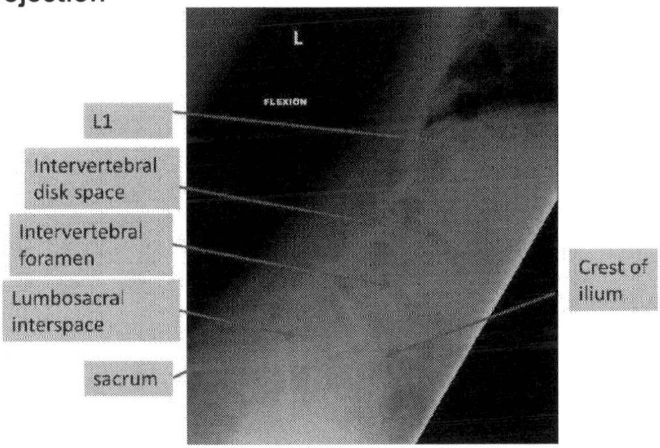

Scoliosis–Lateral hyperextension projection

Spinal fusion series

- 40 inches (100 cm). Grid. 85-95kVp @ 7.5-12.5 mAs or AEC. Gonadal & Breast shielding

Patient/part position

- Erect or supine

Specific part/body position or rotation

- Have patient arch back bringing shoulders and legs backwards

Direction and point of entry of CR

- L3

Fig. 157a. Position. Scoliosis – Lateral Hyperextension projection

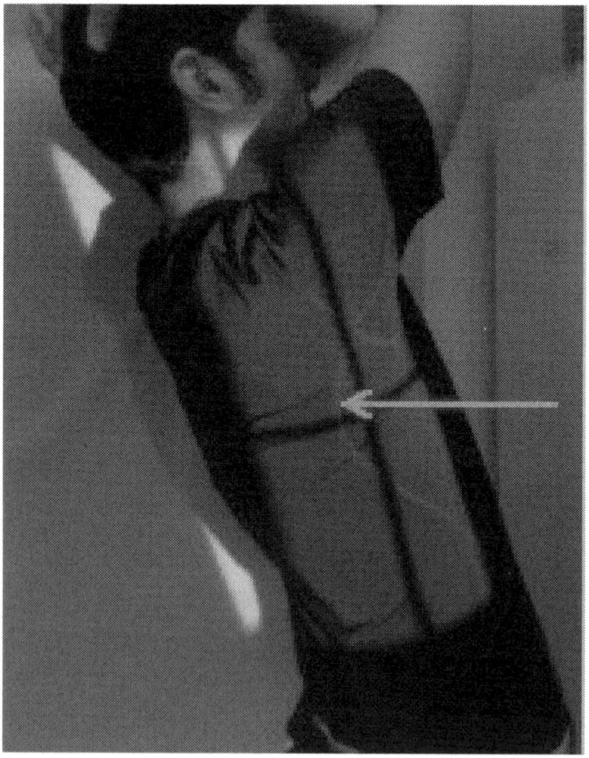

Collimation to include or structures demonstrated

- Bottom edge of IR at level of ASIS, to include 1inch (2.5 cm) of crest

Breathing Instructions

- Arrested expiration

Image evaluation

- Vertebral bodies appear boxlike
- Intervertebral disk spaces and pedicles clearly seen

Notes

- This position best demonstrates mobility of intervertebral joints
- Can be used in cases of disk protrusion to localize the involved joint

Fig. 157b. Radiograph. Scoliosis – Lateral Hyperextension projection

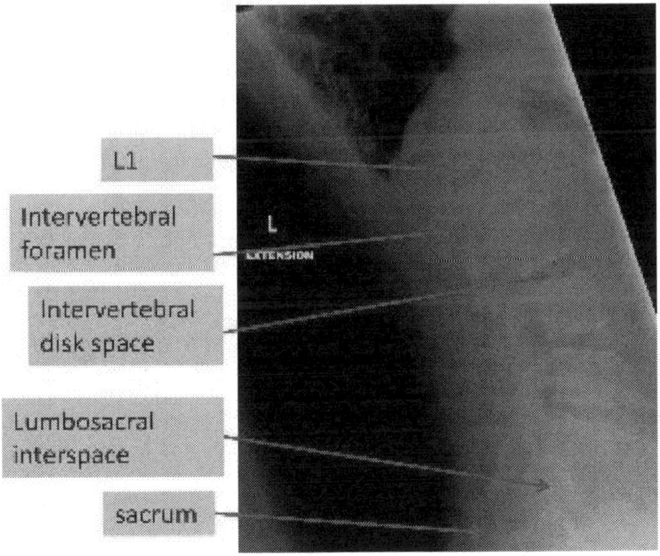

Imaging the Skull, Sinuses and Facial Bones

The two division of the skull

- Cranial
- Facial bones

The two divisions of the cranium

- Calvarium (skull cap) has 4 bones (flat bones with curved outer surface)
- Floor has 6 bones - (irregular shaped bone + portions of 2 calvarium bones

Fig. 158a – lateral skull

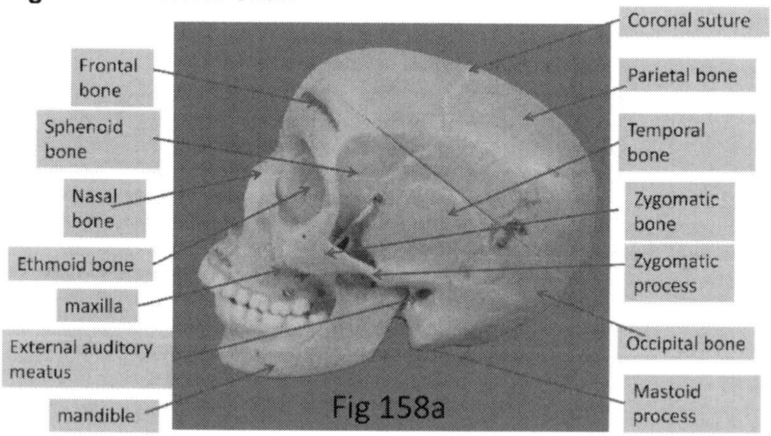

Bones of the face (14)

- 2 nasals
- 2 lacrimal
- 2 maxillae
- 2 malar/zygoma
- 2 palatine
- 2 inferior nasal conchae
- 1 vomer
- 1 mandible (only moving

Fig. 158b. AP skull

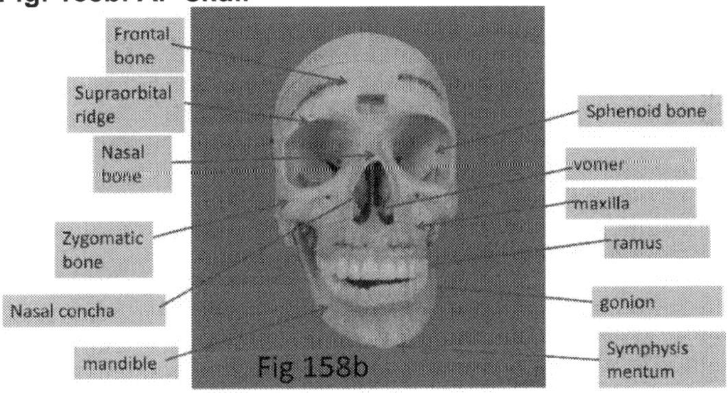

Location of bones of the skull

Bones of the cranium (8)

Calvarium/floor *(small portion)*	1 frontal
floor	1 ethmoid
floor	1 sphenoid
calvarium/floor *(small portion)*	1 occipital
calvarium	2 parietal
floor	2 temporal

Fig. 158c Basal skull

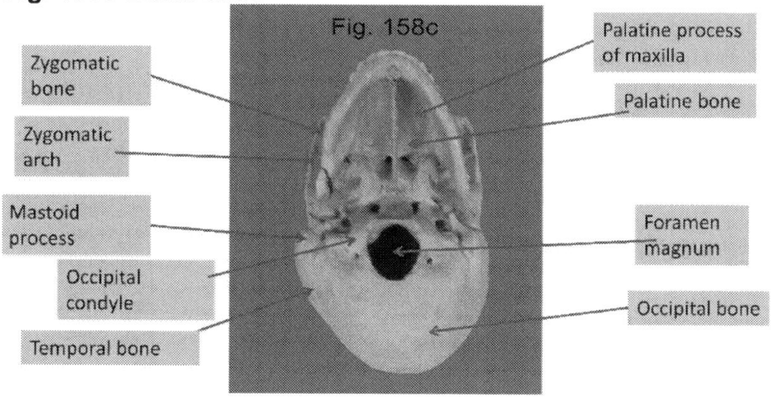

Skull–Planes and Baselines

- Midsagittal plane (MSP)–divides the body into equal right and left halves
- Midcoronal plane (MCP)–divides the body into equal anterior and posterior halves
- Base plane of skull/ anthropological plane or Frankfort horizontal plane–Line formed by connecting lines from inferior edge of orbits to EAM. Similar to IOML (starts a bit lower and ends a bit higher)
- Occlusal plane–Horizontal line formed by biting surfaces of the upper and lower teeth with jaws closed
- Parietoacanthial projection–CR enters the cranial parietal bone and exits ate the acanthion (junction of nose and upper lip)
- Acanthioparietal projection–CR enters the acanthion and exits at the cranial parietal bone
- Submentovertex (SMV)–CR enters below the chin or mentum and exits at the vertex or top of skull
- Verticosubmental (VSM)–CR enters top of skull and exits below the mandible

Fig 158d AP skull showing Baselines

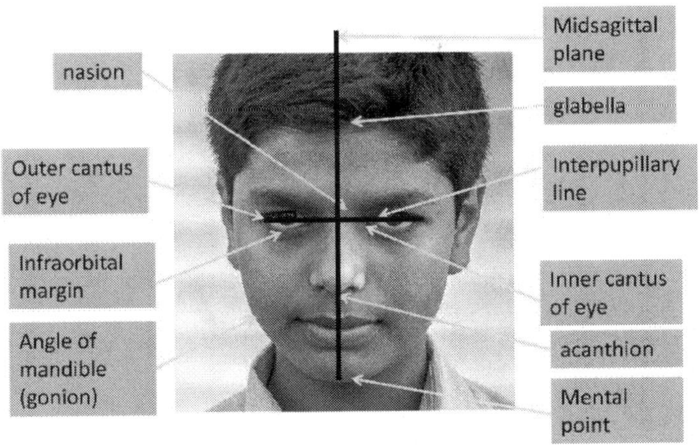

Skull–BASELINES

- OML, orbitomeatal line or canthomeatal line–radiographic base line–from the EAM to outer canthus of eye.
  (There is an 8° difference between the OML and the GML)
- GML, glabellomeatal line–from EAM to glabella
- There is a 15 ° difference between the GML and the IOML
- IOML, infraorbitomeatal line–from the EAM to the infraorbital margin
  (There is a 7° difference between the OML and IOML)
- Anthropological plane/baseline–imaginary line from infraorbital margin to upper border of the EAM–i.e. similar to the IOML (*it starts a bit lower and ends a bit higher.)
- AML, acanthomeatal line –from the EAM to the acanthion
- IPL, interpupillary line–(or interorbital line) line connecting the two pupils or outer canthi of the eyes
- GAL, glabelloalveolar line–from glabella to anterior part of the alveolar process of the maxilla at the midline–(for tangential projections of the nasal bones)
- MML, mentomeatal line–from EAM to mental point
- LML, lips to meatal line–line from the lips to the EAM

Fig. 158e. Lateral Skull showing baselines

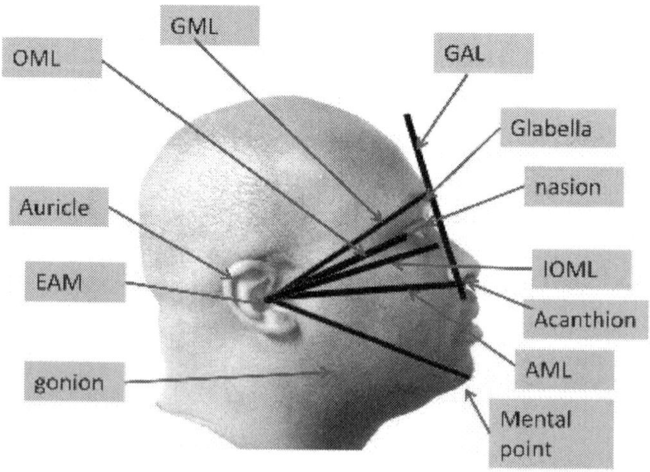

Skull–LANDMARKS

- External auditory meatus (EAM)–external opening into ear canal
- Glabella–superior to the bridge of nose and between the eyebrows
- Nasion–depression on bridge of nose. (Junction of frontal and nasal bones)
- Acanthion–midline junction of upper lip and nose
- Mental point–midpoint of chin. (In bony area called the mentum)
- Outer and inner canthus–junction of upper and lower eyelids (lateral & medial)
- Supraorbital margin/ridge–superior ridge (rim) of orbital base
- Infraorbital margin or ridge–inferior ridge of orbital base
- Vertex–superior point of head (where parietal bone joint with frontal)
- Inion–prominent bump, midline at the back of head (external orbital protuberance)
- Gonion–lower posterior angle on each side of jaw (mandible)
- Tragus or auricular point–small flap of cartilage projecting over the EAM
- Auricle (pinna)–ear
- TEA–top of the ear attachment

Skull–Lateral

SID, Technical factors, Shielding

- 40 inches (100 cm). Grid. 70kVp @ 10mAs or AEC.

Gonadal shielding

Patient/part position

- Erect or recumbent, semi prone
- If semi-prone, affected arm down, unaffected up, unaffected knee flexed

Specific part/body position or rotation

- MSP parallel to IR, IPL perpendicular to IR

Direction and point of entry of CR

- Perpendicular, 2 inches(5cm) above EAM

Fig. 159a. Position. Skull – Lateral

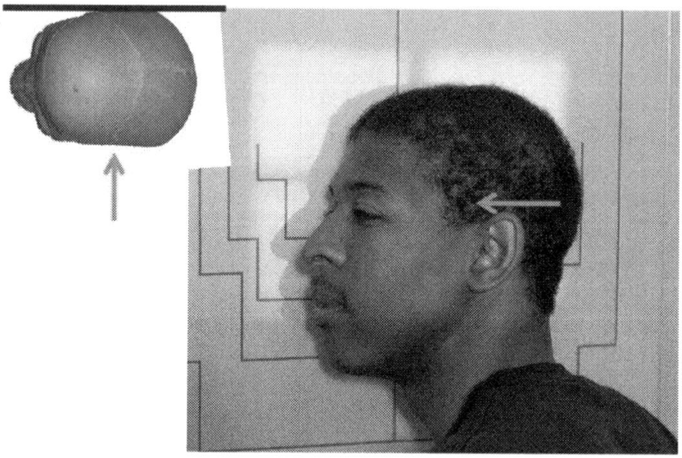

Collimation to include or structures demonstrated

- Entire cranium
- Supraorbital margins superimposed/EAM & TMAs superimposed
- Sella turcica seen in profile

Image evaluation

- Entire cranium without rotation or tilt
- Supraorbital margins superimposed/EAM & TMAs superimposed

Note:

To demonstrate the stella turcia, direct the CR ¾ inch (1.9 cm) superior and & ¾ inch (1.9 cm) posterior to EAM

Fig. 159b. Radiograph. Skull – Lateral

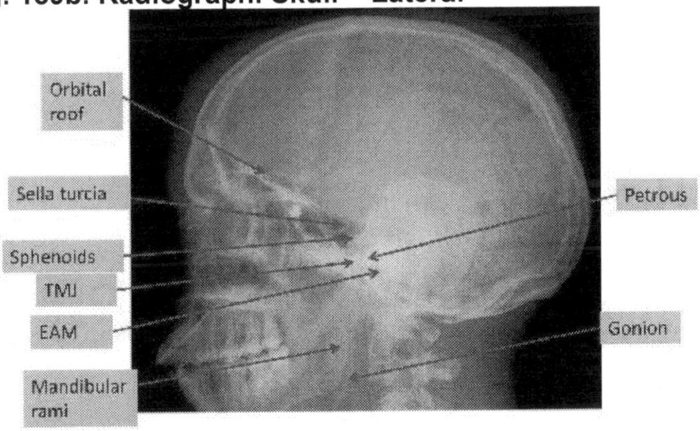

Skull–Posteroanterior (PA) axial projection
Caldwell method

SID, Technical factors, Shielding

- 40 inches (100 cm). Grid. 80kVp @ 12.5 mAs or AEC.

Gonadal shielding

Patient/part position

- Erect, PA or recumbent, prone. Shoulders on same transverse plane

Specific part/body position or rotation

- MSP Perpendicular to IR, OML perpendicular

Direction and point of exit of CR

- 15°caudal exit at nasion

Fig. 160a. Position. Skull- Posteroanterior (PA) Axial projection

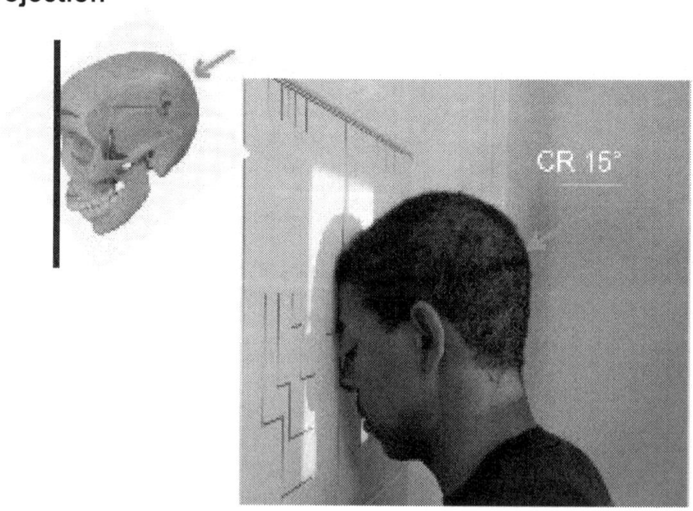

Collimation to include or structures demonstrated

- Entire cranium
- Petrous pyramid in lower1/3 of orbits

Image evaluation

- Equal distance between lateral border of the orbits and lateral skull

Note:

- The AP projection would magnify the facial bone and increase radiation dose to eyes.

Fig. 160b. Radiograph. Skull- Posteroanterior (PA) Axial projection

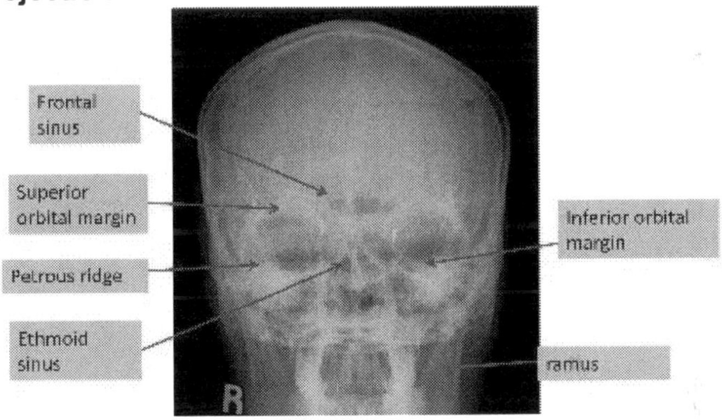

Skull–Posteroanterior (PA) projection

SID, Technical factors, Shielding

- 40 inches (100 cm). Grid. 80kVp @ 12.5 mAs or AEC.

Gonadal shielding

Patient/part position

- Erect, PA or recumbent, prone. Shoulders on same transverse plane

Specific part/body position or rotation

- MSP and OML perpendicular to IR

Direction and point of exit of CR

- CR perpendicular, 0° angle. CR exit at nasion

Fig. 161a. Position. Skull- Posteroanterior (PA) projection

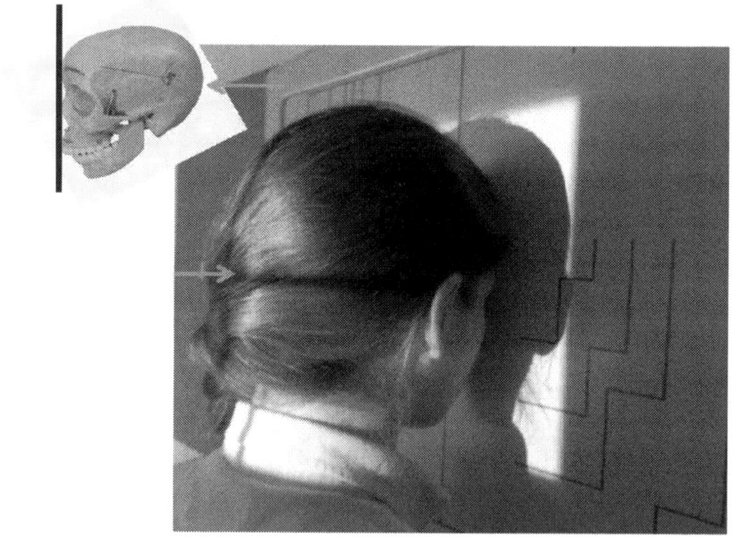

Collimation to include or structures demonstrated

- Entire cranium
- Petrous pyramids fills orbits

Image evaluation

- Equal distance between lateral border of the orbits and lateral skull

Note:

To demonstrate the superior orbital fissures

- Use 20-25°caudal angulation CR directed to **mid orbits**
- The petrous will be demonstrated below orbits

To demonstrate the foramen rotundum

- Use 25–30° caudal angulation. CR exits at the nasion
- The petrous seen in mid maxillary sinuses below the orbits

Fig. 161b. Radiograph. Skull- Posteroanterior (PA) projection

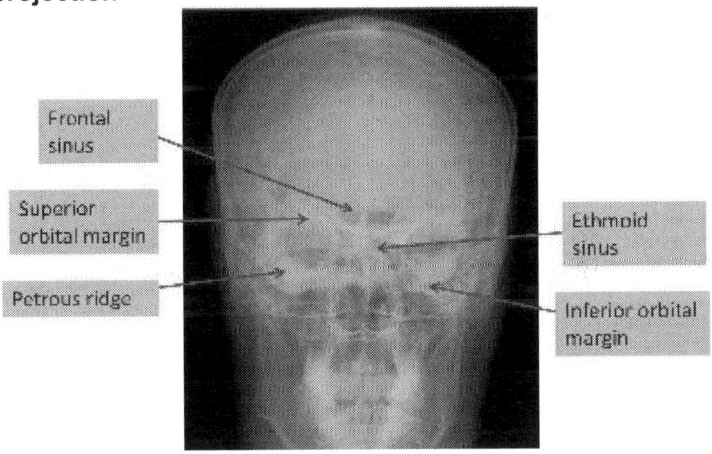

Skull–Anteroposterior (AP) axial projection
Towne/Grashey method

SID, Technical factors, Shielding

- 40 inches (100 cm). Grid. 80kVp @ 12.5 mAs or AEC. Gonadal shielding

Patient/part position

- AP recumbent or erect. Shoulders on same transverse plane

Specific part/body position or rotation

- MSP and OLM perpendicular to the IR

Direction and point of exit of CR

- 30° caudal tube angulation if OML perpendicular to IR
- CR to 2.5inches (6.4cm) above level of superciliary arches or glabella. Exit at foramen magnum

Fig. 162a. Position. Skull- Anteroposterior (AP) Axial projection, Towne/Grashey method

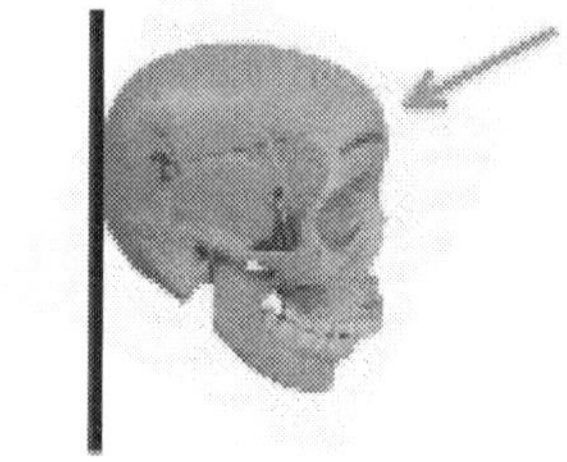

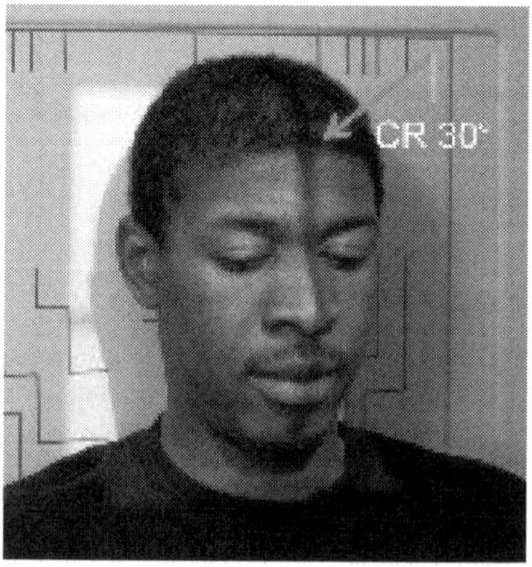

Collimation to include or structures demonstrated

- Entire cranium
- Dorsum sella, occipital bone and posterior clinoid process within the foramen magnum

Image evaluation

- Symmetrical petrous pyramids
- Equal distance between lateral orbital margins and lateral skull

Note:

- If patient is unable to tuck the chin down position the IOML perpendicular to the IR and use 37° caudal tube angulation

Fig. 162b. Radiograph. Skull- Anteroposterior (AP) Axial projection, Towne/Grashey method

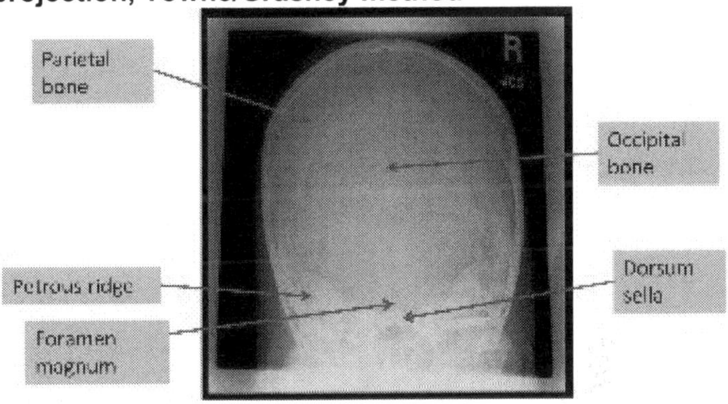

Skull–Posteroanterior projection (PA) axial

Haas, nuchofrontal method

SID, Technical factors, Shielding

- 40 inches (100 cm). Grid. 80kVp @ 12.5 mAs or AEC. Gonadal shielding

Patient/part position

- Recumbent, prone or erect PA, shoulders at side

Specific part/body position or rotation

- MSP and OML perpendicular to IR

Direction and point of exit of CR

- 25°cephalic angulation directed 1.5inches (3.8 cm) inferior to inion, exit 1.5inches (3.8 cm) above nasion

Fig. 163a. Position. Skull- Posteroanterior (PA) Axial projection, Haas or nuchofrontal method

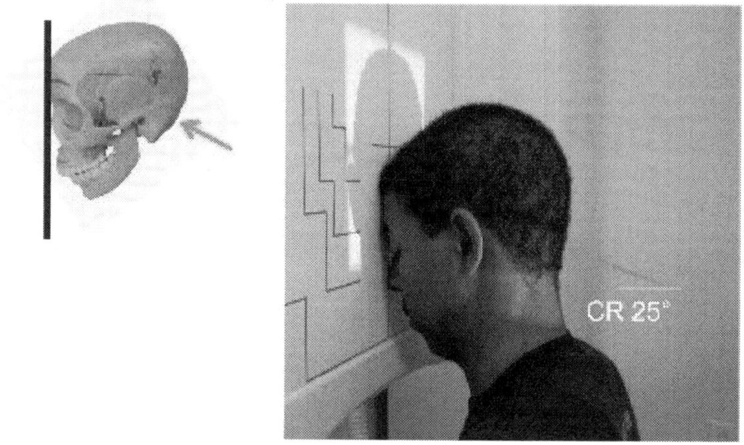

Collimation to include or structures demonstrated

- Entire cranium
- Dorsum sella, occipital bone and posterior clinoid process seen in foramen magnum

Image evaluation

- Symmetrical petrous pyramids
- Equal distance between lateral orbital margins and lateral skull

Fig. 163b. Radiograph. Skull- Posteroanterior (PA) Axial projection, Haas or nuchofrontal method

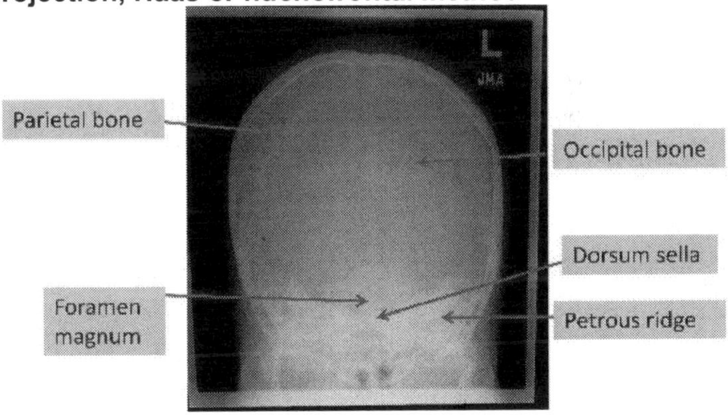

Imaging the Sinuses

There are four paranasal sinuses. They are lined with mucus membrane and all drain into the nasal cavity. In order to demonstrate air-fluid levels, erect is the preferred position when imaging the sinuses

Cleanliness, infection control
Wash hands before & after positioning patient
Clean surface or Bucky, tabletop or IR that will touch the patients' face
Cleaning should be in front of patient

External patient preparations
Removal of dentures, hairpins, glasses, hair braids/clips, chains etc.

Tube angulation rule
Horizontal central ray is always used in sinus imaging in order to demonstrated fluid levels.

Largest of the sinuses–maxillary
Location of the sinuses
Cranial bones–frontal, ethmoid, sphenoid
Facial bones–maxillary

Development of the sinuses in age order

- Maxillary–infant
- Sphenoid, ethmoid & frontal–6-7 years
- Ethmoid–17-18yrs.

Other names for the maxillary sinuses –maxillary antra; antra; antra of Highmore

Structure of the sinuses

- Frontal—rarely symmetrical
- Maxillary—most symmetrical

Fig. 164a.Location of the paranasal sinuses

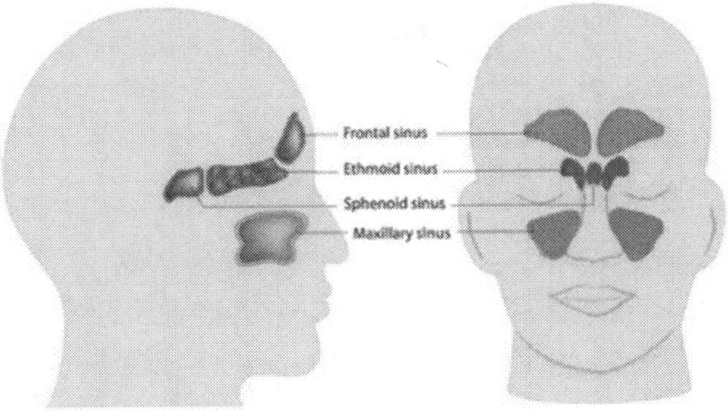

The modified Caldwell projection is used to avoid tube angulation. Either by positioning the OML at 15 degrees to the horizontal or by angulation the IR

Horizontal central ray is always used in sinus imaging in order to demonstrate fluid levels

Fig. 164b Imaging Sinuses – using a horizontal ray with patient angulation. (OML 15 degrees with detector vertical)

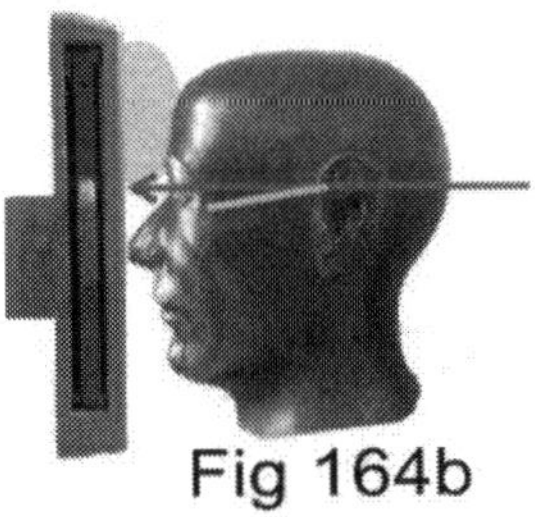

Fig 164b

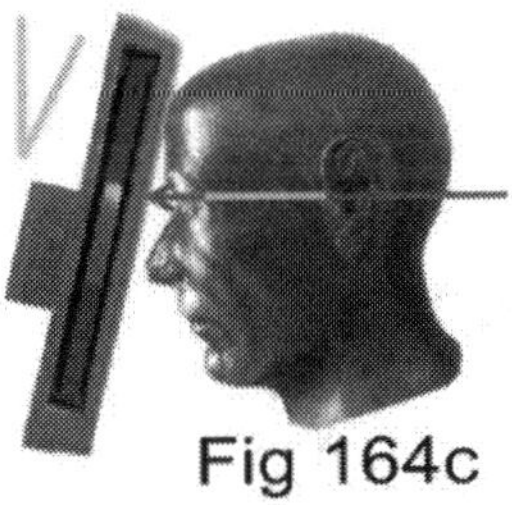

Fig 164c

Fig 164c. Imaging Sinuses – using a horizontal ray the Bucky angulation. (OML 90 degrees with detector 15 degrees

Sinuses–Lateral projection

SID, Technical factors, Shielding

- 40 inches (100 cm). Grid. 65kVp @ 10mAs or AEC.

Gonadal shielding

Patient/part position

- Erect

Specific part/body position or rotation

- MSP parallel to IR. IPL perpendicular to IR

Direction and point of entry of CR

- Perpendicular, ½-1inch (1.5-2.5 cm) posterior to the outer cantus of eye

Fig. 165a. Position. Sinuses- Lateral projection

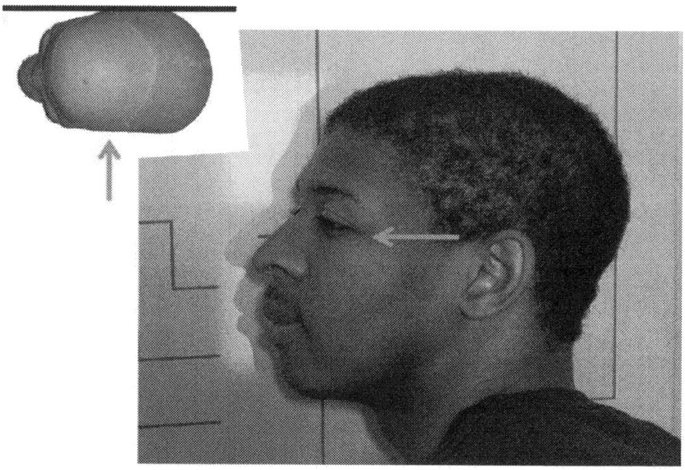

Collimation to include or structures demonstrated

- Close collimation to include all four sinuses
- Sinuses are superimposed
- The sphenoids and ethmoids seen clearly

Image evaluation

- All sinuses seen
- Supraorbital margins and base of skull superimposed

Fig. 165b. Radiograph. Sinuses- Lateral projection

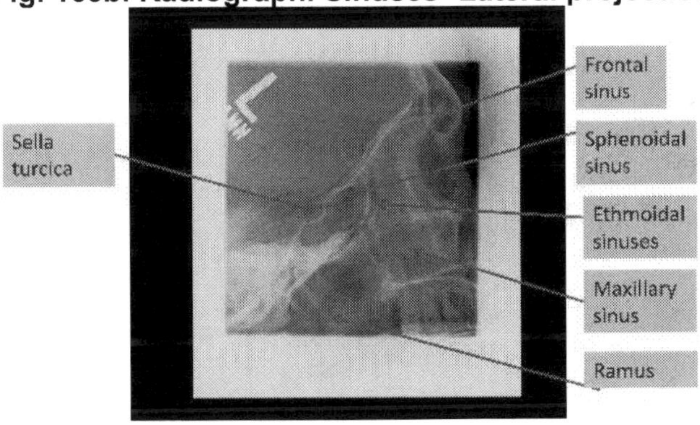

Sinuses–Posteroanterior (PA) axial projection
Modified Caldwell method

SID, Technical factors, Shielding

- 40 inches (100 cm). Grid. 75kVp @ 10mAs or AEC.

Gonadal shielding

Patient/part position

- Erect

Specific part/body position or rotation

- MSP perpendicular to IR
- OML 15° with horizontal. (OML will not be perpendicular to IR)

Direction and point of exit of CR

- Nasion

Fig. 166a. Position. Sinuses – Posteroanterior (PA) Axial projection, Modified Caldwell method

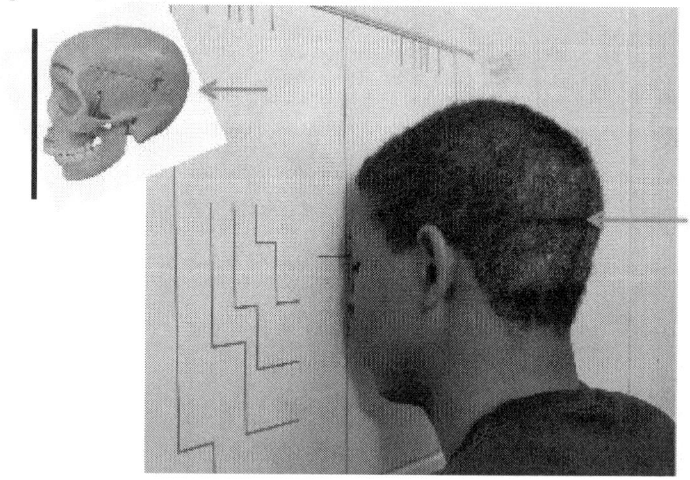

Collimation to include or structures demonstrated

- Close collimation to include the frontal, and anterior ethmoid sinuses
- Frontal sinuses clearly seen. Anterior ethmoid seen below the frontal sinuses
- Sphenoids & superior portion of maxilla will be obscured

Image evaluation

- Petrous pyramids seen in lower ½ to 1/3 of orbits
- Petrous symmetrical with equal distance between lateral orbital margins and lateral skull borders

Notes:

- IR angulation can be used instead of patient angulation. Tilt the IR down to form an angle of 15° from the vertical.

Fig. 166b. Radiograph. Sinuses – Posteroanterior (PA) Axial projection, Modified Caldwell method

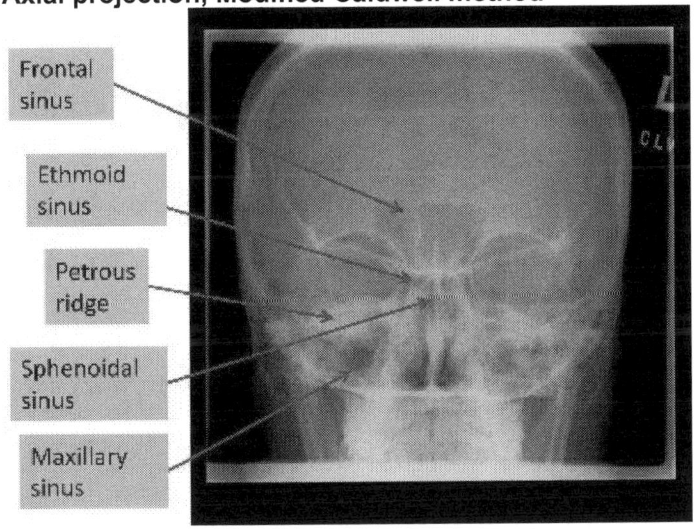

Sinuses–Parietoacanthial projection

Water's method

SID, Technical factors, Shielding

- 40 inches (100 cm). Grid. 75kVp @ 10mAs or AEC.

Gonadal shielding

Patient/part position

- Erect

Specific part/body position or rotation

- MSP and MML perpendicular to the IR, OML 37° to IR

Direction and point of exit of CR

- CR to the parietal bone, entry above inion, exit at acanthion

Fig. 167a. Position. Sinuses – Parietoacanthial projection, Water's method

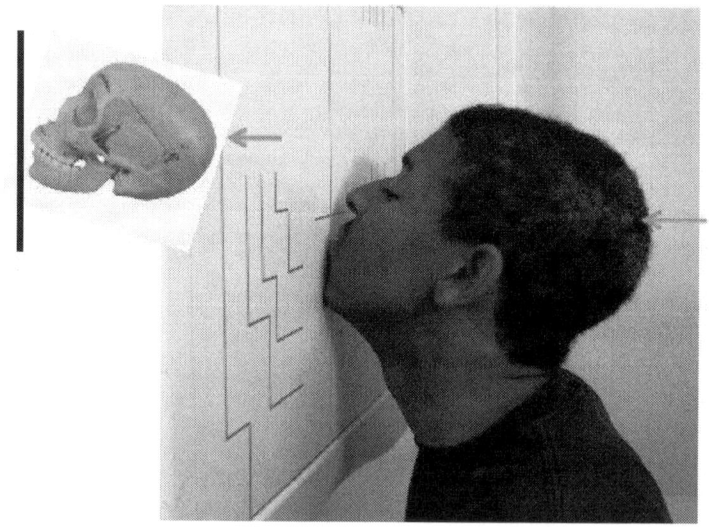

Collimation to include or structures demonstrated

- Close collimation to include the frontal & maxillary sinuses
- Maxillary sinuses clearly seen
- Frontal & ethmoidal sinuses distorted
- Foramen rotundum may be seen

Image evaluation

- Petrous pyramids seen below maxillary sinuses
- Lateral orbital wall to cranial wall symmetrical

Note

- With improper chin position the maxillary will not be clearly seen—too much extension will project teeth in maxillary sinuses. With too little extension, the maxillary will be foreshortened and the petrous will project in the sinuses

Fig. 167b. Radiograph. Sinuses – Parietoacanthial projection, Water's method

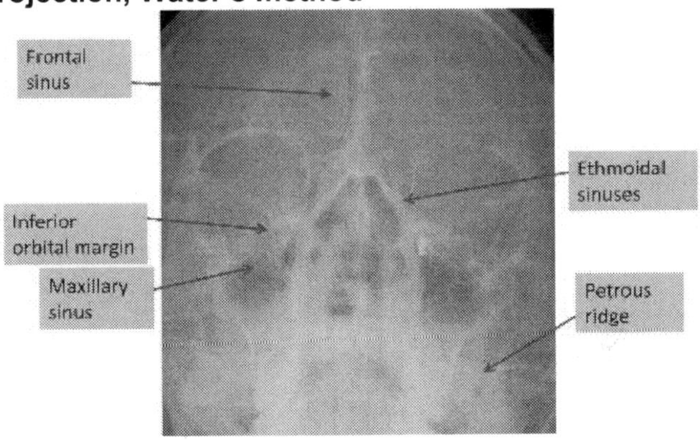

Sinuses–Parietoacanthial, Open Mouth projection

Open Mouth Waters method

SID, Technical factors, Shielding

- 40 inches (100 cm). Grid. 75kVp @ 10mAs or AEC.

Gonadal shielding

Patient/part position

- Erect

Specific part/body position or rotation

- MSP and MML perpendicular and OML 37° to IR
- After opening the mouth the MML will not be perpendicular

Direction and point of exit of CR

- CR enters the parietal bone, exits at acanthion

Fig 168a. Position. Sinuses-Parietoacanthial, Open Mouth projection

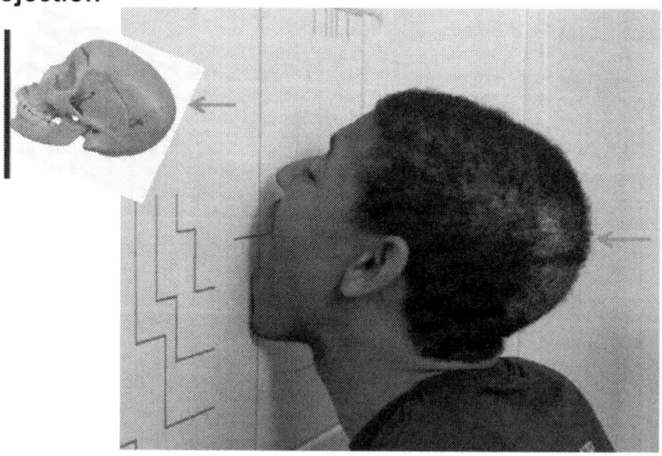

Collimation to include or structures demonstrated

- Close collimation to include the maxillary, frontal and sphenoidal sinuses
- Sphenoidal sinuses visualized in open mouth.
- Maxillary sinuses seen above the petrous

Image evaluation

- Lateral orbital wall to cranial wall symmetrical

Note

- This projection can be used to demonstrate the sphenoids if patient cannot maintain the SMV projection.

Fig 168b. Radiograph. Sinuses-Parietoacanthial, Open Mouth projection

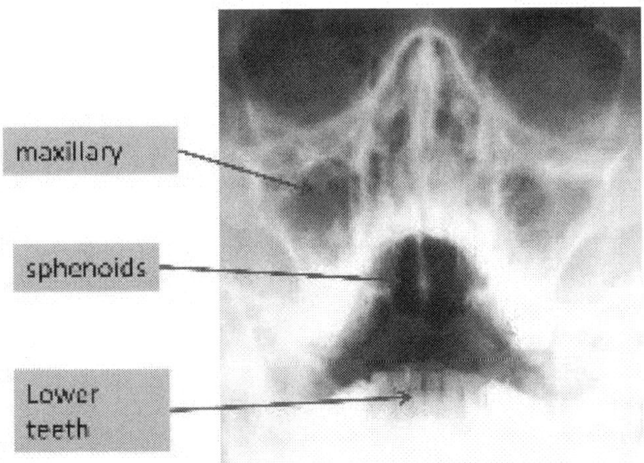

Sinuses–Submentovertex (SMV) projection

Schüller or basal method

SID, Technical factors, Shielding

- 40 inches (100 cm). Grid. 85kVp @ 12.5 mAs or AEC.

Gonadal shielding

Patient/part position

- Erect

Specific part/body position or rotation

- IOML parallel and MSP perpendicular to IR with vertex of head resting on IR

Direction and point of entry of CR

- CR perpendicular through coronal plane passing ¾ inch (1.9 cm) anterior to EAM & perpendicular to IOML. CR should pass 1½ in (3.8cm) posterior to mentum

Fig. 169a. Position. Sinuses – Submentovertex (SMV) projection, Schüller or Basal method

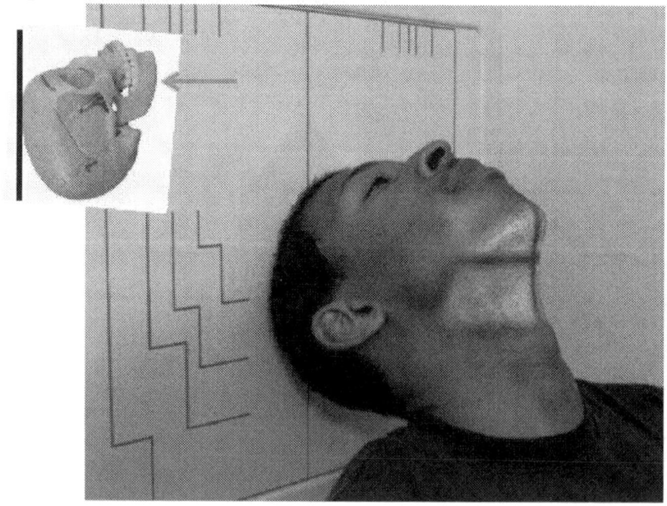

Collimation to include or structures demonstrated

- Close collimation to the sinuses
- Sphenoids and posterior ethmoids well demonstrated

Image evaluation

- Mandible condyles anterior to petrous pyramid with distance between condyles and lateral margin of skull symmetrical
- Petrous symmetrical

Note:

- Keep IOML parallel with the IR

Fig. 169b. Radiograph. Sinuses – Submentovertex (SMV) projection, Schüller or Basal method

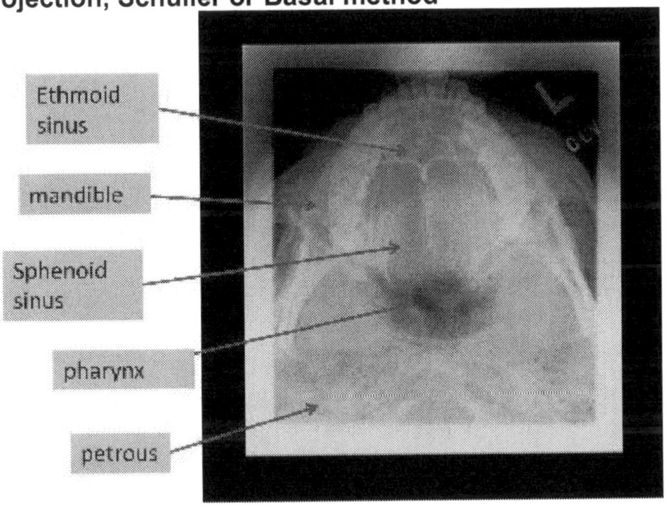

Facial Bones–Lateral projection

SID, Technical factors, Shielding

- 40 inches (100 cm). Grid. 70kVp @ 10mAs or AEC.

Gonadal shielding

Patient/part position

- Semiprone obi, affected side down or erect

Specific part/body position or rotation

- MSP and IOML parallel with IR.
- IPL perpendicular

Direction and point of entry of CR

- CR perpendicular to mid zygoma or mid between outer canthus and EAM

Fig. 170a. Position. Facial Bones - Lateral projection

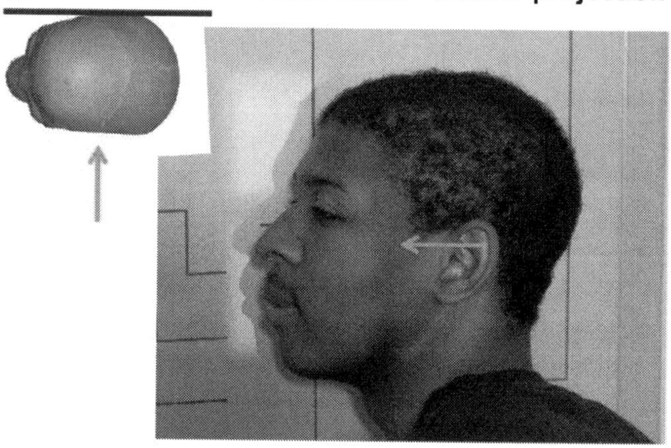

Collimation to include or structures demonstrated

- Close collimation to within 1 inch (2.5 cm) of the facial bones
- Right and left sides superimposed
- Orbital roof and sella turcica demonstrated

Image evaluation

Superimposed orbital margins, sella turcica, zygoma and mandible

Fig. 170b. Radiograph. Facial Bones - Lateral projection

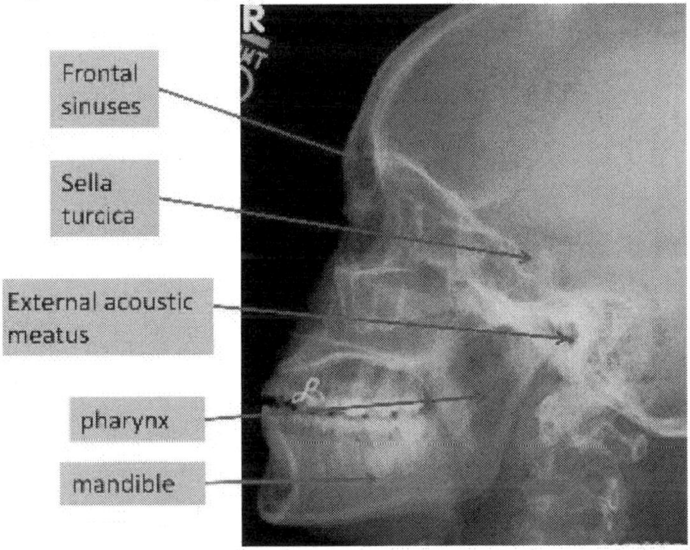

Facial Bones–Parietoacanthial projection

Water's method

SID, Technical factors, Shielding

- 40 inches (100 cm). Grid. 75kVp @ 10mAs or AEC.

Gonadal shielding

Patient/part position

- Prone MSP perpendicular or erect
- Chin on tabletop or erect stand, shoulders in same transverse plane

Specific part/body position or rotation

- OML 37° to IR. MML perpendicular

Direction and point of exit of CR

- Perpendicular CR to exit at acanthion

Fig. 171a. Position. Facial Bones- Parietoacanthial projection, Water's method

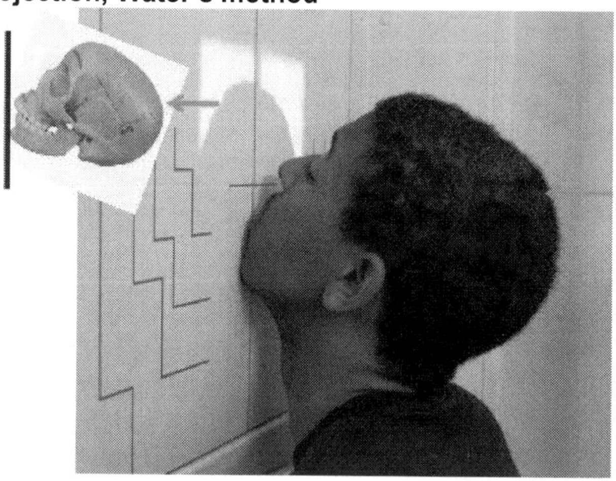

Collimation to include or structures demonstrated

- Close collimation to within 1 inch (2.5 cm) of the facial bones
- The orbits, maxillae and zygomatic arches seen

Image evaluation

- Distance between lateral border of skull and orbits equal on each side
- Petrous ridge below the maxillary sinuses

Note

- This is the best single projection of facial bone

Fig. 171b. Radiograph. Facial Bones- Parietoacanthial projection, Water's method

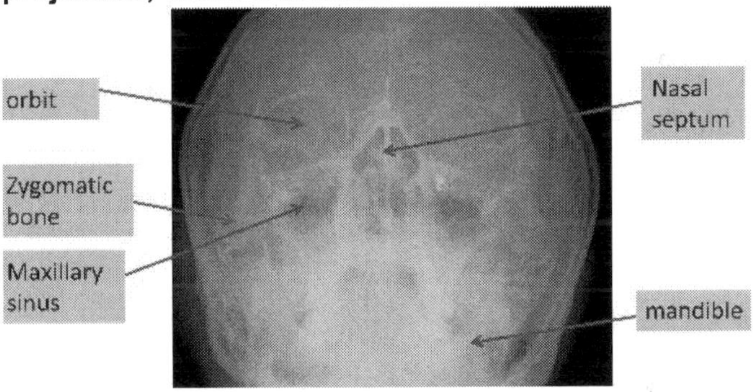

Facial Bones–Acanthioparietal (AP) Axial projection
"Reverse Water's"

SID, Technical factors, Shielding

- 40 inches (100 cm). Grid. 75kVp @ 10mAs or AEC. Gonadal shielding

Patient/part position

- Patient supine with head extended or erect

Specific part/body position or rotation

- MSP and MML perpendicular to IR

Direction and point of entry of central ray (CR)

- CR enters at acanthion parallel to the MML; exits 2 inches (5 cm) above inion

Fig. 172a. Position. Facial Bones – Acanthioparietal (AP) Axial projection, "Reverse Water's"

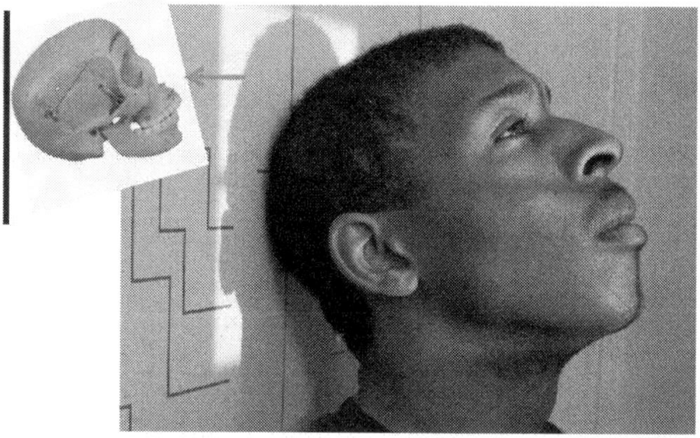

Collimation to include or structures demonstrated

- Close collimation to within 1 inch (2.5 cm) of the facial bones

Image Evaluation

- Distance between lateral border of skull and orbit equal on each side
- Petrous ridge below the maxillary sinuses

Notes

- Image is similar to the Parietoacanthial projection but facial structures are magnified
- This projection is used on trauma patients or if patients is unable to extend neck or lie prone.

Fig. 172b. Radiograph. Facial Bones – Acanthioparietal (AP) Axial projection, "Reverse Water's"

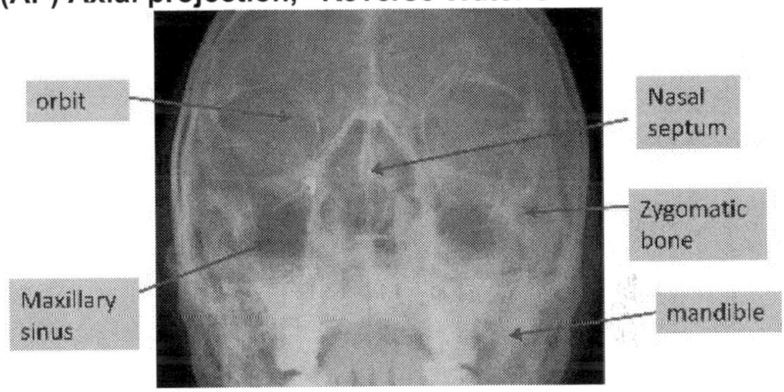

Facial Bones– Parietoacanthial projection

(Modified Water's method)

SID, Technical factors, Shielding

- 40 inches (100 cm). Grid. 75kVp @ 10mAs or AEC.

Gonadal shielding

Patient/part position

- Patient prone with head extended, MSP perpendicular.

Chin rest on erect stand or table Bucky. shoulders in same transverse plane

Specific part/body position or rotation

- OML 55° to IR with LML perpendicular

Direction and point of exit of central ray (CR)

- CR exits perpendicular at acanthion

Fig. 173a. Position. Facial Bone- Parietoacanthial (PA) projection, Modified Water's method

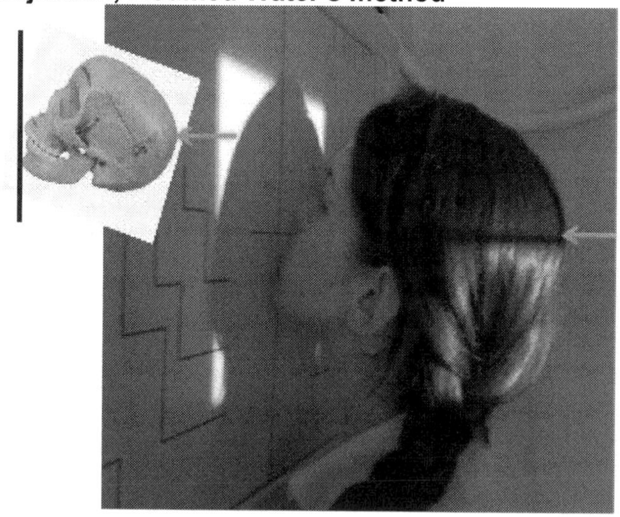

Collimation to include or structures demonstrated

- Close collimation to within 1 inch (2.5 cm) of the facial bones

Image Evaluation

- Petrous ridge projected immediately below the inferior border of the orbits midway through the maxillary sinuses
- Orbits, maxilla & zygoma seen

Note:

- Trauma patients or if patients is unable to extend neck or lie supine.

Fig. 173b. Radiograph. Facial Bone- Parietoacanthial (PA) projection, Modified Water's method

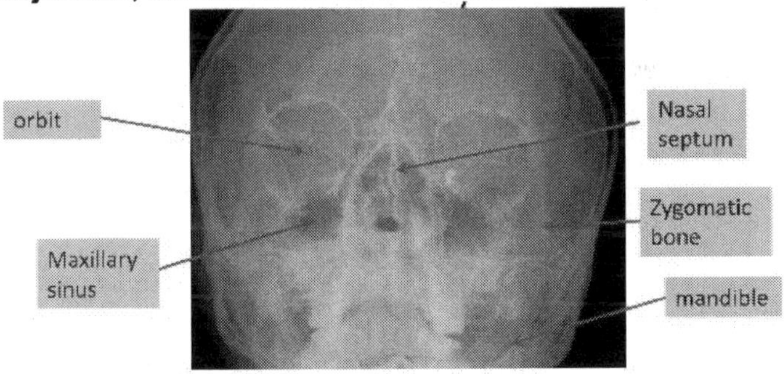

Facial Bones–Posteroanterior (PA) 30-degree Axial projection

SID, Technical factors, Shielding

- 40 inches (100 cm). Grid. 80kVp @ 12.5 mAs or AEC. Gonadal shielding

Patient/part position

- Prone, forehead and nose on table, shoulders same transverse plane

Specific part/body position or rotation

- MSP and OLM perpendicular to IR

Direction and point of exit of CR

- 25-30° caudal angulation
- CR exits at nasion

Fig. 174a. Position. Facial Bone- Posteroanterior (PA) 30-degree Axial projection

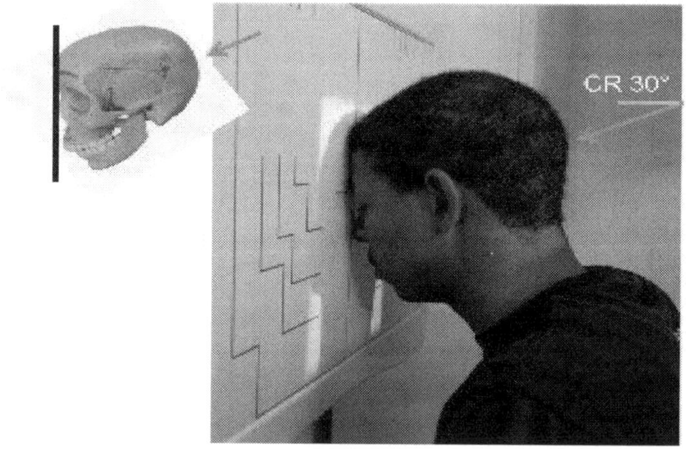

Collimation to include or structures demonstrated

- Close collimation to within 1 inch (2.5 cm) of the facial bones

Image evaluation

- Petrous seen below the orbits
- Petrous symmetrical with equal distance between lateral orbital margins and lateral skull borders

Notes

- To demonstrate mandible rami use a perpendicular CR, exiting at the acanthion. Petrous is visualized within the orbits

Fig. 174b. Radiograph. Facial Bone- Posteroanterior (PA) 30-degree Axial projection

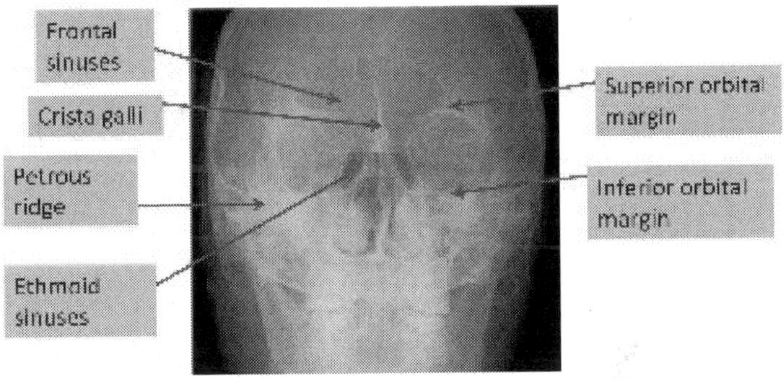

Facial Bones, Zygomatic Arches–Submentovertex (SMV) projection

SID, Technical factors, Shielding

- 40 inches (100 cm). Grid. 75kVp @ 12.5 mAs or AEC.

Gonadal shielding

Patient/part position

- Erect or supine with neck extended

Specific part/body position or rotation

- MSP perpendicular to IR, IOMP parallel

Direction and point of entry of CR

- Perpendicular to IOML, enters midline between gonia at the level of zygomatic arches, 1-inch (2.5 cm) posterior to outer cantus of eye or 1 ½ inch (4cm) posterior to mentum

Fig. 175a. Position. Facial Bones, Zygomatic Arches-Submentovertex (SMV) projection

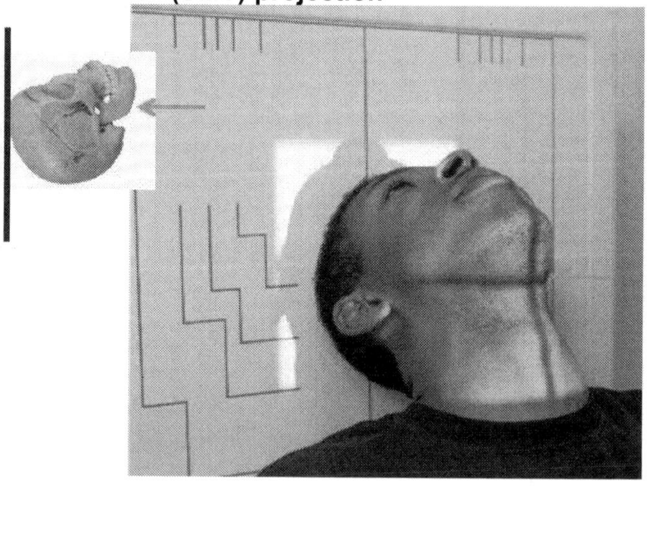

Collimation to include or structures demonstrated

- Close collimation to the outer margins of the zygomatic arches
- Zygomatic arches free of superimposition

Image evaluation

- Zygomatic arch symmetrical

Note

Lower kVp used to avoid over penetrating thin zygoma

Fig. 175b. Radiograph. Facial Bones, Zygomatic Arches-Submentovertex (SMV) projection

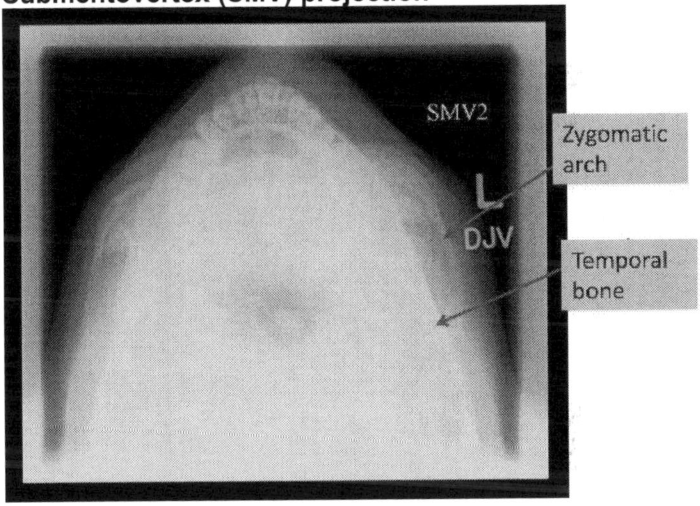

Facial Bones, Zygomatic Arches–Oblique Inferosuperior

or Tangential projection

SID, Technical factors, Shielding

- 40 inches (100 cm). Grid. 70kVp @ 10mAs or AEC. Gonadal shielding

Patient/part position

- Erect or supine with neck extended
- MSP perpendicular to IR, IOML parallel

Specific part/body position or rotation

- Rotate patient's head to side of interest to position the MSP 15° to the side of interest (tilt head and chin to affected side.

Direction and point of entry of CR

- Horizontal at level of zygomatic arch or 1-inch (2.5 cm) posterior to the outer cantus of the eye

Fig. 176a. Position. Facial Bones, Zygomatic Arches-Oblique Inferosuperior or Tangential projection

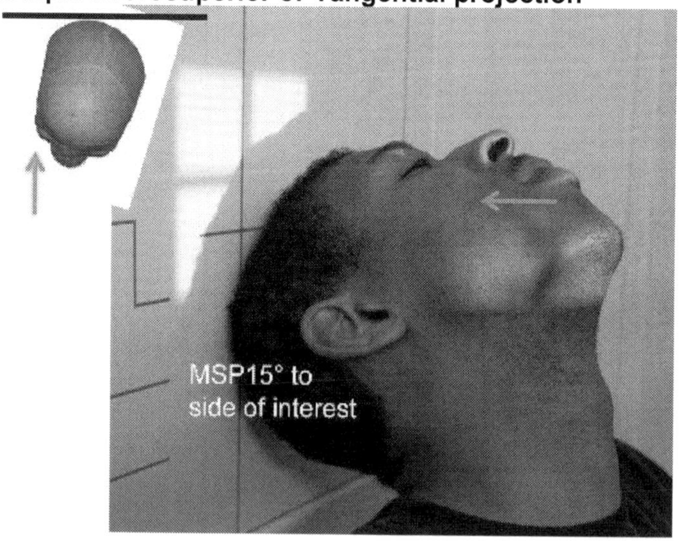

Collimation to include or structures demonstrated

- A single zygomatic arch free of superimposition

Image evaluation

- High contrast image of the zygomatic arch

Note

- Useful with patients with "flat-cheek bones" and to demonstrate depressed fracture.

Fig. 176b. Radiograph. Facial Bones, Zygomatic Arches-Oblique Inferosuperior or Tangential projection

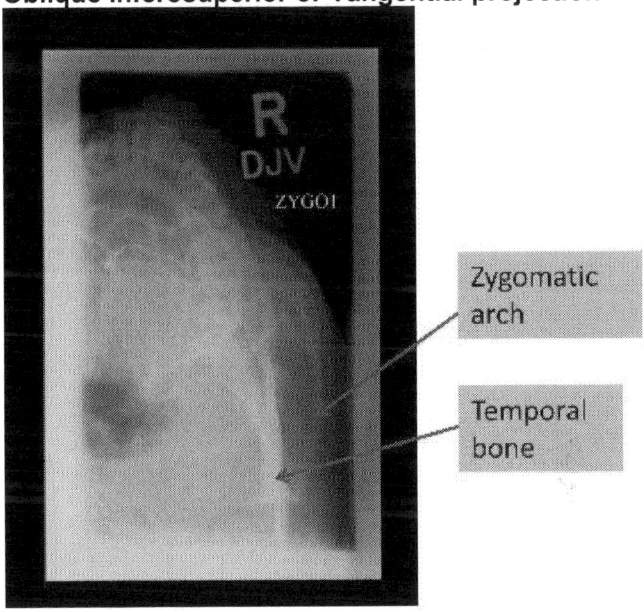

Facial Bones, Mandible–Posteroanterior (PA) projection

SID, Technical factors, Shielding

- 40 inches (100 cm). Grid. 70kVp @ 10mAs or AEC. Gonadal shielding

Patient/part position

- Erect PA, or prone

Specific part/body position or rotation

- MSP and OML perpendicular to IR

Direction and point of exit of CR

- Perpendicular exit at acanthion

Fig. 177a. Position. Facial Bones, Mandible-Posteroanterior (PA) projection

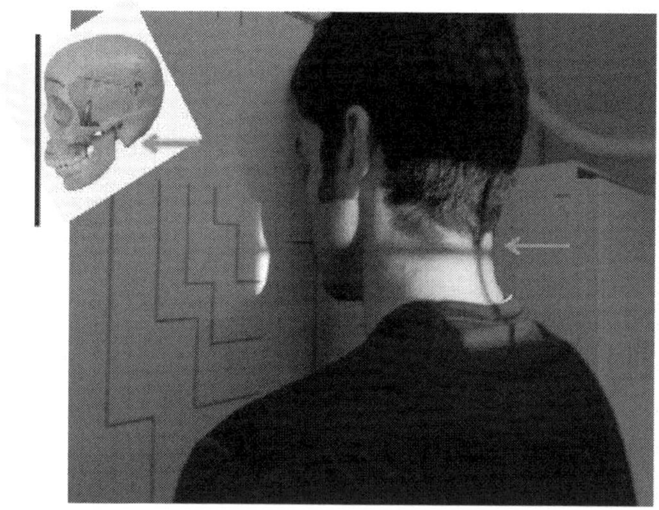

Collimation to include or structures demonstrated

- Entire mandible including mandibular body and rami

Image evaluation

- Symmetrical appearance of the mandibular rami and body

Fig. 177b. Radiograph. Facial Bones, Mandible-Posteroanterior (PA) projection

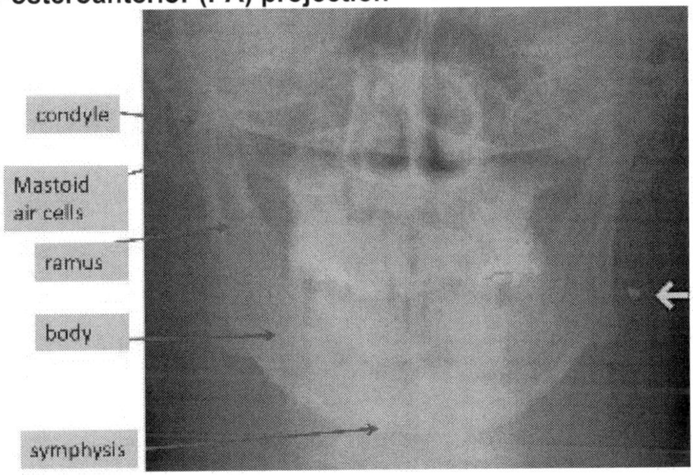

Facial Bones, Mandible–Posteroanterior (PA) axial projection

SID, Technical factors, Shielding

40 inches (100 cm). Grid. kVp @ 10 mAs or AEC. Gonadal shielding

Patient/part position

- PA

Specific part/body position or rotation

- MSP perpendicular (⊥) & OML perpendicular or IOML perpendicular

Direction and point of entry of central ray (CR)

- 20-25 degrees cephalic to exit at the acanthion between the TMAs

Fig. 178a. Position. Facial Bones, Mandible-Posteroanterior (PA) Axial projection

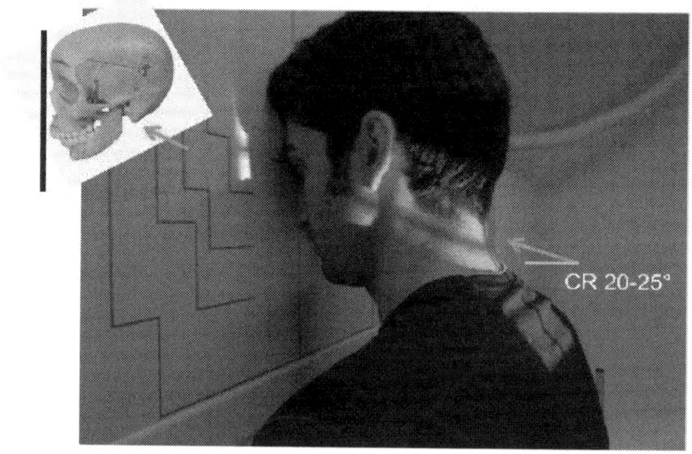

Collimation to include or structures demonstrated

- Entire mandible including mandibular body and rami

Image evaluation

- Include soft tissue and bony trabecular detail of mandibular body and rami

Note

- This projection can demonstrate medial or lateral displacement of fracture fragment of rami

Fig. 178b. Radiograph. Facial Bones, Mandible-Posteroanterior (PA) Axial projection

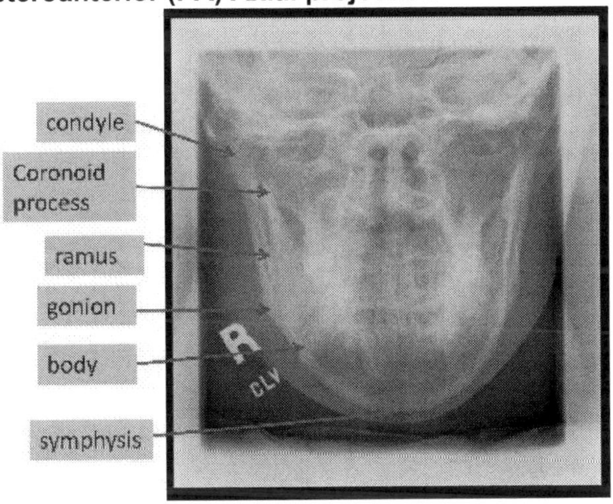

Facial Bones, Mandible–Axiolateral Oblique projection

Part 1 of 3 projections

SID, Technical factors, Shielding

- 40 inches (100 cm). Grid. 70kVp @ 10mAs or AEC.

Gonadal shielding

Patient/part position

- Lateral with neck extended (to prevent superimposition of ramus on C-spine)

Three projections taken depending on area of interest.
Part 1: No rotation, patient remains true lateral.
Part 2: Rotate head 30° to IR.
Part 3: Rotate head 45° to IR

Specific part/body position or rotation for part 1

- Patient remains true lateral with IPL perpendicular to IR and MSP parallel to IR

Direction and point of entry of CR

- 25 ° cephalic angulation through the ramus

Fig. 179a. Position. Facial Bones, Mandible-Axiolateral Oblique projection. No rotation – Ramus

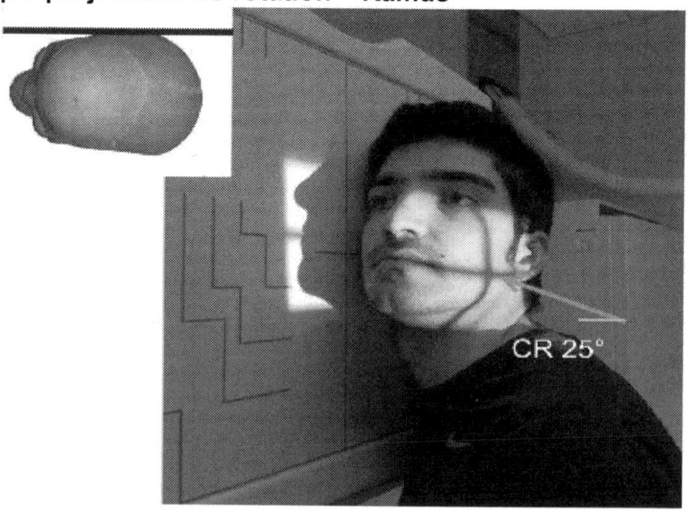

Collimation to include or structures demonstrated

- The mandibular ramus without foreshortening or elongation.

Image evaluation

- The region parallel to the IR will be seen clearly.
- No overlap of the ramus by opposite side of the mandible
- No superimposition of cervical spine on ramus

Fig. 179b. Radiograph. Facial Bones, Mandible-Axiolateral Oblique projection. No rotation – Ramus

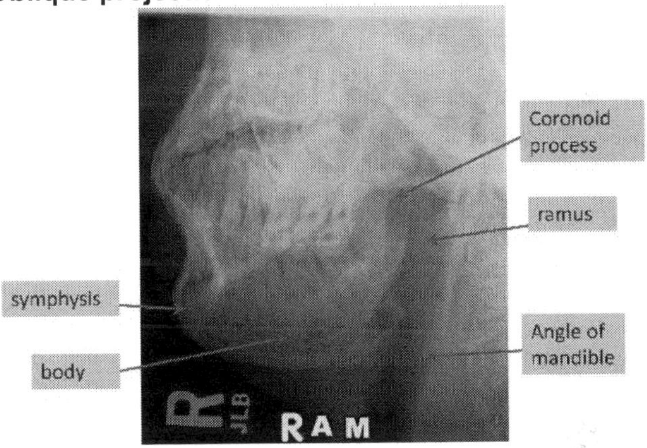

Facial Bones, Mandible–Axiolateral Oblique projection

Part 2 of 3 projections

SID, Technical factors, Shielding

- 40 inches (100 cm). Grid. 70kVp @ 10mAs or AEC.

Gonadal shielding

Patient/part position

- Lateral with neck extended (to prevent superimposition of ramus on C-spine)

Three projections taken depending on area of interest.

Part 1: No rotation, patient remains true lateral.

Part 2: Rotate head 30° to IR.

Part 3: Rotate head 45° to IR

Specific part/body position or rotation for part 2

- Patient is positioned true lateral with MSP parallel to the IR.
- Head is then rotated 30° to IR

Direction and point of entry of CR

- 25 ° cephalic, through the mandibular body

Fig. 179c. Position. Facial Bones, Mandible-Axiolateral Oblique projection. 30-degree rotation- Body

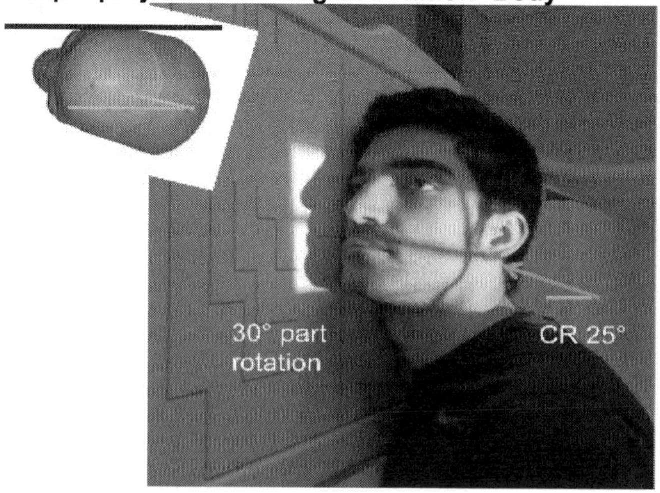

Collimation to include or structures demonstrated

- The body without superposition of the opposite side

Image evaluation

- Body demonstrated without foreshortening or elongation

Fig. 179d. Radiograph. Facial Bones, Mandible-Axiolateral Oblique projection. 30-degree rotation- Body

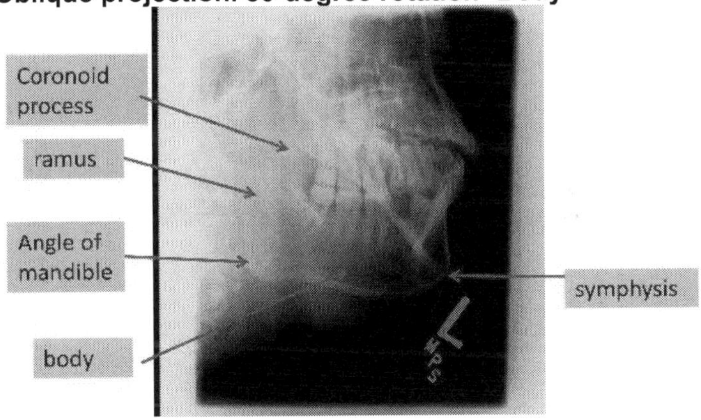

Facial Bones, Mandible–Axiolateral Oblique projection

Part 3 of 3 projections

SID, Technical factors, Shielding

- 40 inches (100 cm). Grid. 70kVp @ 10mAs or AEC.

Gonadal shielding

Patient/part position

- Lateral with neck extended (to prevent superimposition of ramus on C-spine)

Three projections taken depending on area of interest.

Part 1: No rotation, patient remains true lateral.

Part 2: Rotate head 30˚ to IR.

Part 3: Rotate head 45˚ to IR

Specific part/body position or rotation for part 3

- Patient is positioned true lateral with MSP parallel to the IR .
- Head is then rotated 45˚ to IR
- Direction and point of entry of CR
- 25 º cephalic, through the mentum

Fig. 179e. Position. Facial Bones, Mandible-Axiolateral Oblique projection. 45-degree rotation- Symphysis

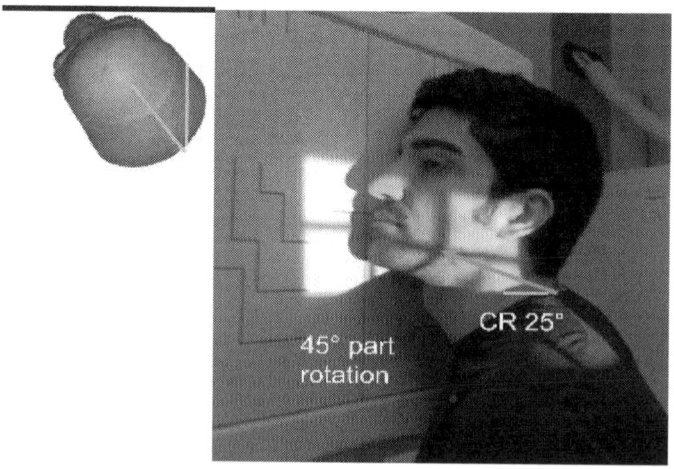

Collimation to include or structures demonstrated

- The symphysis mentum free of overlap
- Image evaluation
- No foreshortening or elongation of the mentum

Fig. 179f. Radiograph. Facial Bones, Mandible-Axiolateral Oblique projection. 45-degree rotation- Symphysis

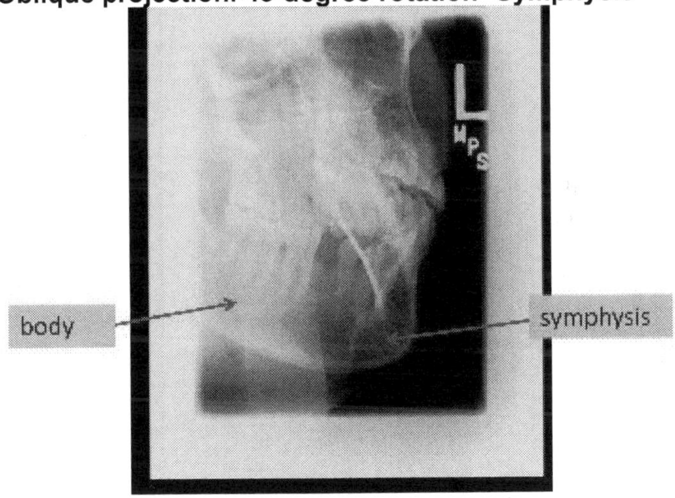

Facial Bones, Nasal–Lateral projection

SID, Technical factors, Shielding

- 40 inches (100 cm). No Grid. 52kVp @ 1.3 mAs or AEC.

Gonadal shielding

Patient/part position

- Patient in true lateral

Specific part/body position or rotation

- MSP and IOML parallel to IR

Direction and point of entry of CR

- ½- ¾inch (1.5-1.9 cm) inferior to nasion

Fig. 180a. Position. Facial Bones, Nasal- Lateral projection

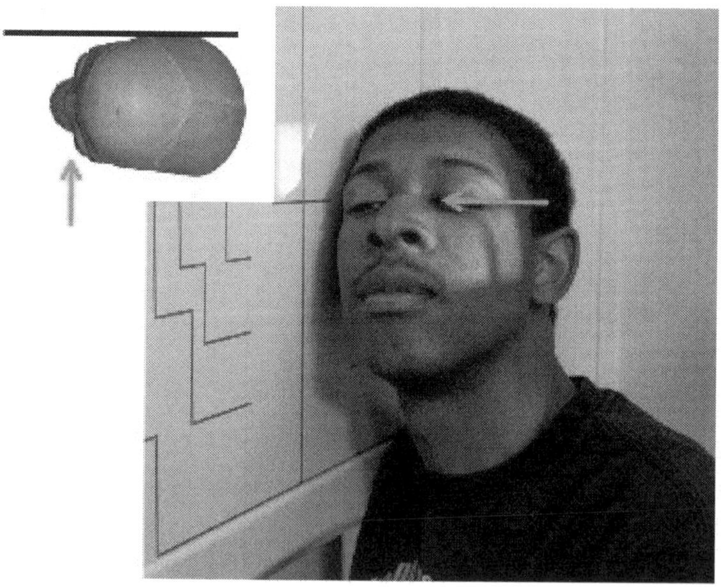

Collimation to include or structures demonstrated

- Lateral nasal bone from the nasofrontal suture to the tip
- Glabella and acanthion included in collimated field

Image evaluation

- No rotation of the nasal bone

Notes

- Both sides done for comparison
- In addition to the lateral the parietoacanthial projection with close collimation is also taken for a complete evaluation of the nasal bones

Fig. 180b. Radiograph. Facial Bones, Nasal- Lateral projection

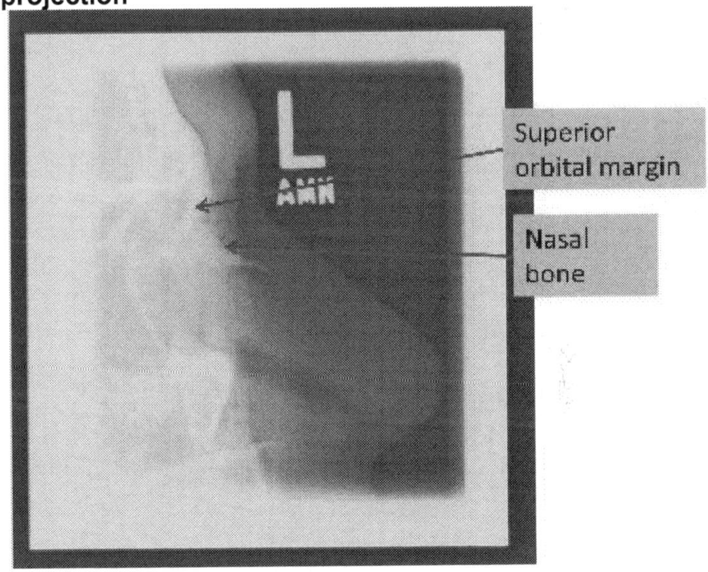

Facial Bones, Temporomandibular Articulations (TMA)–Anteroposterior (AP) axial

SID, Technical factors, Shielding

- 40 inches (100 cm). Grid. 75kVp @ 10mAs or AEC.

Gonadal shielding

Patient/part position

- Supine or erect patient AP

Specific part/body position or rotation

- MSP and OML perpendicular to IR

Direction and point of entry of CR

- 35 degrees caudal
- Center midpoint between the TMAs–3inches (7.6 cm) above the nasion.
- CR passes 1inch (1.5 cm) anterior to TMAs or 2 inches (5 cm) anterior to EAM)

Fig. 181a. Position. Facial Bones, Temporomandibular Articulations (TMA) Anteroposterior (AP) Axial (closed mouth)

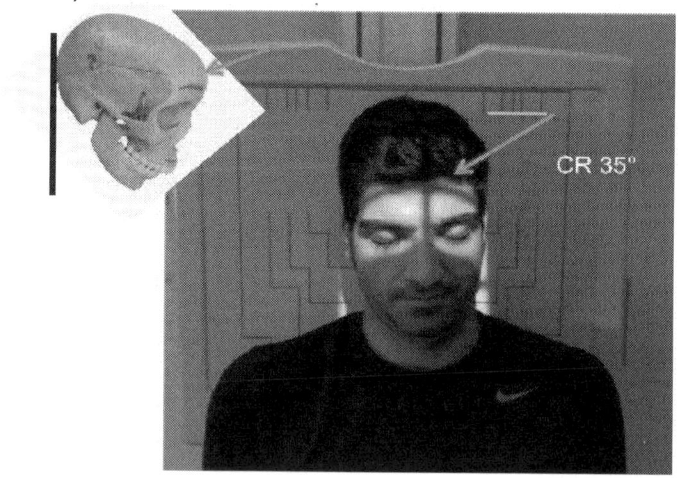

Collimation to include or structures demonstrated

- Mandibular condyles lateral to the cervical spine

Image evaluation

- Condyles slightly superimposed on petrous in closed mouth position and below the petrous with mouth open.

Notes

- Open and closed mouth projections taken
- If IOML is perpendicular increase CR angulation by 7-degrees (42-dgrees)

Fig. 181b. Radiograph. Facial Bones, Temporomandibular Articulations (TMA) Anteroposterior (AP) Axial (closed mouth)

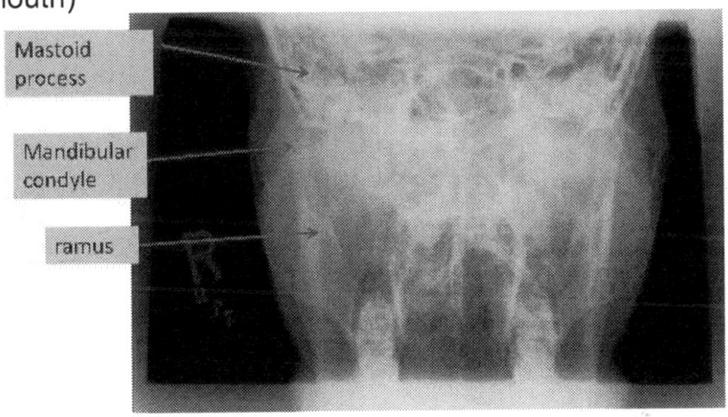

Facial Bone, Temporomandibular Articulations (TMA) –Axiolateral projection

SID, Technical factors, Shielding

- 40 inches (100 cm). Grid. 75kVp @ 10mAs or AEC.

Gonadal shielding

Patient/part position

- Patient Lateral, affected side closest to IR

Specific part/body position or rotation

- MSP parallel and IPL perpendicular to IR.

Direction and point of entry of CR

- 25-30 degrees caudal angulation. CR ½ (1.5 cm) anterior & 2 inches (5 cm) superior to the up side EAM

Fig.182a (closed mouth TMJ) **& 182b** (open mouth TMJ). **Position. Facial Bone-Temporomandibular Articulation (TMA) – Axiolateral projection.**

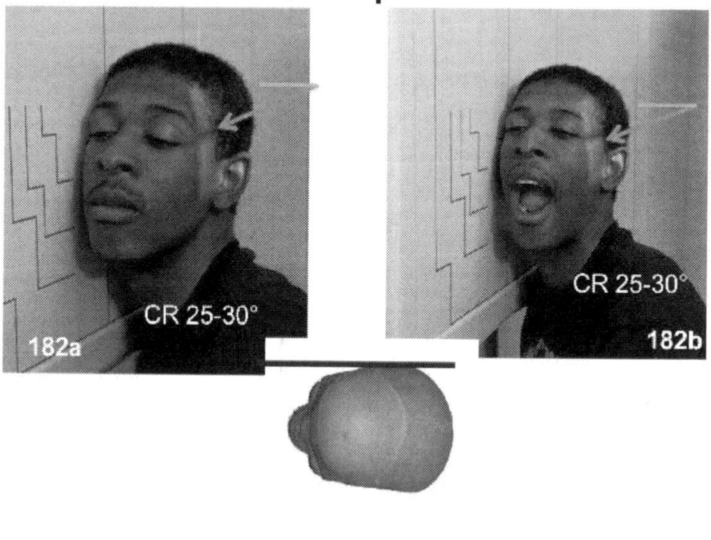

Collimation to include or structures demonstrated

- Temporomandibular articulation anterior to the EAM

Image evaluation

- Condyle in the mandibular fossa in the closed-mouth position
- Condyle inferior and anterior to the fossa in the open-mouth position

Notes

- Open & closed bilateral images taken for comparison
- This projection will demonstrate fracture of the neck and condyles of ramus.

Fig.182c (closed mouth TMJ) **& 182d** (open mouth TMJ). **Radiograph. Facial Bone-Temporomandibular Articulation (TMA) – Axiolateral projection**

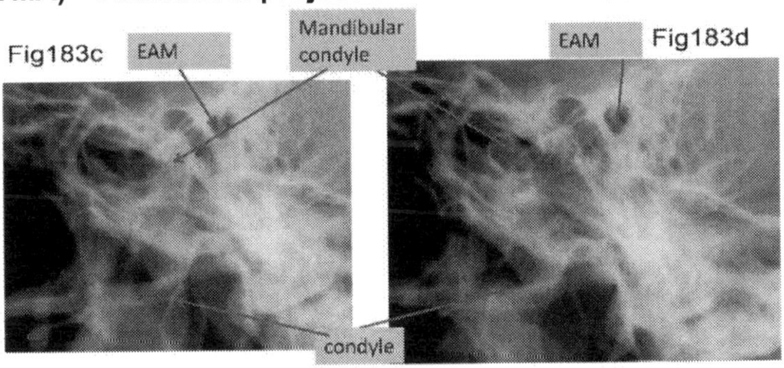

Facial Bones, Petrous portions–Axiolateral projection

Modified Law method–using single tube angulation

SID, Technical factors, Shielding

- 40 inches (100 cm). Grid. 75kVp @ 10mAs or AEC. Gonadal shielding

Patient/part position

- Prone or erect

Specific part/body position or rotation

- Position the patient lateral initially
- Turn the MSP 15° toward table (from the lateral, rotate face to IR)

Direction and point of entry of CR

- 15° caudal angulation
- CR directed 1inch (2.5 cm) posterior and 2 inches (5 cm) superior to upper EAM. Exits at lower EAM

Fig. 183a. Position. Facial Bones, Petrous Portions-Axiolateral projection. Modified Law method- single tube angulation

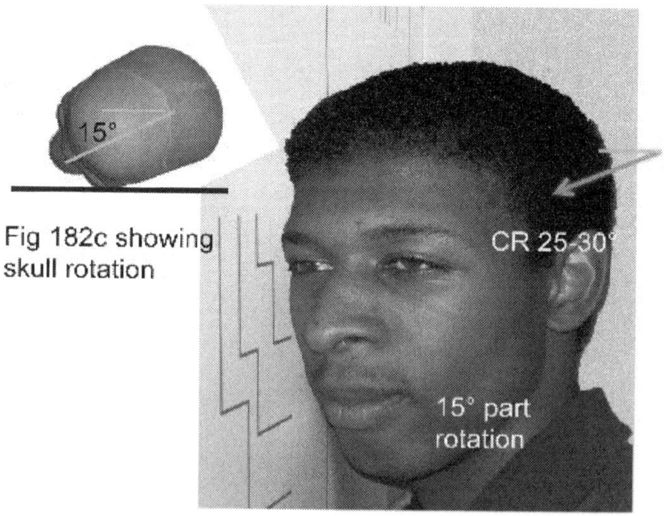

Collimation to include or structures demonstrated

- The TMA nearest the IR is seen clearly
- No superimposition from opposite TMA
- TMA clear of the cervical spine
- Demonstrates mastoid air cells & petrous superimposed on EAM

Image evaluation

- Condyle in the mandibular fossa in the closed-mouth position
- Condyle inferior and anterior to the fossa in the open-mouth position

Notes

- Open & closed bilateral images taken for comparison
- Fold and tape auricles forward to prevent dense shadows over the petrous

Fig. 183b. Radiograph. Facial Bones, Petrous Portions- Axiolateral projection. Modified Law method- single tube angulation

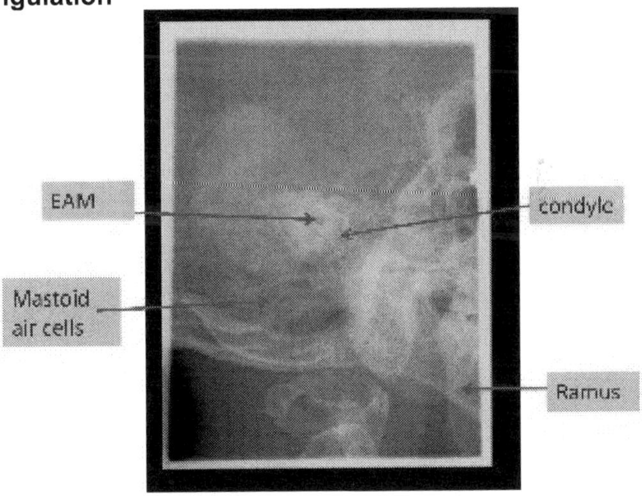

Facial Bones, Optic Canals–Parieto-orbital projection

Rhese method

SID, Technical factors, Shielding

- 40 inches (100 cm). Grid. 80kVp @ 12.5 mAs or AEC. Gonadal shielding

Patient/part position

- Prone or erect

Specific part/body position or rotation

- Start with MSP perpendicular to the IR with patient centered
- Turn affected orbit down with zygoma, nose and resting on IR to rotate head with MSP 53° to IR or 37° to CR
- AML perpendicular to IR

Direction and point of entry of CR

- Perpendicular to affected orbit, 1 inch (2.5 cm) superior and posterior to TEA of raised side

Fig. 184a. Position. Facial Bones - Optic Canals, Parieto-Orbital projection. Reese method

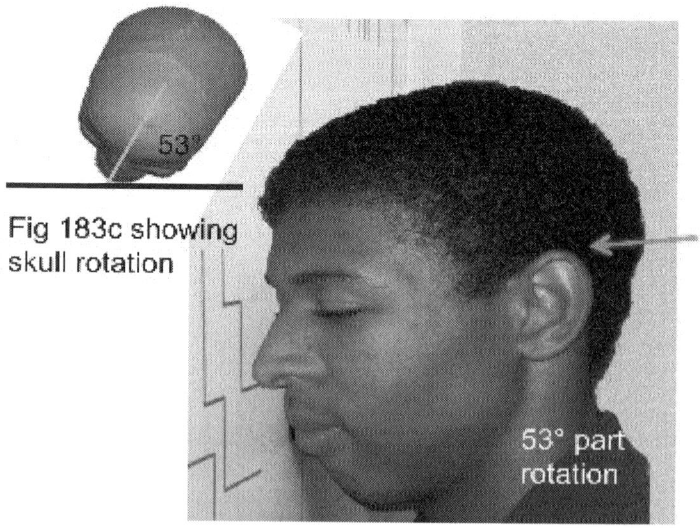

Collimation to include or structures demonstrated

- Include the margins of the orbit
- Optic foramen seen in the lower outer quadrant of the orbit
- Image evaluation
- Clear visualization of the orbital margin and optic foramen

Fig. 184b. Radiograph. Facial Bones - Optic Canals, Parieto-Orbital projection. Reese method

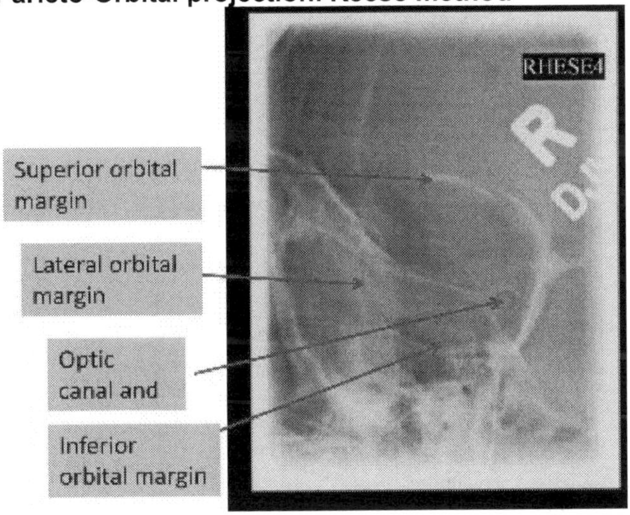

Bibliography

- Long, B.W., Rollins, J.H., Smith, B.J. Merrill's Atlas of Radiographic Positioning and Procedures. 3 Vol. Set. 14th ed. St. Louis, MO: Mosby/Elsevier. 2018

- Lampignano, J.P., Kendrick, L.E. Textbook of Radiographic Positioning and Related Anatomy. 9th ed. St. Louis, MO: Mosby/Elsevier. 2017

- Tortora, G.J., Derrickson, B. Principles of Anatomy and Physiology. 15th ed. John Wiley & Sons, Inc. Hoboken, NJ. 2016

- Adler, A.M., Carlton, R.R. Introduction to Radiologic Science and Patient Care 7th ed. Saunders Elsevier. St. Louis Missouri. 2018

Thank you for purchasing Radiographic Positioning: Pocket Guide.

If this book was helpful, please consider rating this title at the online retailer of your choice. Your ratings and reviews are appreciated by the author and will help other readers find new favorites.

Visit www.opeart.com for details on other titles by Olive Peart.

Works of Fiction by Olive Peart

Fiction

Mind Games
Matthew has the uncanny ability to influence people's thought. To defend himself against the bullies, Matthew is eventually forced to use his special power.

The Starlight Kids, Mystery of the Feather Burglar
With the help of her friends, Shari gets her chance to turn a boring summer vacation into a fantastic action packed adventure.

The Intruders– In This War They Had The Advantage
Six Bronx teens have one thing in common–a thirst for excitement! They get that and more when they set out to explore a neglected track of land in their neighborhood and embark on an adventure of a lifetime. Unfortunately, within weeks, their adventure becomes all too real as brother turns against brother, friends become enemies and people are being killed! This is no longer fun. This is war!

Linked
Same age, same height, same grade—they could have been identical twins, but they were not. Yet they lived in the same imperfect world with overwhelming family problems... One was black and the other was white and they had switched!

Made in the USA
Middletown, DE
23 December 2020

27025760R00239